The Complete Dentist

Positive Leadership and Communication Skills for Success

Barry Polansky, DMD, CAPP

Private dental practice
Cherry Hill, USA

Visiting Faculty at the Pankey Institute
Key Biscayne, USA

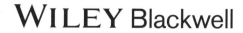

This edition first published 2018
© 2018 John Wiley & Sons, Inc.

The right of Barry Polansky to be identified as the author of this work has been asserted in accordance with law.

Registered Office
John Wiley & Sons, Inc., 111 River Street, Hoboken, NJ 07030, USA

Editorial Office
111 River Street, Hoboken, NJ 07030, USA

For details of our global editorial offices, customer services, and more information about Wiley products visit us at www.wiley.com.

Wiley also publishes its books in a variety of electronic formats and by print-on-demand. Some content that appears in standard print versions of this book may not be available in other formats.

Library of Congress Cataloging-in-Publication Data

Names: Polansky, Barry, author.
Title: The complete dentist : positive leadership and communication skills for success /
   by Barry Polansky.
Description: Hoboken, NJ : Wiley, 2018. | Includes bibliographical references and index. |
Identifiers: LCCN 2017031780 (print) | LCCN 2017033910 (ebook) | ISBN 9781119250814 (pdf) |
   ISBN 9781119250821 (epub) | ISBN 9781119250807 (pbk.)
Subjects: | MESH: Dentists–psychology | Leadership | Communication | Interpersonal Relations
Classification: LCC RK60 (ebook) | LCC RK60 (print) | NLM WU 21 | DDC 617.6/0232–dc23
LC record available at https://lccn.loc.gov/2017031780

Cover Design: Wiley
Cover Images: (Left) © andresr/Gettyimages; (Right) © Hero Images/Gettyimages

Set in 10/12pt Warnock by SPi Global, Pondicherry, India
Printed in Singapore by C.O.S. Printers Pte Ltd

10 9 8 7 6 5 4 3 2 1

The Complete Dentist

Contents

Prologue

"Transformation is a process, and as life happens there are tons of ups and downs. It's a journey of discovery – there are moments on mountaintops and moments in deep valleys of despair."

Rick Warren

"We are at our very best, and we are happiest, when we are fully engaged in work we enjoy on the journey toward the goal we've established for ourselves. It gives meaning to our time off and comfort to our sleep. It makes everything else in life so wonderful, so worthwhile."

Earl Nightingale

On December 29, 1973, President Richard Nixon signed bill S.14 into law. That statute, known as the Health Maintenance Organization Act, provided for a trial federal program to promote and encourage the development of HMOs. Some might consider this the beginning of the end for what many call the "Golden Age of Dentistry." Six months prior to that, in May of '73, I graduated from the University of Pennsylvania School of Dental Medicine. The changing health profession landscape was the last thing on my mind.

I knew I needed to hone my skills, so I joined the US Army to practice, and I mean practice in every sense of the word, on enlisted soldiers coming back from Viet Nam. Once I felt that I was competent enough not to cause damage, I couldn't wait to get out and make some money. After all, the reason I became a dentist was to make a lot of money, be my own boss and make my own hours. That's the way it was.

I opened my first practice in Medford Lakes, New Jersey, in 1975. I had $25 000 in guaranteed school loans and another $25,000 in start-up costs. I was on my way. I had no idea about HMOs, PPOs, or any other third party involvement. I hung up my shingle, as they used to say, and waited for patients to come. And they came, to the tune of 30 new patients per month. Dental insurance, the indemnity type, was new. Like most of my colleagues, I welcomed dental insurance. It helped people to accept my treatment recommendations. It was easy, and I quickly learned to speak the language. It wasn't long before I learned the dark side of third parties.

I loved the business of dentistry in those days. It didn't take long to build a full-time practice. Within five years, I grew so much that I opened a second practice in Cherry Hill, New Jersey. I was unstoppable. But I began to lose patients in my Medford office. I was losing them to a brand new HMO that opened a few miles away from my office. It seemed unfair that good families were leaving my care to go to another office, based on being in a network that I didn't belong to. Union workers from teachers and retail clerks were also leaving, because I didn't belong to their "closed panel" network.

I didn't panic, because I still had plenty of patients, but it certainly annoyed me, because I was a purist about work and business. After all, I had grown up believing in meritocracy, a belief that advancement and success is based on individual ability or achievement. I felt cheated, because I had worked so hard to develop relationships with people and, overnight, they were gone. I was getting the "can you send my records to the doctor down the street" phone call, way too often. It hurt.

I always took dentistry seriously. I wanted to make a difference in the lives of my patients. It wasn't just about making money for me. I believed that dentistry was a noble profession. By noble, I mean it had qualities of high moral character. I was proud to be part of a profession that was regarded as one of the highest on most trust barometers, yet I believed that dentistry could provide a very comfortable life as well. It was the ideal profession. Early in my career, this is what I found. Through the years, things began to change.

I was finding conversations with patients becoming difficult. People were becoming dependent on their insurance plans. Over the next few years, professional advertising became acceptable. Some dentists maintained that they would never advertise, while others began to advertise shamelessly. The moral character that I mentioned earlier was beginning to dissolve. Most dental schools back then preached adherence to the American Dental Association's honored Code of Ethics. I began to sense that it was becoming meaningless. After ten years of practice, I became dissatisfied. I was earning a good living, yet I wasn't happy with my life. I was suffering from burnout.

I didn't know what burnout was, but mentally and emotionally I was suffering. Eventually, it affected me physically. I had heard rumors of dentists having the highest suicide rate, but I never believed that to be true. Patients were leaving my practice, and I couldn't get patients to accept the cases I enjoyed doing, so I spent my time doing what I never wanted to do: drill and fill. Although I never felt depressed, I was. I always considered myself a highly sensitive person. I could not tolerate feeling so lousy. I believed the answer to my problems was to become a better dentist. I took course after course, looking for the answers, but to no avail. Then I got lucky.

I heard that the Pankey Institute in Key Biscayne, Florida, taught the philosophy of a Dr. L.D. Pankey. Although the Institute had a reputation for teaching occlusion, as part of its continuum of courses, a philosophy of practice was covered that discussed the very same issues I was having back in my practice: how to create happiness and fulfillment in dentistry. I was hooked. I committed to learning and applying Dr. Pankey's philosophy, which included both technical, as well as behavioral, dentistry.

Pankey's career included the same difficulties I was going through. He developed his philosophy after returning from Europe, where he met Dr. Daniel Halley-Smith, who had a practice in the Place Vendóme in Paris. He knew, then, that he would have to master certain skills in order to practice dentistry on his own terms. Those skills included occlusion, examination, diagnosis and treatment planning. When he returned home, he began to study those disciplines in addition to taking courses in general philosophy. After reading *What Men Live By*, a book written by Dr. Richard Cabot, a professor of medicine and social ethics from Harvard Medical School, Dr. Pankey developed his own philosophy, based on the teachings of Aristotle and Dr. Cabot's book.

Cabot, in his book, described how to create a life where work is not burdensome. It was an early version of how to live a life worth living. This was especially appealing to me at this point of my career. Dentistry was becoming drudgery, and that had to change. I had invested many years of my life and had financial obligations. Something had to change.

Richard Cabot was a disciple of William James, the Harvard professor and the father of modern psychology, who was devising the principles of the philosophy known as pragmatism, which taught that an idea was only as good as its effect on conduct or behavior. In other words, a philosophy was meaningless unless you could demonstrate its impact on human behavior. Richard

Cabot was a brilliant lab researcher, who wrote the first English language textbook on hematology, yet he gave up research because he was more interested in the human side of medicine and face-to-face treatment. According to Mitch Horowitz, author of the book One Simple Idea [1], "he believed that physicians were assuming an inappropriately distant and inflated role in the new century, and were neglecting the experience, emotions, social problems, and fears of the patient."

Cabot's own father was an intimate friend of Ralph Waldo Emerson and Henry David Thoreau [2], who believed that to be a philosopher is not merely to have subtle thoughts, nor even to found a school – it is to solve some of the problems of life, not only theoretically, but practically. To merely have a philosophy without practical use is what separated the Transcendental philosophers of New England from the others of the day. L.D. Pankey combined both the knowledge and wisdom of Aristotle with the pragmatism of Richard Cabot, William James, and the Transcendentalists, to develop his own philosophy, which he codified in his famous Cross of Dentistry.

By the time I got to the Pankey Institute, Dr. Pankey was gone. I got the feeling he was his era's version of a self-improvement addict. I felt that I shared with him the character trait of being a highly sensitive person. I identified with the general thinking of the new people I was meeting at the Institute, like Dr. Irwin Becker, Dr. Sam Low, and Dr. Peter Dawson, among others. I sensed that what was important about dentistry was the meaning it brought to people's lives. I began to understand the connection between everything we do and how it brought meaning to my patients, my staff and, most, importantly to me. I had never been exposed to this model of learning before. This went way beyond my dental school experience, or even my experiences with continuing education. It seemed to bring all of dentistry together in a much more integrated way, in contrast to the fragmented manner in which dentistry was being taught, and still is taught today.

In reading Dr. Pankey's original philosophy, I came across words that were unfamiliar to me in everyday usage. He used the same language that Aristotle used in Ancient Greece. I could never understand the practical meaning of words like *virtues, ethos, pathos, logos*, and *eudemonia*. I understood words like character, morality, happiness, relationships, and success. This was more the language of our times. By studying a bit of Aristotle, I realized that the principles were timeless and ageless. Aristotle was helping his students with the very same issues that I was facing at the time, and the same issues that drew dentists to the Pankey Institute. Eventually, I came to realize that these concepts fell under the heading of leadership. I became a student of leadership.

Applying the principles of the Pankey philosophy is no easy task. The technical components that deal with the dentistry are more easily understood and applied by most dentists. It's the self-evident softer principles that stop most dentists. I tried mightily to develop systems that would help me to apply the soft skills that were necessary for success. I read everything I could find on leadership and communication. In 2003, I wrote a book titled *The Art of the Examination*,

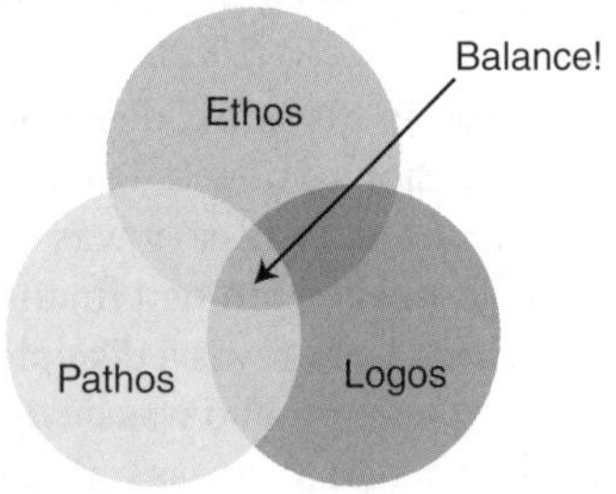

Figure P.1 From Aristotle: Ethos, Pathos and Logos.

which was well received by the dental community. It was my way to bring together all of the principles I had learned through the examination process. I followed that book up in 2013, with *The Art of Case Presentation*, which dealt more with clearly expressing and communicating the examination and diagnostic findings. I am convinced that examination and diagnosis, as well as clear expression, can help dentists to succeed.

Throughout my career in dentistry, I learned many lessons along the way. By far the most important lesson, and the one that is most difficult to apply, is that "people are people are people." In other words, the more things seem to change, consistent human universal principles [3] will always take precedence over any *management principle du jour*. Those principles which will always withstand the test of time include: empathy, generosity, sadness and humor, music and aesthetics, fairness and reciprocity, pride, story, and leadership. I will continue to make the point throughout this book that "people are begging to be led." It's part of the human story, and lies within our deepest nature.

I feel that my dissatisfaction with my work and my working conditions originated from being in opposition to my basic human nature. I found out, as I will explain, that money can't buy happiness, as the cliché tells us. Through my research and my experiences, I came to understand the truth in that saying, and researchers in behavioral economics, cognitive psychology, and social and positive psychology, have backed that up. In other words, what Aristotle, Richard Cabot, and L.D. Pankey intuitively felt can now be backed up through research.

What I am suggesting is that all businesses will see change, as I and my contemporaries have witnessed over the past 40 years. Because these changes are so personal, and affect us on such a deep level, we believe it only happens in our industry. Sweeping changes have occurred, and continue to occur, in all industries throughout the world. From retail to healthcare, the concept of work and what it means to the human remains the same – people are people are people. In dentistry, we have seen changes in technology, in delivery, in payment options, dental insurance, models of practice, implantology, cosmetics, and the newest trend – corporate dentistry.

Corporate dentistry is a natural outgrowth of our times. Baby Boomers like myself, who are retiring or slowing down, are selling their practices at reduced prices to corporate entities. Younger dentists, saddled with high loans, are having a difficult time opening their own practices as I did many years ago. Dental insurance has morphed into mostly networked plans. Dental insurance companies put pressure on dentists to join their networks at reduced payment schedules. The cost of dentistry has risen beyond the ability of the average wage earner in this country to afford.

Technology is a paradox. We can do wondrous things, but many of those procedures are beyond the reach of many patients. They are also beyond the reach of many practitioners. These changes seem to be a natural evolution of what was once a very different profession. No one can deny that beginning a practice in dentistry in these times can be quite challenging. That is why I wrote this book; because, through the principles of leadership and communication, we can appeal to our humanity and write our own story.

Dental education has not caught up. There are some schools that teach these principles but, for the most part, dental educators are technophiles, who believe that more proficiency in technical dentistry will create success. There is still an overemphasis on technical courses in school, which was true back when I attended. I had to learn about leadership and communication on my own. Dentists still have a reluctance to take leadership courses, and the ones they take are very general and non-specific to dentistry. General principles will only get you so far. As I mentioned before, the purpose of philosophy is practicality, so applying general philosophical principles is just not, well – pragmatic. I believe, and I will say it repeatedly throughout this book, that the changes must begin in the dental schools. It is there that we can begin to write the story of our careers.

Dentistry attracts students who enjoy the challenge of technology. They pride themselves in being good with their hands. Many who choose dentistry think they are choosing a field of work that will make use of hand skills. Many choose dentistry because they want to avoid fields like sales, which require much more human connection and, hence, leadership and communication skills. Little do they know they are choosing dentistry while still pursuing a career in sales. A large component of the work of dentistry is persuading people to do things they would rather not do. Their job is to motivate people and to influence them, and that's what leaders do.

Technically oriented people tend to depend on formulas and algorithms to get results. Predictable dentistry is dependent on systems thinking. When it comes to people, though, many of the answers to our patient's problems is, "it depends." Scripts, policies, algorithms, and rules have a big problem with *"it depends."* Leaders must find new ways to communicate and influence if they want to be successful. I had to learn this, too. Through trials and revelations, I created a new story for my career. It's a story I am proud to share with dentists, because I think the entire profession can benefit by exposing this elephant in the dental school lecture room.

If your experiences in dentistry resonate with my story, then this book will help to apply timeless, ageless, universal leadership and communication principles for the present times. Times have changed since 1973. The slow changes in healthcare, the free market, and the economy have created times that can seem hopeless. Leadership and communication skills are needed now, more than ever. As leadership guru Marshall Goldsmith wrote, "What got you here won't get you there." I hear, from many young dentists who attend the Pankey Institute, that the principles don't work for these times. I disagree. My practice and life have continually improved since I hit rock bottom many years ago. I also believe that if Dr. Pankey were alive today, he would have no problems in sustaining a very rewarding dental practice. I will show you that these skills can be learned, and that everyone has the potential to lead. That it is our moral obligation to lead.

References

1 Horowitz, Mitch (2014). *One Simple Idea*. New York: Crown Publishers.
2 Ibid., pp. 116–122.
3 Brown, Don (1991). *Human Universals*, 1st edition. McGraw-Hill Humanities/Social Sciences/ Languages.

Introduction

"Philosophy does not claim to get a person any external possession. To do so would be beyond its field. As wood is to the carpenter, bronze to the sculptor, so our own lives are the proper material in the art of living."

Epictetus, *Discourses*, 1.15.2

We need a map. After practicing dentistry for 44 years, I have come to realize that the one thing that will serve every dentist in their quest for a better career and a better life is to have a map. Our profession suffers from too much morbidity; too much depression, too much burnout, too many broken relationships and, lately, way too many dental career derailments. There is a better way.

I was told many years ago, by a dentist whom I respect very much, that my quest to teach dentists about philosophy was futile. "It just doesn't sell," he told me. Dentists are just trying to make a good living by fixing teeth. They want to learn techniques. That dentist, ironically enough, taught *philosophy* to dentists. I always wondered why teaching a philosophical approach to any field was so challenging to teach. It all looks good on paper. The problems arise in the application. A good philosophy must be practical.

As you will read in this book, I, too, searched for ways to *practice* that would contribute toward a rewarding career. Many years later, I can say that I have had some success, but the early years were filled with many obstacles. There were times when I felt like quitting. There were times that my physical and emotional life was in turmoil. I suffered through many of the same problems that still exist today. But I was lucky.

I was lucky, because I entered dentistry at a time when it was easy to make a good living and build a career. I was lucky, because I found the right mentors, whom you will read about in this book. Mostly, I was lucky because I realized that, if I was going to have a great and long career, I would need to have models and maps. I found those maps by studying philosophy. Not dental philosophy, because that might lead me to better dentistry. What I really wanted was a better life. I needed a philosophy that would teach me how to live, because work is part of life.

Everybody needs a philosophy. Everyone needs to answer the question that has been asked since the beginning of time: "How to live?" Many of us learn from our parents, others from our religious background, and some of us just wing it. I never gave it a second thought until after dental school, when I had to make something of my career and raise a family as well. All of a sudden, things became complicated. I realized that I needed to examine my life and develop a philosophy.

I was first introduced to a philosophical approach to dentistry at the Pankey Institute. I was immediately captivated by Dr. Pankey's original philosophy. I learned everything I could about how he developed his philosophy by studying the Greeks. So I, too, studied the Greeks, specifically Aristotle and the concept of eudemonia, or the virtuous life. It was hard work. Most of the students who went to the Institute were interested in Pankey's restorative dentistry philosophy: how to treatment-plan, and design cases. Of course, that was very valuable for a dental education, but I was mostly interested in the practical side of making the philosophy work – or, as they say, how to get our best dentistry off the shelf.

I found the *softer skills*, the leadership and communication skills, much more challenging than the technical skills. This book is about how I used Aristotle's concept of *ethos, pathos and logos* to develop the skills necessary to practice successfully. As I stated earlier, most philosophies and religions have been trying to answer the question of *how to live* since the dawn of man. This book combines the ancient Greek practical wisdom with the burgeoning new science of positive psychology. The book explains the work of Dr. Martin Seligman, using his Well-Being Theory as the basis of living the life worth living.

The book discusses the current situation in dentistry. I discuss how a philosophy of practice is more important than ever, and how positive leadership and positive communication may hold the answers for creating a very fulfilling and satisfying career. My hope is that, by acknowledging the well-being of our health care providers, they will create a map for future career and life satisfaction.

Part I

The Problem

"How we see the problem is the problem."

Stephen Covey

"Leadership is solving problems. The day soldiers stop bringing you their problems is the day you have stopped leading them. They have either lost confidence that you can help or concluded you do not care. Either case is a failure of leadership."

Colin Powell

"We cannot solve our problems with the same thinking we used when we created them."

Albert Einstein

We live storybook lives. Just like in the movies, there is a pattern – a formula, if you will – that can determine whether we will succeed or fail. Many of us see our graduation from dental school as an ending when, in reality, it is just another scene change. In all likelihood, it is just the end of Act I, and now the real adventure begins. Act II, as in the movies, is where most of us get to fight the dragons that will determine whether we get to the places of our dreams. It is in Act II where we get to apply everything we learned up to that point. Every era has its own set of issues that must be confronted, or not. Are you prepared for this journey?

For me, Act II was a series of trials and revelations. There was a time when I denied that I had a problem. I lived in the world of "shoulds." You know that world. It is what some call the just-world fallacy, as proposed by Melvin Lerner [1]. That theory is a cognitive bias that a person's actions are inherently inclined to bring morally fair and fitting consequences to that person. In other words, the just-world hypothesis is the tendency to attribute consequences to – or expect consequences as the result of – a universal force that restores moral balance. For many dentists, the just-world hypothesis can be interpreted as becoming the very best technical dentist one can become, and everything will take care of itself. This idea can be illustrated by the commonly used belief of "you build it and they will come."

For the early part of my career, I believed that to be true. As a matter of fact, I was told that from my parents and teachers, growing up to my very favorite mentors in dental school and beyond. It was only through my own experiences that I realized I would have to work out the solutions to the problems that seemed to have no answers, or only very vague answers. When I brought my problems to those closest to me, I only received advice that fell back to the "shoulds." It was frustrating. Not solving these problems began to create pain. The pain showed up in various forms. I still hear dentists, young and old, speaking about the pain. Throughout this book, I will interview dentists at certain points along their journey; some have achieved success, while others are still in pain. When you hear their voices, as I do, you will share many of their feelings. Their pain, as was mine, flows from not clearly defining the cause or the problem.

Albert Einstein once said, "If I had an hour to solve a problem, I'd spend 55 minutes thinking about the problem and five minutes thinking about the solution." Navigating a career in dentistry is like solving a giant complex problem. This Part of the book is about seeing the problem from all sides – figuring out where to start the solution, and where the solution will take us. As the three wise men I have quoted above tell us, leadership is first deciding what the problem *is*. How we clearly and simply define the problem is how we attack it. The problems we define today may not be the same as I faced, while some of the problems will be exactly the same – certainly, the pain is the same. In Part I, I will discuss some of the problems that effect us all at an individual, organizational and even an industry-wide level.

Reference

1 Lerner, M.J. and Montada, L. (1998). An Overview: Advances in Belief in a Just World Theory and Methods. In: Leo Montada and M.J. Lerner (eds). *Responses to Victimizations and Belief in a Just World* (1–7). Plenum Press: New York.

1

The Many Faces of Dentistry – A Fragmented Field

"He that breaks a thing to find out what it is has left the path of wisdom."
J.R.R. Tolkien, from *The Fellowship of the Ring*

"Human science fragments everything in order to understand it, kills everything in order to examine it."
Leo Tolstoy, from *War and Peace*

"The whole is greater than the sum of its parts."
Aristotle

What is Dentistry?

If you ask the above question to any number of people, from general dentists, to patients, to dental educators, dental technicians, and specialists, you will get different answers. There is an old Indian story which has spread through many cultures over the ages. In the story, six blind men are asked to describe an elephant. Each man is told to feel a different part of the elephant, but only one part, such as the leg or the tusk. Predictably, each man offers a vastly different assessment. One says an elephant is like a rope (tail), while another says it's like a pillar (leg), or a fan (ear). They argue. Each man is convinced that his experience is the correct one.

All of the men are correct. Each part is described in explicit detail. The problem arises when each individual point of view is mistaken as describing the whole truth. By taking too narrow a focus, we can miss the forest through the trees. The problem comes when people become attached to their very narrow points of view.

This parable is a great example of one of dentistry's biggest problems … fragmentation. Dentistry is not unique in this regard. Many industries are compartmentalized and reduced to their individual components. How we define something determines how we treat it. As they say, in order to tame it, you must name it. Since this is a book about leadership in dentistry, I will explain how fragmenting this profession can be a source of major problems for a dentist.

Most dentists know that patients truly don't understand dentistry. Most, when asked, will tell you it is the science of teeth and gums. The language that patients use is enough to know that even the most astute patient doesn't have a firm grasp of dentistry. Their dental IQ is generally insufficient to understand the entire scope of dentistry.

The Complete Dentist: Positive Leadership and Communication Skills for Success, First Edition. Barry Polansky.
© 2018 John Wiley & Sons, Inc. Published 2018 by John Wiley & Sons, Inc.

Dental offices regularly take calls from patients asking for a cleaning when they need much more involved treatment. Barbara R. called the other day, reporting to my front desk person that she had a cavity. We asked her how she knew she had a *cavity*, and she reported that she was having some pain. When Barbara came in for her appointment, we determined that she had a abscess under an existing crown. Barbara, like many patients, does not understand dentistry or its language. What they do understand is what concerns them. They understand what dentistry means to them: cosmetics, comfort, health, cost, fear, time. Those are the general benefits of dentistry and the main objections to dentistry. Patients depend on us for our leadership to guide them toward better health, hygiene and cosmetics. Yet dentists who lack leadership and communication skills get caught up in more confusing scenarios.

There are others parties whose points of view affect the way dentistry is practiced. Insurance companies and dental service organizations claim that their view of dentistry always puts the patient first. Veteran dentists who have worked with third parties and have had disputes about treatment know that fees and covered services are what drive the third parties. Their view of dentistry is driven by the business side of dentistry, but dentistry, as you will see, has a human side as well. When any business only looks at the financial side, rather than the human side, something must suffer – especially when it comes to health care.

Then there is the government. They, too, have an agenda. The government's role is to help all people have access to health care. Obviously, this has not worked very well, considering all of the bickering that has been going on in Washington. Dental educators want their students to graduate on time with the skills necessary to do a good job. With all of these varying points of view, it's no wonder that dentists truly don't understand what dentistry is all about.

Take the National Football League as an example of an organization that falls under the heading of professional sports. Once again, there are many points of view about football. Fans, like patients, have their own selfish way of looking at football. Players have their points of view, and the way some football players conduct themselves these days, it's a good thing that there are higher powers. Those higher powers would be the owners and the NFL Commissioner. Hopefully, these leaders are there to protect the integrity of the game, for the future of the game. In other words, leaders are mostly concerned with integrity and long-term values.

The Latin root of the word *integrate* is *integrare*, which means "to make whole." One of the themes of this book is that dentistry is a complex field. Psychologist Mihalyi Csikszentmihalyi [1] tells us that evolution has always favored complexity. By complexity, he means highly differentiated and integrated at the same time. If the components are not highly differentiated and integrated, then the result is too simple and not destined to hold up over time. If the components are not integrated, or do not properly communicate with one another, then the result breaks down due to being overly complicated. If dentistry is to survive as a dignified and noble profession, it can only do so with integrity – organizational integrity, as well as individual integrity. I will discuss how to deal with this issue throughout this book. The very best leaders think in terms of sustaining values through integrity.

Wholism vs. Reductionism

In the Prologue, I mentioned that my entire world changed when I was exposed to the Pankey Philosophy. The question to ask is, what made my world change? Was it that I was understood dentistry a deeper level? That I understood the role of occlusion and that, for the first time, I could treat disorders that I could not even diagnose before? Or was is that I now took a more comprehensive approach to dentistry? Maybe it was all of those things, or maybe it was that I now had a model to look at that I could copy. The model or paradigm that I was exposed to was the first model of dentistry that I had ever been exposed to, and it made me feel comfortable. It put an order to what I was doing where none had existed before. Things made more sense to me. That's what paradigms do.

One of the most influential books ever written on leadership is Stephen Covey's *7 Habits of Highly Effective People*. Coincidentally, this book was published just as I was going through my deepest issues in my life and dentistry. Covey questioned the way we think, or our lens of perception [2].

Some of the greatest thinkers of our time were systems thinkers. Einstein, Leonardo and the great Greek philosophers like Plato, Socrates and Aristotle were big picture thinkers, who started with mental models that clarified their thought processes. These models, perceptions, or frames of references are known as paradigms – the way we see the world, as Covey says, "not in terms of our visual sense of sight, but in terms of perceiving, understanding, interpreting."[3] For me, this is a starting point. My whole career up until that point was compartmentalized into subjects like form and function of the masticatory system (otherwise known as occlusion), periodontics, pedodontics, and endodontics. There was a strong focus on learning technique in order to get enough credits to graduate.

When I graduated from Penn Dental School in 1973, I entered the US Army as a captain in the dental corps. I found the same approach to dentistry as I learned in dental school – specialization. As a general dentist, my job was to filter the patients and direct them toward either other general dentists or specialists. There seemed to be a disconnect in communications. I remember one of my earliest patients at Penn: Robert G. was a middle-aged man who came to me in the middle of treatment from a graduating dental student. His file was thick and heavy, almost a burden to carry into the clinic. I remember him needing numerous root canals, and having many broken and missing teeth. He desperately wanted to save his teeth. This was long before the public and the media put such a high value on cosmetic dentistry. Robert just wanted to save his teeth.

Robert came to the dental school's clinic because he couldn't afford to go to a private practice in his hometown in New Jersey. On the days he had appointments, Robert would take off from work and travel into Philadelphia to get his dental work completed. Even as a young dentist, I remember looking over his chart and thinking to myself, how futile, how frustrating this must be. It had been years of treatment by numerous students, who had long gone into their own private practices, yet Robert G. continued to make his weekly treks – and no significant dentistry was completed. All under the eyes of dental school instructors who were paid *per diem* and left every day to go back to their own private practices.

Years passed. I graduated, and had my own experiences, just like those students and dentists I spoke about above. One day, while practicing many years later in my office in Cherry Hill, a new patient came in – Robert G., fifteen years later. He didn't remember me. I could understand that, as he had seen so many young dentists through his years at Penn. But I remembered him. I was elated to see him on the one hand, yet so disappointed that he was coming in for a consult about having complete dentures. There truly was no alternative. He had very few remaining teeth at this point, and what was left was beyond repair. What I noticed even beyond his dental condition was that he was a broken and depressed soul. He admitted to me that his experiences at Penn had not only left him without teeth, but had also taken its toll mentally and emotionally. He blamed Penn. At first, I did, too.

This encounter exposed a hole inside of me – pain, if you will. At this point in my career, I knew that so much of my dentistry lacked meaning. The story of Robert G. clearly exposed this problem. What's the point of dentistry if we can't make a real difference in people's lives? It exposed one of the human universals I wrote about earlier: empathy. Although I didn't know it at the time, doing meaningful work is a major component of our well-being. My well-being was at a low point in my life at that time. Stepping back and looking at the big picture allowed me to assess that I needed a new way of thinking. A new map, model or paradigm of dentistry that was not being taught in dental schools, nor being practiced in the military or the private sector.

Rewriting Robert's story is impossible. Writing a new story would require starting with myself. I knew that in order to have a career I could be proud of would require a new way of thinking. A way that encompassed not only proficiency of technical skills, but how to apply them in order truly to make a difference in the lives of my patients, my staff and myself. One of the first things I noted when I went to the Pankey Institute was their mission statement: "*to inspire dental professionals to narrow the gap between what is known and what is practiced.*" That is a huge mission, and now, after thirty years, it seems that mission is needed more than ever. When I think about my own history, and listen to the pain of young dentists and their stories, I think of what psychologist Carl Rogers, founder of the humanistic psychology movement and client-centered therapy, once said, "What is most personal is most universal."[4] And it all starts with a *paradigm shift.*

A fundamental shift in thinking can make huge differences in the results we obtain. It can affect the technical results, as well as the results we get in our relationships, and health care, above all, is about human relationships. My "Aha" experience came at my first visit to The Pankey Institute. That experience is what was first described by Thomas Kuhn, in his landmark book *The Structure of Scientific Revolutions*, as a paradigm shift. Although many dentists through the years have been exposed to the thinking processes at The Pankey Institute, we have still not experienced a paradigm shift in dentistry. As a matter of fact, we have seen more of the typical way of thinking that created the problem: an overemphasis on highly technical dentistry and a decrease in the stress on human factors and big picture thinking. More reductionistic thinking vs. wholism.

Many dentists have heard of holistic dentistry. That is not what I am referring to when I use the term "wholism". Of course, you notice the "w" in my word usage. According to Wikipedia, holistic dentistry – also called biological dentistry, biologic dentistry, alternative dentistry, unconventional dentistry, or biocompatible dentistry – is the equivalent of complementary and alternative medicine for dentistry. Holistic dentistry emphasizes approaches to dental care said to consider dental health in the context of the patient's entire physical as well as emotional or spiritual health in some cases. Although that may sound like a more comprehensive belief system, it is not the paradigm shift that I had experienced.

The wholism I am describing is a way of thinking about systems. Think about a football team: teams are composed of offensive, defensive units and special teams. Each component team has various coaches, and each team has individual positions that function separately, but with the total team structure. Each team has a quarterback. Yes, the defense has a quarterback. It is the job of the quarterback to communicate with every player, on every play, what the objective is. The coaches play the same role by communicating to the quarterbacks what needs to be done in order to carry out the mission. That mission is the long-term value of winning. The best teams are the ones who have the best coaches and quarterbacks, who can communicate, at a very high level, what the big picture is all of the time. That's the main role of leadership.

It is only human to focus on the individual parts. The complexity of wholism can seem overwhelming at times. That is what separates the leaders from others. Reductionists believe the world can be understood by understanding the component parts, as exemplified by the story of the elephant and the six blind men. The wholist understands that the whole can be greater than the sum of its parts. Leaders apply this thinking to everything they do. I have nothing against holistic dentistry, nor the recent popularity of the oral-systemic connection. Both of those disciplines can actually be practiced using reductionistic thinking. Reductionism is not necessarily a bad thing. Reductionist thinking has been responsible for many breakthroughs in scientific research through the years.

Wholism and reductionism are not opposing thought processes. We need both. The key point is that wholism *encompasses* reductionism. Remember, each of the blind men were correct in their description of the parts, but none of them could describe the whole elephant. Reductionistic thinking has been the rule in many aspects of our lives, from science to how we are taught. In dentistry, we see many examples of this. The separation of all of our courses in school, as mentioned earlier; the over-specialization in private practice; the over-emphasis on technique and technology; the lack of courses in leadership, communication and human relationships; the over-dependence on scripting instead of courses in motivation and creative expression.

The examples are too numerous to mention, but you get the point. Reductionist thinking, although very necessary, has lead the profession into a black hole. Reductionist thinking fails when dealing with complexity. Thinking differently is a starting point. Dentistry is a profession, but it is essentially a form or work, a way and a vehicle not only to earning a living, but a way to create a life as well – and life is very complex.

Fragmented Dental Education

Where do we learn leadership and communication skills? I think most dental schools assume that these key skills are either learned before professional school, or they don't feel it is their responsibility, and that when the student graduates they will learn how to navigate the world. They teach the bare technical essentials; however, most would agree that the bare essentials are not enough in today's world. I believe, through my own experiences and study, that leadership and communication skills are best learned in context. There is an entire leadership community out there ready and willing to teach methods of standard leadership practices that are difficult to apply within the context of dentistry. I realized this many years after graduation, when I wrote *The Art of the Examination.* That book was about a process, but after writing it I realized that the examination process was an excellent way to learn and apply leadership skills. In dental school, the examination is taught as a way to collect data – dead and empty data that needed a human face.

I often hear from young dentists these common complaints:

- *"How come they never told us this in dental school?"*
- *"If I would have known how difficult this was going to be, I would have chosen another field ... who knew I would have to actually sell dentistry?"*
- *"How do they expect me to make a living working for these reduced fees?"*
- *"I was trained to do serious dentistry and all I ever get to do is fillings and root canals ... I'm getting sick of this."*
- *"I owe a fortune in dental school loans ... how will I ever work for myself, do the dentistry I love to do and stop working nights and weekends?"*

Dental school does not prepare dentists for the real world. I also hear of dentists who are leaving dentistry because they are so frustrated that they can't earn a living on their own terms, or that they are being controlled by patients and insurance companies. This takes great courage, because of the sunk costs in time and money they have invested. I never dreamed about leaving dentistry although, I will admit in my early years, I did wish for a way out.

A few years ago I attended an alumni meeting of The Pankey Institute. A young dentist pulled me aside and told me she had been through the entire continuum at the Institute. She said – and I believed her because I knew a little about her character – that she was trying to apply everything she learned. She had also read my book on the examination, and applied that as well. Of course, reading how to do something in a book is just a very early step to mastery. Her frustration was palpable. Having gone through similar experiences, I certainly felt her pain.

I have been haunted by that conversation. Because of the changing landscape in dentistry, I didn't feel as if I had given her an adequate answer. I think about my own career journey and I know how I did it. I thought about Dr. Pankey and read about his personal journey. I thought about many of the successful dentists I know, some of which I have interviewed for this book. I kept returning to leadership, and how it needs to be addressed in dental schools. It's the missing link.

Let's take a look at the history of dentistry. Before 1850, dentistry could best be described as a craft with no requirements to enter the field. It was mostly filled with craftsmen who were good with their hands and enjoyed working with small tools.

Formal dental education in the United States began in 1840 with the opening of the Baltimore College of Dental Surgery. Other dental schools slowly began to emerge, gradually displacing the traditional preceptorship method of training for dentistry. The period of the late 1800s saw a surge in the number of dental colleges in the United States. These schools were largely proprietary in nature, meaning that they were not affiliated with major universities, were private, were of a commercial nature and were, usually, established to benefit their owners. As the trend toward affiliation of dental schools with universities gained impetus at the beginning of the 20th Century, and with the establishment of the Dental Educational Council of America, the trend continued.

Dentistry mirrored medicine in many ways. Early dentistry was considered a sub-specialty of medicine. By 1850, there were two types of dentists in America: uneducated craftsmen who held that dentistry was a mechanical profession; and those with an understanding of science and biology. This much smaller group of "medical men of high character, broad intellectual interests, engaging personality and special influence" led the way toward the much more organized and dignified profession as we know today [5].

Two physician leaders who helped bring about these changes were Chapin Harris, the founder of the first journal of dentistry, and Horace Hayden, who created the first independent dental school in the US in 1840 – The Baltimore College of Dental Surgery, after many years of having been turned down by Maryland's medical college because they felt dentistry was just not important enough. That all changed in 1868, after Harvard opened its dental school, which led to the first of many Dental Practice Acts. In order to enter dentistry, applicants now needed requirements in anatomy, chemistry, physiology and surgery; just being a dental apprentice was no longer allowed. The field was starting to grow. Still, in 1865, there were only four schools and a total of 369 graduates.

Dentistry, however, was still held in low esteem. In order to improve the profession, reforms were progressively made, and dentistry continued to evolve through dental practice acts, licensing, and the development of associations and specialties. During the 1880s, dental education was slowly becoming a very lucrative business. Medical education was leading the way. Medical education in America was pretty dismal [6], and quacks and charlatans flourished as the professions tried to get organized. These were the times of building the foundations of both the medical and dental professions. These were the times that would define what dentistry would mean as a form of work – a job, a career, a calling, or a profession?

As a response to this confusion, a committee was formed to put some order to the medical field. The Carnegie Foundation created an advisory group led by Abraham Flexner – a teacher, not a doctor. He was charged with improving what was becoming a "plague spot of the country in respect to medical education." He teamed with two of the most prominent doctors of that time, William Welch and William Osler of Hopkins Medical School. All agreed that there could be no nobler work for a university than the promotion of medical studies. The committee set out to reform medical education, which essentially sounded the death knell for the for-profit proprietary medical schools in America. [7]

Flexner's main contribution as an educator was to mimic the German methods of education by placing stringent scientific requirements into a curriculum. He mainly believed in teaching through real-world problem-solving. Interestingly, the physician, Osler, believed that the Flexnerians had their priorities wrong in situating the advancement of knowledge as the overriding aspiration of the academic physician. He placed the welfare of patients and the education of students to that effect as more important priorities, although he reverenced the centrality of scientific knowledge. Osler's voice, however, was silenced by those who were more interested in the finances of the medical schools. Osler moved back to Europe and became silent, as William Welch, The Carnegie and Rockefeller foundations and Flexner completed their report in 1910.

Nowhere in the report is evidence of the Oslerian wisdom [8] regarding the primacy of patient beneficence. "Patients were primarily viewed as serving the academic purposes of the professor." In the end, the Flexner Report set the way for American dental education for many years to come. The positives were that the report led the way for advancement and scientific discovery, which undoubtedly improved the lives of most of us in America. The negative, as Osler warned, has created numerous issues in the 20th and 21st centuries in the deliverance of healthcare. Let me reproduce Thomas Duffy's words in his review of the *Flexner Report – 100 Years Later*:

> "There was maldevelopment in the structure of medical education in America in the aftermath of the Flexner Report. The profession's infatuation with the hyper-rational world of German medicine created an excellence in science that was not balanced by a comparable excellence in clinical caring. Flexner's corpus was all nerves without the life blood of caring. Osler's warning that the ideals of medicine would change as "teacher and student chased each other down the fascinating road of research, forgetful of those wider interests to which a hospital must minister" has proven prescient and wise. We have learned that scientific medicine must travel linked to a professional ethos of caring that has been in place in our oaths and aspirations. Cross-talk must occur between the two with a bi-directional bedside to bench dialogue. This creates the frisson that animates the quest for breakthroughs in a medical realm. The revisions in medical education that are now taking place are re-claiming the rightful eminence of the service component of medicine – the centerpiece of the doctor-patient relationship. The Flexner model remains in place, the foundation of the magnificent edifice that is American medicine."

The parallels to today's current state of the dental industry are nothing short of amazing. Sir William Osler, the physician who was ignored, was a wholistic thinker who warned, "*The future is today.*" How prophetic? Reading Osler's biography [9] and many of his quotes is a great example of how wholism thinking in healthcare is timeless. Even today, with supposed ethical codes and stringent licensing regulations, "if you are persuasive enough, articulate enough or even attractive enough, if you have an interesting enough, uplifting story, or some combination of these traits, you are or can be a very successful" [10] dental educator or coach/consultant to dentists who are starving for guidance in what is still not taught in dental schools. In my years in dentistry, I have seen dentist after dentist throw money at imposters and frauds who teach dentists unproven management and leadership techniques, in order to "sell" more dentistry, rather than doing what is right for patients.

I have seen successful dentists who have created careers out of training dentists to repeat persuasive and manipulative scripts meant to sell dentistry, divorced from the actual science of diagnosis and treatment planning. The field is filled with these coaches, consultants and even dentists. Yet there is hope, because there are dentists who teach ethical, comprehensive ways to successful careers. I found some, as mentioned at the Pankey Institute. The good news is that this idea is becoming a trend.

Finding thinkers who believe that *"scientific medicine must travel linked to a professional ethos of caring that has been in place in our oaths and aspirations"* is the job of the medical and dental communities. In medicine, one such man is Dr. Toby Cosgrove, MD, the president and CEO of The Cleveland Clinic. As a modern day Osler, Cosgrove is leading a revolution actively going on in medicine right now. His approach to treating people is more effective and more humane – two traits that require more leadership training at the level of the educational institutions. One of his issues is improving caregiver-patient communication [11].

Cosgrove realized that, in order to fix medicine, it had to be built from the ground up, so he started with medical school reform. In 2002, the Cleveland Clinic opened a new college of medicine, with the goal of reinventing the medical school from top to bottom. One of the first question he asked was, "How can we make this school the ideal medical education experience?" His answer was to protect the young people from medical school debt. He understands that students leaving school with strangling debt restricts them from following a more rewarding career path. Many take jobs and work long hours solely to pay off their debt. This is a current problem that dental school graduates are facing as more and more take jobs with corporate dental practices, and is a problem that, at the very least, must be recognized if the work of dentistry is to continue to be rewarding in every regard.

Another trend Cosgrove advances is training medical students to become better communicators, and more empathetic in general. He understands that addressing this in medical school is important, because there have been studies that show physicians in training actually become *less* empathetic. I remind myself of my dental school experience with Robert G. As part of their training, Cleveland Clinic has incorporated training in the humanities as part of their curriculum, to teach professionalism and communication.

This is the exact type of thinking I encountered at the Pankey Institute five years ago. Dr. Pankey, when asked about how a patient should choose a dentist, used three words: care, skill and judgement. Skill refers to a dedication to the science and technology of dentistry – a commitment to quality and excellence. Care and judgement imply empathy and wisdom. It is interesting to note the current trends in dentistry. The extraordinary attention to hand skills, technical dentistry and digital dentistry has placed care and judgement at the heels of technical skills. The masses have come to believe that dentistry is just about beautiful cases and cosmetic dentistry, ignoring the human component. Dental technicians are becoming dentistry's go-to experts. The time of the craftsman is here. Yet we are ignoring the human side of dentistry.

There is no doubt that the nature of our work is changing. The problems discussed up to this point – a need to focus more on wholism, and training dentists from the beginning in leadership and communication – lead me to the even bigger problem of what is actually at stake. For that, let's turn to the nature of work and why some of these issues truly go against our nature.

The Why of Work

When I was a kid I wanted to work with animals. I loved dogs and horses. As an adult, after I became a dentist, I worked with dogs as a hobby. I breed and show boxers. My parents wanted me to become a doctor – that's what all parents wanted for their kids in the fifties and sixties.

The work of a doctor offered the chance to make a lot of money and do work that wasn't physically demanding, offered the chance to make your own hours, and came with the mantle of respect and dignity. But are those the driving forces of work? I wondered.

As a child and young adult, I constantly asked myself, "What will I do when I grow up?" I remember my own children struggling with the same question. Invoking the Carl Rogers formula that I mentioned earlier, *"that whatever is most personal is most universal,"* I knew that the *what* of work was secondary to the *why* of work. Not many of us get to play third base in a Major League ballpark or perform at Carnegie Hall. Regardless of what the success literature tells us, finding success at that level is not for the masses. No, the masses, I felt, were not looking for the "perfect vocation" but, rather, looking for something much less visible: meaning and purpose.

It is true that making a lot of money, taking vacations, and driving a nice car can provide some degree of meaning for people. I have seen people quite happy just from making a good living, but fulfillment and well-being, as I will explain later in this book, are obtained through engagement in work, purpose in work and meaning in work [12]. I truly believe that what young people are searching for, beyond a good job, is meaning. Dave and Wendy Ulrich, in their book *The Why of Work*, call meaning the object of a nearly universal search. Great thinkers like psychologists Sigmund Freud and Viktor Frankl agree.

Freud was famous for saying that the two things a person in good mental health should be able to do well are "to love and to work" ("lieben und arbeiten"). Looking at Freud's own career path in medicine verifies how he came to that conclusion. As a young man who was not independently wealthy, he chose to go to medical school. He was in love with his future wife, Martha Bernays, and wanted to build a life together. He admitted later [13] that he chose medicine in order to make enough money to survive and build a family. Like most of us, he needed to find a way to earn a respectable living so he could marry Martha. He followed medical school by going into private practice. In practice, he created solutions for many of his patients. At the time, those solutions were groundbreaking, even though most have not held up. Freud worked right up until his death. In the context of his whole life, Freud chose a career path that allowed him to pursue both his family and professional goals, which led him to conclude that love and work, as he stated, were the key elements to mental health and a happy fulfilled life.

Viktor Frankl was a disciple of Freud's. His life wasn't quite the same. Frankl was studying psychology just as World War II broke out. His story is well documented [14], and is a highly recommended read. Before the war, Frankl was working on a system of psychotherapy based on our need for meaning. His own life became a living experiment as he survived the Nazi death camps by using his own theories about surviving, by providing meaning in his own life. His story is exquisitely described in his best-selling book, which has sold over nine million copies worldwide, *Man's Search for Meaning*. Both Freud and Frankl gained insight through their own experiences about the importance of meaning in our lives.

I have always been interested in the concept of work. As a young child, I wondered if there was more to work than just making a living. I grew up in New York City and remember people trudging off to work every morning, sitting in god-awful traffic every night, only to come home and do it again the next day. I wondered how people could do this for years and years and still suffer through the long days at work. Would that be my fate too?

While in dental school, I read the influential book, *Working* [15] by Studs Terkel, the late Pulitzer Prize-winning author. In that book, Terkel repeats the conviction that our universal search is the one for meaning. Terkel calls our jobs a search as well: "for daily meaning as well as for daily bread, for recognition as well as for cash, for astonishment rather than torpor; in short, for a sort of life rather than a Monday through Friday sort of dying." The book is composed of interviews of people with many various jobs. The common attribute in all of the interviews is "meaning to their work well over and beyond the reward of a paycheck."

I recently re-read parts of *Working*. I was particularly interested in the dentist, Dr. Stephen Bartlett, who at the time had practiced in a Detroit suburb for nineteen years. The interview could have been done today. Bartlett's complaints about dentistry were that it was physically demanding, that most patients were under stress, that he had to deal with cancellations and, mostly, that only he knew when he did a good job. He also spoke about what was appealing to him: that he could practice dentistry as he liked (autonomy), that he had the opportunity to play a role in the lives of his patients by changing their appearance (meaning), that he was his own boss and could make his own hours. I thought how similar the job is today but, like Frankl, that the landscape has changed. It has become more difficult to practice with meaning. We must make our own meaning. *Leaders are meaning makers.*

The work of dentistry truly has not changed much since I began to practice. Bartlett complained of standing all the time but, in 1973, four-handed sit-down dentistry was coming into vogue. I practiced sit-down dentistry for forty-two years. In re-reading the Bartlett interview, I came to realize that patient interaction hasn't changed at all. People still come to the dentist for the same reasons, and still have their prevailing objections. The human factor has never changed; technology has changed, and the context within which we practice has changed. Insurance, advertising and the 2008 economic meltdown changed the landscape so much so that dentists today struggle much more to create and maintain meaningful work scenarios. But it can, and still must, be done for the sake of the profession.

The context in which we see our work is important. As Stephen Covey reminds us, "how we see the problem is the problem." In other words, what is driving you is important. I opened this segment by saying that I raised dogs as a hobby. More recently, I have taken up yoga. I never considered doing either of these things to make a living. I dabble. I could earn a living doing either, but would I truly be happier if my and my family's well-being depended on making a living from these two endeavors? I chose dentistry 42 years ago, and it has always been a great way to provide for my family. A much better way than most forms of work. Somewhere along the line, I had to make an adjustment. I had to see dentistry as more than a job, and that's a problem. We need to re-frame the way we see our work. We need to see the big picture – another leadership trait.

There is an old story that many writers in the leadership industry use to bring out the differences between a job, a career, and a calling. There are many versions of the story, but I want to emphasize that if you are a dentist reading this, you are already in a career. If you choose to see your work as a job, as many do, there will be the consequence of forfeiting meaningful work. On the flip side, not all dentists have been called upon to fix teeth. Let's interpret the story:

> "One day a traveller, walking along a lane, came across three stonecutters working in a quarry. Each was busy cutting a block of stone. Interested to find out what they were working on, he asked the first stonecutter what he was doing. 'I am cutting a stone!' Still no wiser the traveller turned to the second stonecutter and asked him what he was doing. "I am cutting this block of stone to make sure that it's square, and its dimensions are uniform, so that it will fit exactly in its place in a wall." A bit closer to finding out what the stonecutters were working on but still unclear, the traveller turned to the third stonecutter. He seemed to be the happiest of the three and when asked what he was doing replied: "I am building a cathedral."

The story illustrates many lessons in leadership:

1) Knowing not just how and what to do, but knowing why.
2) Viewing the whole and not just its parts.
3) Seeing a vision, a sense of a bigger picture.

4) Having the ability to see significance in work, beyond the obvious.
5) Understanding that a legacy will live on, whether in the stone of a cathedral, or in the impact of other people.

I will come back to this throughout the course of this book. I see the second option as a problem in dentistry. If a person sees dentistry as a job that only provides him or her with a way to make a living, then it will be difficult to convince them to see otherwise. If the person sees dentistry as a calling, then their only problem will be how to make a living at doing something they truly love. I find, as in my case, that the difficult thing is to create a career that is balanced. I come back to this in the next chapter.

I know that the idea of the third stonecutter can make us a bit depressed if we truly weren't called upon to do dentistry but, as leaders, we must take a bigger picture if we want to satisfy our need to find meaningful work. When work becomes simply a means of earning a living, it becomes drudgery – the same word the Richard Cabot used in developing his philosophy. Another issue that I see today is the over-emphasis on the dentist as the grand hero of the story. Social media and advertising have taken the shine off of the true purpose of dentistry – the patient – and have placed it on the dentist. I will have a lot to say about being other-focused in a later chapter. One more issue that may seem to be a reach is that all of the self-focus that comes with seeing dentistry as a job has helped to create this *fragmented* profession that behaves unilaterally, rather than as a community.

Peter Senge, author the classic book, *The Fifth Discipline, The Art and Practice of a Learning Organization* [16], tells us: "the responsibility of a leader is not just to share a vision but to build a shared vision." I would add that to do that is to build meaning everyday. Charles Handy, author of *The Hungry Spirit* [17], repeats this thought about changing our thinking which has been a theme of this chapter by saying, "We may not need any more cathedrals, but we do need *cathedral thinkers*, people who can think beyond their own lifetimes." The original founders of what once was organized dentistry were cathedral thinkers – leaders like Chapin Harris, Horace Hayden and L.D. Pankey. Where have they gone?

Another big problem with work these days is a lack of engagement. With those who do not find meaningful work, it is not difficult to see that they spend most of their days unengaged. Many studies have shown this to be true. Job satisfaction, in all areas, has been on the decline for many years. A national survey conducted by the Nielson Company reported that fewer than one-half of employees (47.2%) reported being satisfied with their jobs. That survey showed a decrease in job satisfaction from 61.1% in 1987 to 47.2% in 2015. In another study, conducted in 2012 by Right Management, it was reported that only 19% of people were satisfied with their jobs. *Forbes Magazine* recently reported on a survey conducted by Mercer, the human resource consulting firm, that out of some 30 000 workers worldwide, between 28–56% of employees wanted to leave their jobs [18].

The Gallup Organization collected data on actual job engagement in 2012. They determined that only 30% of the US workforce was engaged and inspired at work, with 20% of people reporting they were *actively disengaged*. In another Gallup study of 142 countries worldwide, only 13% of employees were engaged at work, with 24% actively disengaged. There are many other studies that support the same idea, that we have a problem: people are becoming more dissatisfied with their work and disengaging from their jobs [19].

The dental community is not immune to these statistics. Although there is no study that I know of that has been done in dentistry, I can only surmise that, as humans, we are all suscep-tible to job dissatisfaction and disengagement. It is interesting to take note of a blog post [20] written by Dr. Laura Brenner, who calls herself the expert who loves to hate dentistry, about the reasons she left dentistry. The post practically went viral. Over 80,000 hits and 260 comments were written by dentists and dental students applauding her courage in making the decision to leave dentistry. Many books are beginning to fill the shelves in bookstores advising young people to take the leap, or to jump ship to find a more fulfilling job [21].

Laura has obviously struck a nerve with blogs posts titled, *Escaping the Cult of Dentistry*, and *10 Reasons Your Dentist Hates You Too* [22]. Of course, not everyone has the luxury of just picking up their toys and leaving the sandbox. The decision to leave a profession is a difficult one that is more dependent on the circumstances than just having the determination of the Peter Finch character in the movie Network when he screams out of the window, "I'm mad as hell and not going to take this anymore." Workplace drama at its best.

The idea of leaving dentistry in spite of the sunk costs involved may be an expression of the dissatisfaction that underlies the profession but it may be a generational idea as well. A large number of Millennials are openly expressing a desire to leave the profession. Unlike my generation, the younger generation has traded money for meaning, and are not willing to "sell out." Their dental school dreams of autonomy and freedom are less realistic after graduation. It is my belief that the dissatisfaction is another expression of reductionist thinking. Our tendency is to blame the profession for our unhappiness and dissatisfaction. There is nothing inherently wrong with the profession of dentistry that a practice of leadership, communication and wisdom will not cure.

When there is a lack of autonomy, meaning, and purpose, a lack of control of our own time and work, and a general dissatisfaction with our work environment, it is difficult to become engaged in our work, as the studies reveal. In the next chapter, I will discuss a concept known as *flow,* an important element in developing our well-being. When we're truly engaged in a situation, task, or project, we experience this state of flow: time seems to stop, we lose our sense of self, and we concentrate intensely on the present. This feels really good! The more we experience this type of engagement, the more likely we are to experience well-being.

Once again, these problems can be solved through making meaning, developing autonomy, gaining control over our own destinies. Stephen Covey, in his book *The 7 Habits of Highly Effective People* [23], makes a distinction between what lies within our control and things we have no direct control over. He tells us to act within our "Circle of Concerns" rather than acting on our "Circle of Influence". In time, he says, leaders acting on their concerns will stretch that circle and have a greater influence on things that do not appear within their control. I will discuss this leadership character trait in a later chapter. For now, understand that people with a strong *internal locus of control* believe events in their life derive primarily from their own actions, and they have more control of their lives, or they have an external locus of control, meaning that their lives are controlled by environmental factors which they cannot influence – or, worse yet, by chance, bad luck or fate.

This chapter presented some of the problems that are under our control. The book will continue to provide solutions to these problems; however, there are many issues that have created problems for dentists that are seemingly outside of our circle of concern. The problems would be analogous to Viktor Frankl's response to WWII. In other words, although he could not control his circumstances, he controlled his response (an obvious strong inner locus of control). In today's current economic climate, with rising health costs, the high cost of dental education and technology, the influences of government and corporations attempting to control expenses, the shrinking middle class, and income inequality, it is not difficult to see dentists reacting out of fear rather than responding to the conditions as they are. In the next chapter, I will discuss these issues.

References and Notes

1 Mihaly Csikszentmihaly (1997). *Creativity Flow and the Psychology of Discovery and Invention.* Harper Perennial.

2 Stephen R. Covey (1989). *The Seven Habits of Highly Effective People*, p. 18. Fireside Book, Simon and Schuster.

3 Ibid., p. 23

4 Carl Rogers (1961). *On Becoming a Person: A Therapist's View of Psychotherapy.* Mariner Books.

5 Schulein, T.M. (2004). A chronology of dental education in the United States. *Journal of the History of Dentistry* **52**(3): 97–108.

6 Prefer Jeffrey (2015). *Leadership B.S. Fixing Workplaces and Careers One Truth at a Time*, p. VIII. New York: Harper Collins.

7 Thomas P. Duffy (2011). The Flexner Report – 100 Years Later. *Yale Journal of Biology and Medicine* **84**(3): 269–276

8 Ibid.

9 Michael Bliss (1999). *William Osler A Life in Medicine.* New York: Oxford University Press.

10 Pfeffer Jeffrey, p. IX.

11 Cosgrove, Toby (2014). *The Cleveland Clinic Way: Lessons in Excellence From One of the World's Leading Healthcare Organizations*, pp. 100–105. McGraw Hill.

12 Ulrich, Dave and Ulrich, Wendy (2010). *The Why of Work – How Great Leaders Build Abundant Organizations That Win.* New York: McGraw Hill.

13 Lieben und Arbeiten (2012). *Figuring Out Fulfillment.* Blog, January 23, 2010.

14 Frank, Viktor (2006). *Man's Search for Meaning.* Beacon Press.

15 Terkel, Studs (1973). *WORKING, People Talk About What They Do All Day and How They Feel About What They Do.* New York: The New Press.

16 Senge, Peter (2006). *The Fifth Discipline, The Art and Practice of Learning Organizations*, 2nd Edition Revised. Doubleday.

17 Handy, Charles (1999). *The Hungry Spirit, Beyond Capitalism: A Quest for Purpose in the Modern World.* Broadway Books.

18 Susan Adams, (2012). *Americans are Starting to Hate Their Jobs.* Forbes, June 28.

19 Steve Crabtree (2013). *Worldwide, 13% of Employees are Engaged at Work.* Gallup, October 8, 2013.

20 Brenner, Laura (2013). *The Pros and Cons of Dentistry*, Lolabees Blog, January 27, 2013. Lolabees.me/2013/01/27/the-pros-and-cons-of-denytistry/.

21 Two current popular books are: *LEAP:Leaving a Job with No Plan B to Find the Career and Life You Really Want* by Tess Vigeland, and *Jump Ship: Ditch Your Dead-End Job and Turn Your Passion into a Profession* by Josh Ship.

22 Laura Brenner's blog posts can be found at Lolabees.me.

23 Stephen R. Covey (1989). *The Seven Habits of Highly Effective People*, pp. 81–86. Fireside Book, Simon and Schuster.

2

Not the Golden Age of Dentistry

"The ideas of economists and political philosophers, both when they are right and when they are wrong, are more powerful than is commonly understood. Indeed the world is ruled by little else.

"Practical men, who believe themselves to be quite exempt from any intellectual influences, are usually the slaves of some defunct economist."

John Maynard Keynes

"It's the economy, stupid."

James Carville

"The trouble with being in the rat race is that even if you win, you're still a rat."

Lily Tomlin

Did you ever feel like Rip Van Winkle, the main character of a pre-revolutionary fictional story by Washington Irving? Van Winkle fell asleep after drinking moonshine, only to wake up twenty years later, in a new world. Doesn't life feel like that sometimes? Throughout time there have been some watershed moments that have changed the course of history. A watershed moment is an important point of division or transition. In the movies, they call it a turning point. Some of these watershed moments have the potential to change our social attitudes forever, like Pearl Harbor, 9/11 and, the housing and mortgage crisis of 2008. It would have been hard to miss those moments but, in the world of economics and politics, it can be easy to miss a meeting occasionally.

Dentistry has had a few watershed moments that have changed the attitudes of health care providers and patients alike. In 1973, President Richard Nixon signed into law Bill S.14, which set the stage for the intrusion of third parties into dentistry forever. That bill started the ball rolling for people to increasingly become dependent on third parties for payment. What started as mostly indemnity coverage back then has turned into a majority of HMO and PPO plans. In my first book, *The Art of the Examination*, I referred to these seemingly innocent changes in the law as memes, or replicable ideas that eventually go viral and become part of our culture. I practiced in 1973, and slept right through the passage of that bill. Well, we can't un-ring that bill (pun intended). Even if we could see into the future, we never could have predicted the long-term consequences. The conditions were different then and, as Albert Einstein reminds us, *"No problem can be solved from the same level of consciousness that created it."*

In the last chapter, I mentioned Dr. Stephen Bartlett, the subject of an interview from the 1973 book, *Working*. I began my practice in 1973, and there have been so many changes

The Complete Dentist: Positive Leadership and Communication Skills for Success, First Edition. Barry Polansky.
© 2018 John Wiley & Sons, Inc. Published 2018 by John Wiley & Sons, Inc.

since those golden days. Many of those changes have brought on circumstances that we cannot control. Let me illustrate with a story of a patient who recently entered my practice. Because I take the time to get to know every one of my patients, I learned a lot as she told me her story.

Seven months prior to calling my practice, Connie G. broke her upper left lateral incisor (#10). At the time, she didn't have a family dentist. Her tooth broke, so she went to her computer and typed in the words "broken tooth." I know this, because I take the time to learn all of the details of the story. Google led her to an oral surgeon. As reported by Connie, the surgeon was a wonderful person who not only took her tooth out painlessly, but also replaced the tooth the next day with a flipper [1]. Connie was happy until two weeks prior to calling my office.

Two weeks ago, she noticed that the flipper was starting to look different. It is important to add that Connie is 69 years old, very fit and very attuned to new age science and well-being. She is a vegan and she does yoga. Noticing the changes, the first word that came into her mind was "shifting teeth." Back to Google. Guess what those keywords brought up? Orthodontist. So 69-year-old Connie, without a referring dentist, made an appointment with an orthodontist. He proceeded to do a workup – radiographs, photographs and models. He then presented her with a treatment plan. She was agreeable, since shifting teeth wasn't something she wanted. But the orthodontist told her she would first have to get the cavities, broken teeth and gum disease taken care of. She asked for a referral and was handed a list of dentists who were in her network.

Exercising her freedom of choice, she chose one close to her home. That office scheduled her with a hygienist, who immediately told her how bad her gums were, but when the doctor came in she would explain more. After more radiographs and a "cleaning," the doctor came in and told her that, yes, she had gum disease that would probably require surgery. Connie went home and consulted with Google once more. This time she looked for "painless gum surgery," and a new word came up – *laser*.

That's where I came in. I have a laser, so Connie entered my practice. I was the fourth dentist she had seen in less than six months. She was no closer to getting anything done since she visited the oral surgeon. Did Connie need an oral surgeon? I am still not sure because I wasn't there that day. Did Connie need an orthodontist? I concluded immediately that her teeth were not shifting – she was seeing the tissue above the flipper healing and changing form. Did Connie need a cleaning? Probably, but most people need cleanings. Connie needed guidance, needed someone to trust. She needed someone to spend time with her, to understand her and find out what she really wanted because she herself did not know. Connie needed a leader.

How did we reach this point? In 1973, patients did not enter practices like this. The 1973 version of Connie was the same as today's version, except today she can't hear the signal through the noise. She is a victim of what author Barry Schwartz calls the *paradox of choice*, or why having more is less, in his book by the same name. I am sure you can point out numerous points in Connie's story where you wanted to interrupt and explain to her why she could have done things differently, or tried to clarify for her a better outcome. In 1973, it was likely that if Connie had found a wise dentist, she could have been set straight – but today, there are so many voices spouting information, from advertising, to human resource people, insurance companies, and the public at large, that she truly can't hear the signal through the noise.

But Connie is still Connie and the dentist is still the dentist – both human beings trying to get through life any way you can.

There is a famous story by the late author, David Foster Wallace, titled *This is Water* [2]. In the story, there are these two young fish swimming along, and they happen to meet an older fish swimming the other way, who nods at them and says, "Morning boys, how's the water?" The two young fish swim on for a bit, and eventually one of them looks over at the other and says, "What the hell is water?" I am not making a high and mighty point here. It is just that we get so used to living in an environment or culture that evolves through each of our own levels of self-focus that we don't even realize what we truly want or need. We can't see the forest through the trees. And most of it we can't control. Let's take a look at some of the changes that have affected dentistry.

In 1973, when a patient needed a dentist, well, it was just that simple. Call a friend or neighbor, ask someone at work or open the phone book (yesterday's Google, without all of the explanations). There was no professional advertising then. You made an appointment, paid your bill, and either made another appointment, were referred to a specialist, or never followed up. Everything you did was based on your response or reaction to the dentist and his office, the price, and how motivated you were to follow up. Pretty simple.

These days, there are lists. The patient seemingly has a choice of dentists to go to who are on a network. Speaking of networks, there are information networks that provide out of context knowledge that leave it up to the patient to make their decisions. And all of this seems as natural as if it has always been part of the culture. The "water" we are all swimming in is the water we must accept. Insurance, income stagnation and inequality, advertising, and corporate dentistry are not going away. As individuals, we all have an obligation to take care of ourselves first and foremost. That goes for all people. The result is that there are competing forces. each looking out for their own self-interests – a fragmented community. This is a book about leadership, and leaders respond by understanding what is important to them and to all concerned, then creating their own version of water.

So what is all this about self-interest, and why is it important? To answer that question, we have to get a bit philosophical and go way back to the developers of capitalism. It is important to note that capitalism is an ideology. That means it was not discovered as an natural outgrowth of human nature. It was invented, as was its polar opposite, communism, or socialism or statism. Its inventor was Adam Smith, the Scottish moral philosopher best known for his classic treatise, *An Inquiry Into the Nature and Causes of the Wealth of Nations* (1776). He is credited with establishing the discipline of political economics, and is known as the founding father of capitalism.

It is interesting to note that Adam Smith was known as a moral philosopher, rather than an economist, even after writing the classic *Wealth of Nations.* He studied social philosophy at the University of Glasgow, and in 1759 he wrote his first book, *The Theory of Moral Sentiments*, which may be considered the first book written on the popular modern day subject of behavioral economics. Smith realized how important work and material wealth were in regards to creating a path to the good life (or what Aristotle called the virtuous life). He knew that pursuing money alone was futile in the quest to find happiness. His first book on morality and human nature has withstood the test of time, and is still used today by academicians in the fields of social psychology, economics and personal psychology.

One of dentistry's problems is the focus on purely making money, and not understanding its role in creating happiness. Dr. L.D. Pankey was one of the very few dentists who clearly understood this connection and used it to develop his philosophy of practice. In the center of his Cross of Dentistry, he placed the word "*Reward*" to signify the reasons why we work. That word is subdivided into material and spiritual rewards. Although students go through the Institute learning his basic philosophy, understanding the center of the Cross is not fully explained, and dentists rarely get to apply that aspect of the Cross.

Economics helps you understand that money is the only thing that matters in life. Economics teaches you that making a choice means giving up something. And economics can help you appreciate complexity and how seemingly unrelated actions and people can become entangled. An economics professor once said that a student told her that economics is the study of how to get the most out of life. Life is all about choices. Getting the most out of life means choosing wisely and well. And making choices – being aware of how choosing one road means not taking another – *being aware* of how my choices interact with the choices of others – that's the essence of economics [3].

In reading *The Wealth of Nations*, we find that Adam Smith believed that we are grotesquely self-interested. He believed, like the 20th century philosopher Ayn Rand, that the world is driven by selfishness (not the same as selfish). This is known through his most famous quote: "*It is not from the benevolence of the butcher, the brewer or the baker, that we expect our dinner, but from their regard to their own interest. We address ourselves, not to their humanity but to their self-love, and never talk to them of our own necessities but of their advantages.*" Smith recognized this paradox, because he observed that people do not always act out of their own self-interest. He believed in a constant interplay between the ego and what he named the "impartial spectator."

I will continue the discussion of this paradox in the next section, and in Part II on leadership ethos. For now I would like to re-examine a story I told in *The Art of Examination* [4]. It was a story about a young dentist who worked in a practice that did not do high-quality dentistry. In other words, they knowingly did dentistry that was well below the standard of care, as she reported to me. She asked the senior dentist if she should cement a bridge that she knew had poor margins. He said "yes," and she cemented the bridge. She remembered thinking at the time, "God will punish me for this. How can I live with myself?" That is her impartial spectator speaking. This is Smith's moral voice. Awareness of the spectator, the inner critic or whatever you want to call it places you at a crossroad of morality that could lead to a better life.

If you want to get better at what you do, if you want to get better at this thing called life, you have to pay attention. When you pay attention, you can remember what really matters, what is real and enduring, versus what is false and fleeting. Thinking of it as the impartial spectator can help you know yourself, help you become a better boss, a better spouse, a better parent, a better dentist. Thinking of an impartial spectator can help you interact with actual, real-life spectators (e.g., the Jewish mother that provides your guilty conscience) and change how they think of you. That's nice, but Adam Smith argues that it's more than a pleasant side benefit the comes from paying attention to how your behavior is perceived. It can actually lead to serenity, tranquility, and happiness.

How you are perceived is important. Not to others, but how you perceive yourself. Smith claimed that we all want to feel worthy of being loved. He used the word lovely to describe what he meant "to be worthy of being loved." This is a spiritual reward that is not spoken about much in the halls of dental education. If it were, we wouldn't think that all success is dependent on just making more money. Money equals success, and more money equals more success, is an example of the reductionist ideas being promoted in our culture, as well in as our schools. I am not just preaching here. These are *principles of human nature* that were written about by Aristotle and Adam Smith, and only now are being proven in the research labs of cognitive and social scientists.

Awareness is a key factor in who you become. It is quite easy to deceive ourselves. When we lose our autonomy, our discretion and our ability to do meaningful work, it plays on who we are. Adam Smith claimed that when our work causes us to lose something, we become something else [5]. I have seen many dentists change who they were when their working conditions were not conducive to a happy life. In time, these dentists became apathetic toward their work and their patients. I should know – I was one of them. Many dentists burn out, and yet deceive themselves into thinking it's the work.

In a classic article by Melvin Cohn and Carmi Schooler showed that work over which people exercise some discretion and control leads to cognitive flexibility and to an engaged orientation to self and society; in contrast, excessively monitored, oppressively supervised working conditions lead to distress. It takes a strong level of awareness not to fall into the trap of working for "some defunct economist", as mentioned by John Maynard Keynes in his quote at the start of this chapter.

Reading Adam Smith and the foundation of capitalism led me to reinterpret much of the philosophy I had been exposed to – for example, L.D. Pankey's *Ladder of Competency.* Pankey believed that 2% of dentists are masters, 8% are adept, 36% are students and 54% are apathetic. I am not sure if his numbers are true [6]. When I was first exposed to these numbers, my natural reaction was to push myself toward mastery. It is not an easy road. What I believe today is that there are many factors that can cause us to stumble along that road. Dentists who want to achieve mastery must acquire more than knowledge. Dentists who are masters, and even those who are very adept, have more than hand skills and knowledge. They are system thinkers, as mentioned earlier, and have achieved a degree of wisdom which is different from knowledge.

I have an ongoing argument with my wife. Whenever one of our conversations is about someone we know who is successful, she always says they're very smart. Many times, I tend to disagree. I do see a correlation between intelligence and success but not, as they say, the cause of success. I have been reading the success and happiness literature for over thirty years. I am a voracious reader who relied on books to get me through my "burnout years." I have come to covet wisdom much more than knowledge. Wholism and systems thinking is wisdom. Dr. Pankey's Cross of Dentistry infers that knowing yourself, your patient and your work is the key to the reward, a successful life and career in dentistry. I will have more to say about acquiring the knowledge in later chapters. It is the application of the knowledge that is difficult and is what many have trouble with, as the young dentist I met at the Pankey Alumni Meeting, whom I mentioned in Chapter 1.

Webster's Dictionary distinguishes three types of wisdom:

1) *knowledge*, or accumulated philosophic or scientific learning;
2) *insight*, or the ability to discern inner qualities and relationships; and
3) *judgment*, or good sense.

I try to explain to my wife that the emphasis on discernment and good sense highlights the difference between a *wise* person and a *smart* one. We all know people with high IQs who are not successful or happy. They may lack insight about human affairs and display poor judgment in both day-to-day interactions and the larger pursuit of a rewarding and meaningful life. In other words, there are many people who are smart, yet use their intelligence toward only their selfish interests; who not only lack a moral compass, but wisdom about what goals are truly worth pursuing, and the means by which they are best pursued.

I don't want it to seem that I am throwing Dr. Pankey under the bus. His description of what makes a good dentist, and what it takes to have a fulfilling career in dentistry, went way beyond just acquiring the knowledge. He said it was *care, skill and judgment.* Therefore, becoming a skilled wise dentist is the goal of this book. He knew that wisdom, unlike pure intelligence, demands some insight and effectiveness around people.

Let's go back to Connie G., the patient I mentioned at the beginning of this chapter. Each of the three dentists she visited had knowledge in their respective areas of expertise. However, none of them took the time to listen to her story and understand her hopes, fears, passion, desires and drives. Dentistry is not done in a vacuum. All dentistry is done within the context of human beings, and that requires wisdom. In order to be a wise person, you must be wise about people. When L.D. Pankey said he never saw a tooth walk into his office, he was expressing the idea that the content of dentistry (teeth) is forever entwined with the context of dentistry (people).

The road to mastery then is more than just acquiring knowledge. It is having the ability to think differently, without restrictions. The dentist must be able to choose his path wisely, and then execute his march toward mastery, unencumbered. Many dentists believe that having passion alone can drive that journey – yet, as mentioned earlier, that may only be available to those who were "*called*" to dentistry. I would agree that to become a leader takes a high degree of positivity and passion for one's work, but to sustain high levels of passion requires a sense of control – and that is a problem these days.

In a study published in the *Journal of Research Personality*, it was determined that acquiring passion takes time. The study made a distinction between the job, the career and the calling. The study showed that people were split evenly between the three choices of how people view their work. When further asked about a "calling," whether it was innate or could be promoted or amplified, most said it could be developed through more years on the job, that they were there long enough to become good at what they do and have consistent feelings of efficacy and the ability to create relationships. In other words, creating passion, and hence a calling, takes time [7]. The road toward mastery takes time, and I know this was true for me. Many people abandon the road in favor of expediency, distractions, fears and the opinions of others. Wouldn't it be better for the profession if the road were clear?

Robert Greene, in his book, *Mastery*, explains that mastery is wired into our brains. It is built into our human nature to take the time and focus on the depth of our subject of study [8]. Taking this one step further, author Dan Pink reports on a study, *On the Surprising Science of Motivation* [9], which claims humans need three nutriments to feel intrinsically motivated for work: *autonomy, competence, and relatedness.* All of these nutriments refer to having some control over our work. Autonomy is the ability to have control over our time at work and at home. Competence is the feeling of self-capability and self-efficacy. The third nutriment, relatedness, is the feeling of being connected to other people. Dr. Pankey once said, "I never saw a tooth walk into my office." He was expressing the idea that the content of dentistry (teeth) is forever entwined with the context of dentistry (people). In other words, developing a true passion for dentistry, and the ability and desire to help patients at an optimal level, requires much more that acquiring the knowledge. Knowledge equaling success would be a good example of reductionist thinking.

The late psychologist Chris Peterson, from the University of Michigan, was one of the most influential voices in the new science of positive psychology. Positive psychology is the scientific study of the strengths that enable individuals and communities to thrive. The field is founded on the belief that people want to lead meaningful and fulfilling lives, to cultivate what is best within themselves, and to enhance their experiences of love, work, and play. In a manner of speaking, it could be the new science of leadership and communication. My own studies began with the teachings of the positive psychologists, and I would be remiss not to point out the crossover between business, self-help and positive/cognitive psychology. This point can be illustrated in a quote by Peterson: "Good days have common features: feeling autonomous, competent and connected to others." Isn't that a simple explanation of what we are looking for, and what is guaranteed in our Constitution – the pursuit of happiness.

So why the roadblocks?

This book so far has listed ingredients for a fulfilling and successful career. Meaningful work, autonomy, discretion at work, self-esteem and capability, engagement, worthiness (Adam Smith's lovely), control, satisfaction and, of course, money, are just some of the rewards that have been promised (the pursuit anyway) to us by the founding fathers. Yet we find ourselves at a crossroads or a balancing point, if you will. I use the metaphor of the crossroads numerous times in this book. Like the center of Pankey's Cross, it is a crucial place, centrally located where two or more roads meet. Dr. Pankey called it balance, one of the defining traits of mental equilibrium – the place between opposing forces that needs to be mastered.

The balancing point or crossroads we face in dentistry today are the forces that exist between human nature and human design. Human nature is comprehensive and occurs through all cultures throughout time. It is the human condition, over which we have little control. It shows up in our genes. As mentioned earlier, the list of human universals includes empathy, generosity, sadness and humor, music and aesthetics, fairness and reciprocity, pride, story, and leadership [10].

Another authority on what drives human motivation is Abraham Maslow, a psychologist best known for the development of his Hierarchy of Needs [11], a theory of psychological health predicated on fulfilling innate human needs in priority, culminating in self-actualization. At the base of his pyramid, Maslow placed the fundamental needs of all humans – what he called "deficiency needs". If these deficiency needs are not met – with the exception of the most fundamental (physiological) need – there may not be a physical indication, but the individual will feel anxious and tense:

- *Physiological Needs* – the physical requirements for human survival. This explains Adam Smith's logic in saying that the primary motive for work is money and material wealth. Putting food on the table trumps everything, and is the reason why most of us are driven to do things in our careers that we might otherwise not do.
- *Safety Needs* – in the absence of economic safety, due to economic crisis and lack of work opportunities, these safety needs manifest themselves in ways such as a preference for job security, grievance procedures for protecting the individual from unilateral authority, savings accounts, insurance policies, reasonable disability accommodations, etc.
- *Love and Belonging Needs* – according to Maslow, humans need to feel a sense of belonging and acceptance among their social groups, regardless whether these groups are large or small. The largest group in the world is the human race.
- *Esteem Needs* – one of the human universals, we all have the need to be respected. Esteem presents the typical human desire to be accepted and valued by others. People often engage in a profession or a hobby to gain recognition and a sense of value, and to feel that what we do makes a difference.
- *Self-actualization* – Maslow said, "What a man can be, he must be." This quotation forms the basis of the perceived need for self-actualization. This level of need refers to what a person's full potential is, and the realization of that potential

Recent research appears to validate the existence of universal human needs [12, 13]. Study after study throughout time informs us of our basic human needs and desires. It is astounding to me that dentists in the 21st Century are having a difficult time fulfilling their basic human needs. It is because of what is known in the field of evolutionary biology as the Mismatch Theory [14].

As a diabetic, I have an acute awareness of how this theory works in life. The increase in prevalence of diabetes in modern times may also be attributed to mismatch theory. Human diet has changed considerably over the 10 000 years since the advent of agriculture. The evolutionary history of humans has selected for an intense craving for high sugar/high fat food.

In modern human environments, however, sugars and fats are highly attainable. The mismatch hypothesis, via a substantial change in diet and fat/sugar availability, can partially explain the marked increase in diabetes in modern human populations. As a diabetic, I can appreciate the control it takes to overcome what our human design allows, and what is available in the environment. According to Wikipedia: "The essence of mismatch theory is that organisms possess traits (including behavioral, emotional, and biological) that have been passed down through generations, preserved by natural selection because of their adaptive function in a given environment. However, the given environment of the evolutionary period can be quite unlike the current environment. Therefore, traits that were at one time adaptive in a certain environment are now 'mismatched' to the environment that the trait is currently present in."

 The same analogy can be used when viewing our current work conditions, and how much control we can exercise. The dental profession evolved over one hundred years ago to provide dental care to the public, and to provide a level of organization that protected the freedom of choice for all parties concerned. Today, regardless of what we are being told, patients, as well as dental health professionals, are having their freedom of choice compromised. This is where human design comes in. Capitalism is an ideology. It was designed, and its primary designer realized that, although material wealth is the main driver, it also provided a source of well-being and self-esteem through meaningful work.

Today's version of free-market capitalism has evolved to cut off that function of work. The economist Thomas Sowell believes in two visions of human nature – what he calls "constrained" and "unconstrained." The constrained focuses on the selfish, aggressive, dark side of human nature and, as we cannot control human nature, we put constraints on it. Most health professionals are aware of these constraints. The "free market" under these constraining rules can, and does, affect the way work is performed. Sowell explains the unconstrained nature of work as seeing enormous human possibility, and condemns the state for subverting all that is good in human nature.

Dentists who work in the insurance system see evidence of this every day. A few years ago, I sat on a panel set up by the *Huffington Post* to discuss the current state of dentistry. I was the only dentist on the panel. Joining me were two patients who were "wronged" by the dental profession, a lawyer for an insurance company, a health writer and a dental fraud inspector. I remember wondering to myself, "how did we get to this point?" I don't know how to design the future of dentistry, but I do know that the complex circumstances that I am describing need to be addressed. In my practice life, I designed the way I practiced. I designed it by striking a balance between the material rewards doing "good work." The leader's main role, I believe, is to design dental practices and dental workplaces that are more hospitable to doing meaningful work.

In the end, the free market that we all claim is the purpose of capitalism is a myth. We have lost that freedom to government and the corporations. Free market capitalism should generate outcomes that improve the well-being of the vast majority. That is not happening in healthcare today.

Robert Reich in his insightful book *Saving Capitalism* [15], sums it all up. Markets, he says, are designed by human beings. As with any system, there are alternative ways to organize the market. "However organized, the rules of the market create incentives for people. Ideally, they motivate people to work and collaborate, to be productive and inventive; they help people achieve the lives they seek. The rules will also reflect their moral values and judgments about what is good and worthy and what is fair." The rules, as we have seen, have changed over time. The new rules, which have evolved for the benefit of the few, have not been fair. We now have a mismatch.

The result of the mismatch has been to challenge freedom of choice of both doctors and patients, and has created a situation where most of the middle class hasn't had an increase in wages for over 30 years. The dentist is either a worker or a small business owner, both of which have been forced to more work for less money as a result of capitalism going awry. It is no longer true in America that the harder you work, the more successful you will be. Like the weather or traffic, these are problems that we must deal with by designing our own futures, and by making ourselves and the people we lead better.

The Paradox of Duty and Desire

"I don't like the word 'balance.' To me, that somehow conjures up conflict between work and family... as long as we think of these things as conflicting, we will never have happiness. True happiness comes from integration... of work, family, self, community."

Padmasree Warrior

"You are doomed to make choices. This is life's greatest paradox."

Wayne Dyer

"The decisions you make are a choice of values that reflect your life in every way."

Alice Waters

Someone once told me, "You can have anything in the world you want; but you can't have everything." Doesn't that seem the way life is? Don't we all wish life could be more clear cut? That our decisions would be easier? I have used the word "balance" numerous times. The Pankey Institute teaches its students to "keep the Cross in balance." The problem is that in order to stay balanced, we must choose between contradictory or conflicting choices. This is what is known as a paradox – and life is paradoxical.

There are many paradoxes that dentists are confronted with on a daily basis – for example, whether to save a tooth because it is the right thing to do clinically, or to extract a salvageable tooth because the patient can't afford treatment or just wants the tooth out. Clinical situations like that occur frequently in dentistry, and everyday dentists make those choices. Best treatment? Best materials? Best technique? Behind all of these choices is one that I have found the most difficult and the one that can make the biggest difference in the dentist's whole career. I call it "reconciling the paradox of duty and desire." Most people, not just dentists, choose one over the other, and desire usually wins out.

First, let me define the terms, duty and desire. By duty, I mean performing your moral or legal obligation, your responsibility. When one acts out of a sense of duty, one provides the function that goes along with the job, like providing good service for all patients. Dr. Pankey felt dentists were morally obliged to perform complete examinations on patients. That thought, acting out of a sense of duty, is what stirred me to write *Art of Examination*, and to change the way I practiced over 30 years ago. Consistently choosing to do a complete examination on every patient tested my ability and willingness to make that choice every time. A complete exam is the right thing to do. I truly want to say it is the legal thing to do as well because, if there is an issue with a patient, it will always come back to the diagnosis and the initial complete examination.

Desire, on the other hand, is usually the easier choice; after all, it tests all of the reasons we chose dentistry to begin with. Steven R. Covey, in a summary of all of his work, *Primary Greatness* [16], says, "there are two ways to live: a life of primary greatness or a life of secondary greatness. Primary greatness is who you really are – your character, your integrity, your deepest motives and desires. Secondary greatness is popularity, title, position, fame, fortune and honors." The irony, he believed, is that focusing on primary greatness leads to success because it leads to intrinsic rewards, such as peace of mind, contribution and rich and rewarding relationships. Most of us get it backwards – we seek the extrinsic rewards first.

It's like having a devil on one shoulder and an angel on the other, each competing for your attention. Devil or angel, which one will it be?

The choices we make everyday in our work and in our private lives begin with our fundamental drives. All of our choices emanate from "why?" The philosopher Friedrich Nietzsche once said, "He who has a why to live for can bear almost any how." To me this means, at some point, deep within ourselves, deep within our hearts, lie our true motivations. If we never take the time for self-contemplation and self-reflection, we end up living and working for other people, which is becoming more the norm in dentistry. Throughout this book, I will continue to show how the deep drives and human universals that exist within each of us are the keys to a successful and fulfilling life.

So what is the problem with reconciling the paradox of duty and desire, if it is nothing more than taking the time to get to know ourselves? There are volumes written about how to slow down life and become more aware so that we can make better choices. However, knowing that isn't the key. Discovering our motivations is the first step, but aligning them through living is another. The problem is that our culture is geared toward accumulation of material wealth, life is fast, and we don't take the time to understand ourselves. It can get confusing like David Foster Wallace's "two fish" – *what* water?

In *The Art of Examination*, I wrote about the 1996 movie, *The Big Night*. The plot of the film tells the story of two Italian immigrant brothers who open and operate a restaurant called "Paradise" on the Jersey shore in the 1950s. One brother, Primo, is a brilliant, perfectionist chef who chafes under their few customers' expectations of "Americanized" Italian food. Their uncle's offer for them to return to Rome to help with his restaurant is growing in appeal to Primo, because of his attachment to the purity and principles of good authentic cooking. The younger brother, Secondo, is the restaurant manager, a man enamored of the possibilities presented by their new endeavor and life in America. Despite Secondo's efforts and Primo's magnificent food, their restaurant is failing.

The movie illustrates the paradox of the two mindsets that live within us – the devil or the angel that create our mental attitudes, that push and pull at each choice we have to make. It is interesting that the screenwriter gave the names Primo and Secondo to the two brothers to show that they had to reconcile these mindsets in order for the restaurant to succeed. It is up to each of us to decide, based on who we are and what drives us, how we run our practice and our lives. We must choose what comes first and what comes second.

If we decide that we are healers first, before we are businesspeople, then that will be reflected in the way we practice. In his book, *Money and the Meaning of Life* [17], author and philosopher, Jacob Needleman claimed that money is very important for a good life, but he said, "it is secondary." When asked if it is secondary, then second to what, he said, "whatever is primary." Reconciling the ever-present paradox is a starting point that most people rarely see. It starts with answering a few self-evident questions: "Who are you?"; "What do you want?"; "How will you get what you want?"

Another fundamental question to ask ourselves is, "why did we choose dentistry as a profession?"

Answering these questions will help us to reconcile the great paradox. The answers will lead to your true motivations beyond simply making money. It will lead to the reasons you spent eight years in school while others were out making a living after high school or college. Was it to avoid having a job or a career that was boring, repetitive and could lead to daily monotony and drudgery, as Richard Cabot wrote of over 100 years ago? Answering these self-evident questions can result in making dentistry a worthwhile career, that can change our roles from a mechanic of the mouth to a physician of the oral cavity.

There are trends in society today that are making our choices more difficult and, although the factors have always been present, the trends are growing. We are moving away from a society that rewards autonomy, meaning, discretion, challenge, engagement and judgment, toward a culture that is producing the professional equivalent of factory work – the actual thing we stayed in school to avoid.

Current trends in dentistry are leaning toward more dependence on insurance. The shrinking middle class has put pressure on dentists to accept the lower fees offered by the dental networks. When more and more patients become insurance dependent, and dentists join the insurance networks, there is less incentive to create optimal treatment plans. The administrative duties, including marketing and sales, get transferred to trained staff, and the practice of dentistry begins to run on automated systems and algorithms. There becomes an overdependence on systems and scripting, which minimizes the human factor. Whatever communication and leadership skills the dentist uses are reduced to weekend courses and in-house coaching.

Another trend is the overemphasis on the business of dentistry. It seems that most practices are consumed with the idea of daily and monthly production goals, as if these were the only goals available for a practice. Jody Thompson and Cali Ressler developed a concept known as ROWE (*results only work environment*), wherein employees are paid for results, rather than the just their accumulated hours and production bonuses. Dentists can create any number of types of results, way beyond incentives for production. The overemphasis on production goals can backfire and can create insensitivity toward patient's real needs.

A third trend that has been growing since the eighties when the Federal Trade Commission allowed professional advertising is all forms of print, and digital advertising. This has caused advanced commercialism and commoditization of dentistry. Creative marketing has put a emphasis on lowering our fees and increasing the competitiveness of dentists. Advertising certainly has changed the dental landscape. It would have made dentistry's founding fathers roll over in their graves to see what these trends have done to what they tried to create one hundred years ago.

And dentistry is not the only field that has been affected. Medicine, law, and education have had their share of issues as well. Medicine has already lost much of its autonomy. The tendency through the years has been to lessen the odds of creating a career or a calling in all of the professions. The available choices are leaving one option for most: a job. Authors Barry Schwartz and Kenneth Sharpe, in their book, *Practical Wisdom: The Right Way to Do the Right Thing* [18], interview Dr. David Hilfiker, a physician who expresses what many of us are seeing in today's professions:

> "The fee schedule had made procedures much more lucrative than in-depth interviews, counseling sessions, or time taken to comfort a hospitalized patient. There were also many important services I performed which had no charge attached whatsoever: returning telephone calls about a child's fever, giving an emotional support to a family after the death, going to medical staff meetings, to mention only a few. But despite my conscious disagreement with many of the values assigned by price, I noticed that surgery, procedures, hospital admissions, and emergency-room work slowly became a more and more important part of my practice. Dealing with emotionally hurting patients, taking time to educate patients about the course of their disease and the nature of their treatment, even obtaining a comprehensive medical history, became less central. Not that I consciously changed my routines; but money had powerful ways of bending my perceptions.... It is not an exaggeration to say that money seeped into every crack in my life....
>
> Paradoxically, as I did my best to manipulate patients into conforming to the needs of an efficiently run office, it was I who became the object, the machine.... I measured myself at the end of the day by what I had produced.... I certainly recognized the limited power of money to satisfy me, yet since much of my day was structured around charges and costs and since my income level had become emotionally important to me, money was an important value. Patients' diseases and my service became commodities that were bought and sold at a price."

We can see the same thing happening in dentistry. Someone once said we become the products of the times we live in. What happens to us when we succumb to decisions based on a culture of money? When the most important thing in our professional lives is production? Dr. Hifiker hints at the possibilities. Many professionals these days are leaving their respective fields. They go into sales or teaching. What happens is that dentists become apathetic and then unethical, like the young dentist I mentioned earlier. They become unethical a little bit at a time. Not by committing fraud, but more by cutting corners and taking shortcuts. There won't be time to spend with patients to do in-depth pre-clinical and clinical exams. Errors of omission will occur. Drip by drip we become who we never intended, and fall off the road to mastery... toward apathy.

And it starts with making good choices.

It is true that you create your destiny in these quiet moments of decision. We must live our lives going forward. When looking back, we can see whether our decisions made sense. My decision to commit to the principles of comprehensive dentistry by applying sound leadership and communication skills has led to the biggest difference in my career. Recently, I was going through the years and years of photographs of patient cases I completed. I stopped at each one to remember who they were and what happened to each of them. Some left the practice, many stayed, some cases didn't work out the way I planned, and some exceeded all expectations. At the end of that exercise, I felt a great sense of satisfaction. I had truly helped a great many patients. The successes certainly outweighed many of the issues I had to deal with on a daily basis.

I am nearing the end of a long career in clinical dentistry, and I will end it with complete fulfillment and assurance that I truly helped most of the people I served. Each day when the devil appeared, I would face him and make the right choice, based on my well-thought-out values. That devil appears because he is summoned through fear. There are only two basic fears we predominantly deal with: the fear of not being enough and the fear of not having enough. The problem is that our culture feeds these fears everywhere we go.

There is an old story from the Nanticoke Indian culture which describes this choice in The Tale of Two Wolves:

> *One evening, an elderly*
> *Cherokee brave told his*
> *grandson about a battle that*
> *goes on inside people.*
> *He said "my son, the battle is*
> *between two 'wolves' inside us all.*
> *One is evil. it is anger,*
> *envy, jealousy, sorrow,*
> *regret, greed, arrogance,*
> *self-pity, guilt, resentment,*
> *inferiority, lies, false pride,*
> *superiority, and ego.*
> *The other is good.*
> *it is joy, peace love, hope serenity,*
> *humility, kindness, benevolence,*
> *empathy, generosity,*
> *truth, compassion and faith."*
> *The grandson though about*
> *it for a minute and then asked*
> *his grandfather:*
> *"which wolf wins?..."*
> *The old Cherokee simply replied,*
> *"The one that you feed"*
> *"Feed the right wolf and you will reconcile the paradox of duty and desire."*

References and Notes

1 Not being sure who my reader is, I will describe some of the dental terms I use for those who don't understand. A flipper is an all-acrylic removable partial denture, usually used to replace teeth temporarily.

2 Wallace, David Foster (2009). *This Is Water: Some Thoughts, Delivered on a Significant Occasion, about Living a Compassionate Life*. Little Brown and Company.

3 Russ Roberts (2015). *How Adam Smith Can Change Your Life: An Unexpected Guide to Human Nature and Happiness*, p.13. Portfolio.

4 Barry Polansky (2003). *The Art of the Examination*. Word of Mouth Enterprises.

5 Barry Schwartz (2015). *Why We Work*, p. 69. TED Books, Simon and Schuster.

6 Peter E. Dawson (2006). *Functional Occlusion: From TMJ to Smile Design*, Preface, Mosby.

7 Barry Polansky (2013). *The Art of Case Presentation*, p.44. Word of Mouth Enterprises.

8 Robert Greene (2013). *Mastery*. Penguin Books,.

9 Barry Polansky (2013). *The Art of Case Presentation*, p.46. Word of Mouth Enterprises.

10 Brown, Don, *Human Universals*(McGraw-Hill Humanities/Social Sciences/Languages; 1 edition (January 1, 1991)

11 Maslow, A (1954). *Motivation and personality*, p. 236. New York, NY: Harper.

12 Villarica, H. (2011). *Maslow 2.0: A New and Improved Recipe for Happiness*. theatlantic.com, August 17.

13 Tay, L. and Diener, E. (2011). Needs and subjective well-being around the world. *Journal of Personality and Social Psychology* **101** (2): 354–365.

14 Mismatch Theory: en.wikipedia.org

15 Robert Reich (2015). *Saving Capitalism*, p. 82. New York, NY: Knopf.

16 Stephen R. Covey (2015). *Primary Greatness*, p. xiv. New York, NY: Simon and Schuster.

17 Jabob Needleman, Money and the Meaning of Life. (New York, Doubleday), 1994.

18 Barry Schwartz and Kenneth Sharpe (2011). *Practical Wisdom: The Right Way to Do the Right Thing*. Riverhead Books.

3

Dentistry Today

"Your time is limited, so don't waste it living someone else's life. Don't be trapped by dogma – which is living with the results of other people's thinking. Don't let the noise of other's opinions drown out your own inner voice. And most important, have the courage to follow your heart and intuition. They somehow already know what you truly want to become. Everything else is secondary."

Steve Jobs

"Technology is just a tool. In terms of getting the kids working together and motivating them, the teacher is the most important."

Bill Gates

"It has become appallingly obvious that our technology has exceeded our humanity."

Albert Einstein

In 2009, Walter Isaacson, the famed author, journalist and President and CEO of the Aspen Institute, a nonpartisan educational and policy studies organization based in Washington DC, decided, after five years of deliberation, to write the biography of Steve Jobs. It was no accident that Isaacson was personally chosen by Jobs. Isaacson's decision, to write the biography was based on a number of factors. Firstly, Job's story needed to be told while he was still alive. He had just been given his fatal diagnosis. Not only was Isaacson an established best-selling author, but his position in the Aspen Institute "think tank" played a role in Jobs's choice of biographer.

The Aspen Institute was founded in 1950 as the Aspen Institute of Humanistic Studies. The organization is dedicated to "fostering enlightened leadership, the appreciation of timeless ideas and values, and open-minded dialogue on contemporary issues." That mission was undoubtedly appealing to Jobs, since it shared much of the same thought as his 1984 advertising slogan, "Think Different." The ad, if you remember, showed the faces of many iconic figures throughout history who thought differently, like Einstein, Picasso and Edison (wholism thinkers?).

As Isaacson tells the story in the Introduction of the eventual book [1], Jobs said, "I always thought of myself as a humanities person as a kid, but I liked electronics. Then I read something that one of my heroes, Edwin Land of Polaroid, said about the importance of people who could stand at the intersection of humanities and sciences, and I decided that's what I wanted to do." In that moment, Isaacson realized the theme of Job's life was similar to the subjects he had written about before with the biographies of Einstein and Ben Franklin. That theme, Isaacson said, was that, "the creativity that can occur when a feel for both the humanities and the sciences can combine" will be the key to creating innovative economies in the 21st century.

The Complete Dentist: Positive Leadership and Communication Skills for Success, First Edition. Barry Polansky.
© 2018 John Wiley & Sons, Inc. Published 2018 by John Wiley & Sons, Inc.

Yet, we are seeing just the opposite in dentistry today.

Medicine is beginning to see the light. In chapter 1, I mentioned the work of Toby Cosgrove of the Cleveland Clinic. Drs. Nicholas LaRusso, Barbara Spurrier and Gianrico Farrugia are doing similar things at the Mayo Clinic in Rochester, Minnesota [2], and they have developed and implemented a program designed around the needs of their patients. The movement, called *Think Big, Start Small, Move Fast*, is based on reframing the problem of healthcare to be more about the health and healthcare experience. They claim that by focusing on the larger definition of the healthcare experience, they can transform the bigger picture of global health. By starting small and moving fast, they are changing the way the healthcare experience is being delivered.

Dentistry needs to learn the same lesson. For decades, we have seen improvements in materials, and technology, but the dental experience has stayed the same, with a few exceptions in the area of oral sedation and biofeedback. As the three wise men quoted above tell us, technology won't save us; what is missing is the human touch. Issues of character and communication failures permeate all industries. We usually don't discover problems until it is too late. We see it in the newspapers every day, from politicians to football players. We see it in dentistry as well, in the form of people failing their staff, their patients and, mostly, themselves.

Why all of these leadership failures?

Could it be that schools recruit the wrong people? Unethical people? Even the National Football League screens its players for leadership qualities and histories of poor behavior. Yet, many players get through the system on sheer talent alone. Who would argue that the players with the highest ability to lead and communicate go the furthest?

Another way to look at the leadership failures is to explore the systemic processes that produce leaders who often behave differently from what most people might expect. In other words, whose responsibility is it to educate leaders? When I was in dental school, the only exposure to this problem was being told about our school's Code of Ethics. After leaving dental school we were exposed to the American Dental Association's Code of Ethics. The only time we discussed these issues was when someone went out of bounds. Through the years, there have been many examples of these failures through lawsuits, employee grievances and, worse yet, the apathy that sets in and causes unspeakable issues in the secret lives of dentists.

How does the dental industry expect to build leadership? If not in the curriculum, then where and when? Does the dental community assume that these skills can't be taught, or that dentists should have learned them before entering the profession, or that every dentist is on his or her own to find instructors, trainers or coaches after graduation? That doesn't happen, especially when we are being sold on the idea that technology is the key to a successful career.

Leadership can be taught, as we will see in this book. Dentists need to be recruited and celebrated for more than their hands and their technical ability. Skills of the heart and mind play an equal part taking care of people, and this needs to be emphasized at the education level. There should be standards for becoming a dentist that go beyond passing clinical requirements. Not only are these personal skills not taught or even acknowledged – they are ignored over business skills and technical skills. It is not guaranteed that dental students learned these values at home growing up. That wasn't true 40 years ago, and it is less true today.

Today, the coaching industry is booming. Everyone and anyone can be a mentor, coach, even a guru. That's how it was for me. Looking back, I had my share of teachers, coaches and mentors and gurus. They weren't all good. Some were just plain bad. Some were great clinicians, and others practiced with a black heart. There are so many different philosophies of leadership and communication that, just like dentistry, we don't know if we are learning the right stuff. Leadership and dentistry are based on principles.

Principles are rules or laws that hold up over time. Principles are perennial. They aren't based on current trends or fads. They answer questions that dentists have about all situations and circumstances. Stephen Covey, in *The 7 Habits of Highly Effective People*, gives an excellent account of the meaning of principles. He tells a story by Frank Koch from the magazine *Proceedings*, published by the US Naval Institute. The story is about a battleship navigating its way through patchy fog and bad weather. The captain remained on the bridge to keep an eye on all proceedings. All of a sudden, a lookout spotted a light in the distance. The captain surmised that they were about to collide with another boat. He called to the boat to change course. What came back was another order that the battleship should change its course. The captain became angry and said, "I am the captain, this is a battleship, and this is an order."

The next reply came back, "I am a seaman second class, and you had better change course… because this is a lighthouse [3]!"

Covey's point is that principles are like lighthouses. "They are natural laws that cannot be broken…as Cecil B. DeMille observed of the principles contained in the movie *The Ten Commandments*, 'It is impossible for us to break the law.'"

Maybe dental schools assume that we already know how the world works – after all, natural laws have been around for eternity. Aristotle's philosophy was based on natural law, reason and logic, which is why, as you will come to see later in this book, why so much depends on character and ethics. For now, suffice it to say that many have abandoned principles and natural law to find "quick fixes" to everyday problems. These quick fixes and manipulative techniques have become quite popular in the leadership, consulting and coaching industry. So, this problem, like many others, is complex and driven by pressure that comes from the self-interest of others, rather than the intellectual and moral strength of the individual dentist. We are all susceptible to coercion.

We don't know what we don't know.

During the 1970s, Noel Burch, while working for Gordon Training International [4], drafted what he called the "four stages for learning any new skill." His Four States of Competence became a learning model that is used by many educational and leadership institutes throughout the world. Numerous studies have verified that cooperation, communication, interpersonal skills, listening, and summarizing skills are critical to higher-order team success.

In their book, *The Leadership Challenge* [5], Kouzes and Posner write, "Every leader ought to know how to paraphrase, summarize, express feelings, disclose personal information, admit mistakes, respond non-defensively, ask for clarification, solicit different views, and so on." These skills are at the heart of emotional intelligence. Cultivating them in managers and employees is the key to all of the benefits of training and development. An organization that is already able to communicate across levels productively and functionally, and to manage conflicts creatively and beneficially, is prepared for higher-order training and learning that will require those skills for successful implementation.

The skills that Kouzes and Posner are speaking of are leadership and communication skills – the same set of skills that Gordon Training International has been teaching to parents for over 50 years. In other words we, as parents, see the faults of our ways through the difficulties we encounter in raising our kids – leadership and communication, under the guise of parenting. Yet, in working with our patients and staff, we prefer to wing it. We deceive ourselves into thinking we already know what we need to know.

You may recognize yourself in one of the four stages of learning. Understand, that I am speaking of the "soft skills" referenced above by Kouzes and Posner.

The Four Stages of Learning

Stage 1 – The Unconscious Incompetent

This is the stage of not knowing what we don't know. I encounter this stage every day. When I go to the gym just after New Year, I see people who want to get in shape and lose weight, randomly doing exercises and lifting weights without any real instructions. The smarter ones refer to books or get personal training, but many just "wing it." More often than not, when I see someone doing something wrong, I mistakenly stick in my two cents. Sometimes they take my advice, but some just give me a dirty look and go on with their routine, never getting any better. Of course, this is the gym at New Year, so the story plays out in many failures by February for any other number of reasons.

I also encounter the same phenomenon in coaching dentists to do comprehensive examinations and case presentations – much more difficult than doing bench presses. Completing successful exams and presentations require a whole gamut of skills that take years to learn. I find that clients who just never get it never get out of this stage. It's frustrating for me as their coach – even more frustrating than it is for them, because they are under some self-deception that it's easy and self-evident. I don't know if it's just arrogance or ignorance. Hopefully, it is the latter, because then they can be helped.

I remember a client visiting my office for over-the-shoulder training. He spent the day observing me interacting with patients during all clinical circumstances. During the day, he would comment how in his office he "did it just like I was doing." When I asked him why they needed to be coached, they replied that they weren't getting the same results as I was getting. Where was the disconnect?

Others whom I coach through telephone conversations give similar responses. When I try to correct or point out slight nuances about how their patients and staff members are responding to them, they defend their positions. My role as a coach is to be an impartial spectator, but if the student is unwilling to see what is in front of them, they will continue unconsciously to commit incompetence.

I have even heard dentists tell me, after their treatment plans have been rejected, that the patient had no value, and that it was hopeless even to try. One dentist I worked with actually referred to some of his patients as lowlifes when they didn't respond to their liking. I always wondered whether they would have referred to their own children in that manner if they refused advice. I wanted to make a referral to parent effectiveness training (PET).

As you can tell, our general beliefs play a role in what we think we know. I am fond of the Joseph Campbell advice on knowledge: "*He who thinks he knows, doesn't know. He who knows that he doesn't know, knows.*" I think that quote helped me to move out of Stage 1 just at the right time of my life. I find that those who stay at this level are the most susceptible to the quacks and charlatans who promise people results through tricks and gimmicks.

Stage 2 – The Conscious Incompetent

This is when we know what we don't know, and it is a critical moment in the life of any student. Understanding that there is room to learn and grow makes all the difference. It is true that technical errors demand an immediate response. The dentist who continually sees his or her work failing seeks advice right away, or that dentist stops doing certain procedures, choosing the path of least resistance. Carolyn Dweck, Stanford psychologist, and author of the bestselling book, *Mindset: The New Psychology of Success*, believes individuals can be placed on a continuum according to their implicit views of where ability comes from. Some believe their success is based on innate ability; these are said to have a "fixed" theory of intelligence (fixed mindset). Others, who believe their success is based on hard work, learning, training and doggedness, are said to have a "growth" or an "incremental" theory of intelligence (growth mindset). Individuals may not necessarily be aware of their own mindset, but their mindset can still be discerned, based on their behavior.

It is the behavior observed at this critical point, when the student realizes or becomes cognizant, that indicates that there is room for improvement. Dweck believes that the behavior is a response to how the student feels about failure. It is at this point that the one with the growth mindset overcomes any fears of failure, and develops self-esteem. She feels that this turning point can make all the difference between a life lived in stress, and success and ultimate growth.

For many technical procedures, there is little risk. Dental education has prepared students to understand the importance of clinical dentistry, and the entire dental school experience is geared toward learning new techniques and using new materials. For many, this is fun, and most are able to deal with the frustrations. Most dentists will choose the type of dentistry they do because they enjoy it. Leadership skills and communication skills are life skills. We have no choice: in order to succeed, for ourselves and our patients, we must learn, we must grow. Yet many choose not to, even when they become aware.

When a dentist fails to get the desired results because of a lack of communication and leadership skills, more often than not they get discouraged and stop trying to get their very best dentistry *off the shelf*, as we say at the Pankey Institute. This is sad, but what is sadder is that there is no training, either in dental school or post-graduation, that addresses the levels of mastery needed to deal with managing a long and successful career in dentistry. So, once again, although this student is more aware than the Stage 1 student, they still have a problem in finding a course of study or curriculum that teaches the essential abilities and qualities necessary for success specific to the field of dentistry.

Stage 3 – Conscious Competence

Stage 3 is trying the skills out, experimenting and practicing. We now know how to do the skill the right way, but we need to think and work hard to do it. This is why we call it the "practice" of dentistry. Everything can be broken down into steps, methods and procedures. I like to think that everything has a structure or process. I know dentists like the idea of process; it has been said that we like the idea of a "cookbook" method. It is easy to see the application of process when we learn technical skills, yet most dentists fail to see the structure that exists behind leadership and communication skills. I will have a lot more to say about process in the chapters on application of leadership skills.

Most dentists do not practice. Einstein defined insanity as doing the same thing over and over again and expecting different results. Most dentists make business their goal. They practice for years, making the same mistakes over and over again. Most people mistake busyness for actual achievement, especially when it comes to communication. Many years ago, when I first started in practice, I went around to all of the dentists in my area to introduce myself. I found it interesting that most were having the same problems. They were mostly forthright and earnest people, just trying to make a living and do it the right way. I was impressed by this, but felt a subliminal level of disappointment and discontent.

One dentist, in particular, remains in my memory. I was in my first or second year of private practice when George asked if he could come to my office for a heart-to-heart. I was confused, because I normally would be the one to ask for counsel and wisdom. George was frustrated, and I remember him throwing his wallet on the floor and saying something to the tune of, "What do they want? Do they want me to pay for their dentistry?" He was referring to the problems he was having communicating with his patients. This was long before my own burnout years. I remember feeling bad for George, and vowed that would never happen to me. Of course, that was during my "unconscious" time. Within a few years, I would feel the same way.

The irony was that, many years later, I was lecturing in Atlantic City and, at the break, a dentist approached me and asked to have a word with me after the lecture. By now, you realize – it was George. He had aged to the point that I barely recognized him. He had sold his practice long ago and was now working at an HMO. He remembered how, during my "rebel" years, I tried to unite all of the local dentists to fight the HMO movement. He thought, even then, that I was a real leader. George came to my lecture that day to say hello and to ask if I would treat his wife, who was in need of extensive dentistry.

George had survived dentistry. He was still in good health, as far as I could see, and his marriage had survived. But George had not thrived. Leaders thrive – George languished for 30 years. He stayed busy, made some money, but never achieved what he set out to do. Disappointing. Too many of our colleagues follow this scenario and, yes, you may be saying it is just a matter of taking responsibility, but maybe if dentists were exposed to leadership and communication much earlier, then the practice of dentistry might be more rewarding.

Outside of dentistry, I have many hobbies. I do yoga, I raise and show dogs (boxers), and I write. All three of these disciplines share something in common with dentistry. They all require learning a process, and they all require regular practice. It takes years of practice to get better at yoga, showing dogs and writing. Consistent practice will eventually lead to success. Being aware is the first step, but continuous and never-ending improvement, or the ongoing practice of all of the skills necessary for success, is mandatory. It is difficult for me to understand why dental educators do not include the practice of soft skills in their curricula.

Many people confuse the idea of practice. As a noun, it means the actual application or use of an idea, belief, or method, as opposed to theories about such application or use. A dental practice, then is the manner in which we apply what we have learned through our education. In L.D. Pankey's terms, it would be the pinnacle and purpose of all education. We accumulate the knowledge of ourselves, our patients, and our work for the sole purpose of applying the knowledge in our daily practice.

But practice is also a verb, such as in writing, or practicing yoga. As a verb, The *Merriam-Webster Dictionary* says it means "to perform (an activity) or exercise (a skill) repeatedly or regularly in order to improve or maintain one's proficiency." In order to become consciously competent in dentistry, we must both engage in and sustain a practice. When the dentist truly sees dentistry as a practice in order to grow and build his or her practice, that makes all the difference in the learning levels. The dentist will then have the ability to try new things and accept failure in order to grow. This change in perception is a way to go from a fixed mindset to a growth mindset.

Through my years in practice, I have been faced with instituting new techniques, procedures and equipment into my practice. Some that I never learned in dental school included bonding, porcelain veneers, lasers and implants. On the softer side, there was the entire world of computers and, even today, social media. It may seem obvious to you but, as each new technology was introduced, there was a level of fear and a reluctance to change. Most dentists have faced these feelings and have gone on to improve their practices. But not all dentists embrace new technologies. The dental community helps dentists to grow in regards to learning new technical skills, yet I have seen many of my colleagues left behind. Most continuing education programs today do a very good job in helping dentists to keep up.

However, when there is a failure in communication, it usually stops right there. The same desires and motivations to fix these problems and grow seem to be stopped by fears of confrontation, or engagement into psychological areas that dentists would rather leave alone. This is where leadership fails. Practicing dentistry requires the dentist to try new things continually. Each time we try and fail, we learn something that helps prepare us for eventual success. Only in school is there a single correct answer for every problem. That is what makes mastering soft skills so difficult. If you try an approach that doesn't work, try something different.

Maybe I was lucky. Dentistry is a comprehensive and complex discipline. I chose to focus on the examination as the single discipline I wanted to master. The examination encompasses the entirety of dentistry, both in terms of technical and soft skills. In writing my book on the examination I was forced to break it down to every component and all of their distinctions. Then I would practice each component. The soft skills were infinitely more difficult. I was guilty of a *faux pas* every day I corrected myself and slowed down enough to truly reach my patients. I would teach each component to my staff. In time, a culture was born, all based on a practice that was committed to the examination. I don't expect every dentist to do that, but just to understand the meaning of practice, and what it takes to become consciously competent.

Stage 4 – Unconscious Competence

When we continue to practice and apply the new skills, eventually we arrive at a stage where they become easier and, given time, even natural. Yes, there will come a time when practice pays dividends. For those who study the concept of "practice," it is referred to as the 10,000 Hour Rule. Over the last few years, many books, including *Outliers* by Malcolm Gladwell, and *Talent is Overrated* by Geoff Colvin, have referred to the work of Dr. K. Anders Ericsson on the role of deliberate practice in expert performance [6].

Anders tested and conceived the rule by recruiting violinists from the Berlin Music Academy and asking them to record the amount of time each week that they devoted to deliberate practice. He found, by comparing the time journals of all the recruits, that it took 10,000 hours or ten years of deliberate practice to achieve mastery. Since that study in 1993, there have been many theories put forth on the exact amount needed to become a master. My experience has told me that, even more important than the amount of time needed, is the word "deliberate", or focused practice. By consistently repeating the same efforts everyday – by prioritizing what is truly important, whether it be listening better or asking better questions or taking better photographs – daily, consistent, deliberate practice works.

It works because the discipline reaches a certain level of simplicity. I am fond of a quote by the Supreme Court Justice Oliver Wendell Holmes Jr.: "*I wouldn't give a fig for the simplicity on this side of complexity; but I would give my right arm for the simplicity on the far side of complexity.*" Through deliberate practice, we cut through the complexity until we cross over to the other side. There comes a point when what seemed complex, complicated, and overwhelming becomes simple. What started out as demanding and draining becomes energizing, challenging, and engaging. It becomes an unconscious endeavor. Fear dissolves, and you actually look forward to the difficult conversations that were so dreaded in the past.

When I first took on the idea of mastering the examination process, it seemed daunting. I kept thinking more about doing the "big cases," which is what most educational programs focus on. Mastering the technical dentistry was mostly a matter of repetition. Direct bonding, for example, improved by doing more and more. Going to meetings and reading helped me to apply tips and tools. Getting to actually use the sophisticated techniques and tools was another story. But I kept plugging away and practicing things like active listening, asking better questions, storytelling, non-judgment and the technical components like mounting models, taking bite registrations and photography.

Eventually, people started to listen to me. People followed my recommendations. I matured into a leader, and it came naturally, rather than by being a "doctor" and in a position of authority. It was authentic. Albert Einstein once described the five levels of ascending intelligence as [7]:

1) Smart
2) Intelligent
3) Brilliant
4) Genius
5) Simple

One step beyond genius? Simplicity. Yes, most people truly are smart enough even to the point of being genius, but most haven't figured out how make our lives more simple. It is at this level of simplicity that we can truly reach our full potential; when we become unconsciously competent, life gets much simpler. Our ability to create simplicity is based on our power to choose. Each day we are faced with choices that enable us to practice in any manner we like. The problems we must recognize are the ones that interfere with our freedom of choice and our desire to create our own careers with autonomy, meaning and discretion.

I close this section with the words of Buckminster Fuller, the American architect, systems theorist, author, designer and inventor:

"All children are born geniuses; 9,999 out of every 10,000 are swiftly, inadvertently degeniusized by grownups."

Technology – Wagging the Dog

The movie *Little Shop of Horrors* is a comedy, rock 'n' roll, horror musical about a hapless florist shop worker who raises a plant that feeds on human flesh and blood. If you remember the 1986 film, the sadistic dentist, played by Steve Martin, is probably the first thing that comes to your mind. I remember the movie for another reason. In 1986, I had just bought a computer imaging machine. The technology was brand new, and I genuinely thought a $25 000 investment would be a boon to my practice. When it didn't turn out that way, the song from the movie, *Feed Me, Seymour*, kept playing in my head.

In the movie, Seymour, the florist shop worker, discovers a mysterious plant that looks like a Venus flytrap. He names the plant Audrey II, after a co-worker, Audrey, over whom he has a romantic crush. One day, Seymour cuts his finger and the plant licks the blood. Soon the plant comes alive and is craving Seymour's blood. In one scene, the plant sings a comical song that demands more blood from Seymour, and in return he will give him anything he wants and make Seymour's dreams come true.

Sometimes, we purchase technology that promises to change our lives and our practices, but never lives up to its potential. The high cost of learning the technology, combined with the high costs of purchase and maintenance, can make us feel like we bought a man-eating plant that screams "feed me." Technology certainly has its place in dentistry, and much of it has changed the dental world for the better, but we must ask ourselves who is wagging the dog. In other words, is creating more and more technology becoming more significant than allowing dentists to perform their true role? The expression "wag the dog" comes from the saying that a dog is smarter than its tail but, if the tail were smarter, then the tail would "wag the dog."

Is technology wagging the dog?

We certainly live in interesting times. I began practice in 1973. Bonding was the newest technique, and it truly changed dentistry. Acid etching and bonding started what eventually became the cosmetic revolution. At the time, dentists had two choices of composite resins, each having their own bonding systems: Adaptic by Johnson and Johnson; and Concise by 3 M. These were macro-filled resins and, surprisingly, they are still available in the dental marketplace. Their use is very limited, because their properties lead to less than optimal clinical performance, like staining, wear and a poor ability to be polished. Improvement soon followed, and an entire industry was born.

Composite resins have continued to evolve and improve. Clinicians have an overwhelming and unlimited number of choices for just about every clinical situation. Manufacturers have continued to develop categories of composites based on filler size, shades, polishability, flowability, shrinkage, and strength that fill every need a dentist can think of. Even now, 50 years later, this market continues to expand, because dentistry is big business.

Using composite resins is just one example in a sea of products and equipment. Think about the enormous number of implant systems and dental cements. Can you believe there was a time dentists only used zinc phosphate and zinc oxide and eugenol? And equipment? Digital radiographs, lasers (CO_2, Nd-Yag, Erbium, Diode), Cad-Cam (Cerec), digital impression systems, and CT scanners, just to name a few items that dentists have a choice of purchasing to protect and guarantee their success.

Yes...we live in interesting times.

The dental industry has become a gigantic supermarket. Is it any wonder why Einstein believed that the highest level of intelligence is simplicity, which he based on our power to choose? Are all of these choices good? Are they good for our own health and happiness? Is our success and happiness dependent on making the perfect choice when it comes to the vast numbers of available choices? The commercial and business component of dentistry has exploded, as it has in all industries. Technological innovation drives our economy. In order to survive, corporations must develop new products and continue to sell.

Many products are worthy and deserving of praise. Others are not, and most dentists have purchased new technology that disappeared after a short life. We need technology, but it becomes a problem when it becomes a distraction, and we begin to confuse our roles. Dentists get distracted by the "shiny new toys," believing that if they don't have the newest technology, they will not feel good enough. Many dentists, out of a sense of not feeling good enough, will purchase new technology that must be paid for and, like Audrey II, will need to be fed. If we understand our key roles, this may be avoided.

Many of the manufacturers and supply companies fund clinics, dental schools, and continuing education programs. These institutions, in turn, promote the technology, so that young dentists get the message that these products have the potential to make them better dentists. When I first attended the Pankey Institute, it was known that they never accepted donations or gifts from any companies, but through the years, in order to compete, this has changed. Dental manufacturers and supply companies, through subsidies, drive most dental education today. So the question of how dental education is funded becomes an issue as we go into the future, because following the money drives the motivations.

Dental student debt has increased from just over $50,000 in 1990 to almost $250,000 in 2013. This increase has surpassed most other inflationary costs over the same period [8]. Considering that wage increases and fee increases have stagnated since 2008, that puts extra pressure on young dentists in the real world. A major cause of the increase in student debt is a shifting of dental school revenue; individual states have decreased their funding significantly to all forms of higher education. For example, in 1989, revenue from state sources accounted for 52% of total dental school revenue. By 2012, revenue from state sources shrank to only 12% [9]. This significant, but not quite clearly evident, occurrence may be one of the factors creating the manner in which dentistry is practiced today and will be practiced into the future.

Because of the shortfall in state funding, dental schools have been forced to raise tuition. Clinic fees, as most private practitioners realize, cannot account for the ever-increasing costs of running a dental practice, either in the private sector or an educational format. Average tuition for students has risen from $8,867 in 1989 to $41,015 in 2012 [10]. All of these economic changes have shifted the burden of funding dental education from the states to the students. This is a problem that interested parties need to solve. Luckily, there is help, in the shape of corporations that are willing to help fund education. But there is a price.

Merging the issues of expanding technologies, rising tuitions, the rising cost of dental expenditures, the role of third parties and changes in the marketplace, like social media and advertising, the dental landscape has changed significantly since my graduation in 1973. *"The US Centers for*

Medicare and Medicaid Services predicts insurance as a source of dental expenditures will remain relatively stable at 51%, up to 2023. They also estimate out-of-pocket expenditures will decline to 35% and government sources will increase to 13.9% by 2023. This projection estimates government expenditures for dental services more than doubling by 2023 to $26.7 billion [11]."

Clearly, these changes have changed the way dentists have practiced. Admittedly, I came from an era when private practice fee-for-service was the standard model of practice. I would be a fool not to acknowledge the changes, yet through the changes there are many things that have remained the same. The unchanging human factors are what must be preserved, rather than lost in the selfish motivations of corporate America.

The *Journal of the American College of Dentists* created a classification scheme for the way dentistry is being practiced today:

- Traditional: dentist owns and manages practice, provides clinical care.
- Dental Management Service Organizations (DMSO): dentist owns practice and provides clinical care; a service organization provides management.
- Corporate: dentist provides clinical care, with corporate ownership and management.
- Nonprofit: ownership by government agency or educational institution; dental care is provided by employees, students and faculty.

The key element in the classification scheme is *ownership*, because ownership status has implications for the dentist's freedom to determine the course of treatment.

When I hear the word ownership, I hear more than just the legal definition of having the right to possession. I hear the deeper meaning of responsibility, trustfulness, accountability (to oneself and others), reliability and obligation. Ownership is, as I will discuss, a character trait of leadership. As I review the classification, I see that each level differs in the amount of responsibility that needs to be taken. Truly, with all of the issues that young dentists face today, who can blame them for wanting to be "just a dentist?" Yet most dentists still go into dentistry to be the masters of their own destiny, to make their own choices, to be free to treat their patients as they see fit.

In order to solve these issues, we must see through the fog. We must do what Stephen Covey suggests for leaders to become effective: "The main thing is to keep the main thing the main thing." In today's world, this is becoming more difficult. The main thing for me has always been to understand my roles – to myself, to my family, to my staff and to my patients.

Dentists, like most professionals, are service providers. There are differing opinions about what the role of a dentist should be. I like what Albert Schweitzer once said about service in general: "I don't know what your destiny will be, but one thing I know: the only ones among you who will be really happy are those who will have sought and found how to serve."

This may not be your idea of a job description, but the service aspect is shared by many throughout history. The American Dental Association has weighed in on the role of the dentist as well [12]. The following is their description of the dentist's role:

Dentists are doctors who specialize in oral health. Their responsibilities include:

- diagnosing oral diseases;
- promoting oral health and disease prevention;
- creating treatment plans to maintain or restore the oral health of their patients;
- interpreting x-rays and diagnostic tests;
- ensuring the safe administration of anesthetics;
- monitoring growth and development of the teeth and jaws;
- performing surgical procedures on the teeth, bone and soft tissues of the oral cavity.

Many of today's leading lecturers have defined the role of the dentist as a physician of the oral cavity. Although I agree with all of these descriptions, the one that rings of significance for me is the service component. To me service is an essential and fundamental component of all health care providers. Most of today's authorities on leadership like Stephen Covey, Ken Blanchard and Peter Senge are well-known advocates of the servant leadership concept.

Servant leadership is an ancient philosophy that has been referenced in the Tao Te Ching, written by the Chinese philosopher Lao-Tzu sometime between 570 BCE and 490 BCE. Essentially, the concept was best described and named by Robert K. Greenleaf, in an essay he published in 1970, titled *The Servant as Leader* [13]. The essay described the role of the leader as being a servant first before being a leader – to serve before leading. He contended that the leader-first and the servant-first are two extreme types. He believed the servant-first leader's main priority was other people's well-being and growth. For Covey, this would be the "main thing." This should be the purpose of dentistry.

Leonard Berry, professor of marketing at the Mays Business School at Texas A&M, and a senior fellow at the Institute for Healthcare Improvement, is the author of numerous books on service whose work has focused on service delivery in cancer care. Berry's research has concluded that the five most important components of great service are: dependability, reliability, assuredness, empathy and tangible items (hi-tech). It is interesting to note that being reliable, dependable and empathetic all relate to the human side of dentistry while assuredness of competence and tangible items relate to today's newest technology. In other words, what is driving dentistry today diminishes the role of the softer or human side of our profession.

I will have much to say about the elements of servant leadership as the book progresses. For now, understand why the focus is on technology, and how that focus can distract today's dentist from performing at his best and serving the best interests of patients.

Human Interaction Rules

Dentistry is the most intimate and personal of the health professions. A few years ago, I had a minor bicycle accident. I gashed my shin on the bike pedal. The resulting wound took a while to heal. After two weeks, the margins of the wound began to roll, and the center continued to ooze. I visited a dermatologist, because I suspected something serious. He entered the room, looked at the lesion, anesthetized my shin and proceeded to do a shave biopsy. With a scalpel, he took a thin slice off of the top part of the lesion and sent it out to a laboratory for a definitive diagnosis. He told me his differential diagnosis was squamous cell carcinoma, and that it looked bad; he would call me back in a few days with the diagnosis. He never said hello, nor goodbye.

Two weeks later, he called with the results. Two weeks! He told me it was squamous cell carcinoma and it would have to be removed with Mohs surgery, also known as chemosurgery. The procedure was developed in 1938 by a general surgeon, Dr. Frederic Mohs, as a microscopically controlled surgery which removes layers of tissue surface while the patient waits until all signs of cancerous cells are removed. I asked him if he had done many of these procedures. He said he had done his share – so I moved on to a surgeon with more experience.

I found the "best one" in my area. She came highly recommended. My wife accompanied me to the initial visit. I remember the appointment for two reasons. First, the doctor came in, looked at my leg, and never spoke directly to me – she only spoke to my wife. Once again, no greeting. Then, without warning, she stuck a Q-Tip directly into the center of the lesion. She looked at my wife and said, before she did Mohs surgery, she had to make sure it wasn't infected. Tears were rolling down my eyes. I thought at that moment that, in my entire career as a dentist, I probably never had induced more pain. Then she did it again, without warning, to get a second sample.

If she hadn't had those great credentials, I would have left right then.

In Parts III-V of the book, I will give a detailed explanation of the role of trust and trustworthiness in the life of a leader. For now, I will define trust as a blend of character and competence. Both of these elements are necessary to build a culture of trust. We all make character judgments. I questioned the character of both of these doctors, yet chose to do the surgery with the second one. Stephen Covey, in his book, *The 8th Habit*, explains this in a story about his son-in-law on getting into medical school.

During the interview process, his son-in-law was asked about his preference: an honest surgeon who was incompetent, or a competent surgeon who was dishonest. His answer was quite profound. He said, "It all depends on the issue. If I needed the surgery, I'd go for the competent one. If it was a question of whether to have surgery or not, I'd go for the honest one." This is the question I faced with my Mohs procedure.

Dental patients ask these same questions of themselves everyday. Very few dentists distinguish themselves through competence, although this is where most spend their efforts. Many dentists who are very competent send mixed signals in the area of character. I certainly am not judging the character of either dermatologist, but they were both sending mixed signals. This book will teach dentists how to work on character and competence, with the end result being trust.

Reflecting back on the classification scheme of how dentistry is practiced today, as the level of ownership decreases, the incentives to work on the people issues and administrative issues decrease as well. It's just human nature.

When building trusting culture is not a priority, our roles become purely functional. Imagine working in an organization where people only related to one another at a functional level. Better yet, imagine a purely functional marriage or family!

A few years after my dermatologic event, I had another frightful diagnosis to deal with: prostate cancer. At the time, most surgeons concurred that radical prostatectomy was the best solution. After numerous consultations, and facing the same quandary I had faced with my leg, I chose a surgeon who had done over 3000 of these procedures with the DaVinci robot. Things went smoothly. It's been over five years and there has been no evidence of cancer. I guess I made the right decision, although five years later, I understand why there is a debate.

Through the entire process, from my initial appointment to every single follow-up over the next five years, I can only remember meeting the surgeon four or five times. Those meetings were very brief, except for the surgical procedure itself, and I have no recollection of that. Competence worked in that situation.

I am sure you or a family member has had similar experiences with today's health care environment. When extreme competence is the deciding factor, who would question the system? But most medicine today requires a much more intimate and personal touch. Emotions are riding high on every decision. Dentistry cannot follow the medical model. The medical model is being questioned, as I mentioned, in the work of Toby Cosgrove at the Cleveland Clinic.

Medicine and dentistry are not purely functional and technical industries. There is a human side that must be addressed. Our human side is being undervalued, as I reveal later in this book. By not acknowledging the human side of dentistry, we have created the two biggest losers – the dentists and the patients – which will be discussed in the next chapter.

Geoff Colvin, in his book *Humans are Underrated* [14], explains that the skills that will prove to be most valuable in the future are no longer technical, classroom-taught, left-brain skills that advancing technology seems to have insisted upon. He claims while those skills remain important, their importance isn't the same as valuable, because those skills are becoming commoditized and, thus, are "a diminishing source of competitive advantage." According to Colvin, the new high value skills are the ones associated with our deepest nature – the abilities that define us as human beings: sensing the thoughts and feelings of others; building relationships; solving problems together; and expressing ourselves with greater power than logic can achieve. In other words, as leadership specialist Marshall Goldsmith tells us in his book, titled with the same name: "what got you here, won't get you there [15]."

In other words, the big lesson is that human interaction rules our lives. In many ways, it holds the key to our value. Once again, the theme of human universals trumps technology. The question of nurture vs. nature comes into play. It would seem that the environmental forces that helped to create our cultural tendencies would win out over human nature, that humans are a blank slate susceptible to the cultural forces of the day.

This blank slate view has recently been challenged by Harvard psychologist Steven Pinker, in his book, *The Blank Slate: The Modern Denial of Human Nature* [16]. Much of his theory is credited to the human universal theory of anthropologist Donald Brown [17], who said there are human universal traits that are "features of culture, society, language, behavior and psyche for which there are no known exceptions." For our purposes, here are a few that show up in every culture on earth, and are very relevant for this discussion:

- Empathy is universal.
- People everywhere admire generosity and disapprove of stinginess.
- We all cry, we all make jokes.
- All cultures create music with melody. Everyone dances. All societies have aesthetics and create decorative art.
- We all have a concept of fairness, and we all understand reciprocity.
- We all have pride.
- We all tell stories.
- Every society has leaders.

Every one of these universal elements involve human interaction and, in a world that seems to be getting more overpowered by technology every day, it's good to keep these universals in mind.

References and Notes

1 Walter Isaacson (2011). *Steve Jobs*, p. xix. New York, NY: Simon and Schuster.
2 Nicholas LaRusso, Barbara Spurrier and Gianrico Farrugia (2015). *Think Big, Start Small, Move Fast*, xi–xxiv. McGraw-Hill.
3 Stephen R. Covey (1989). *The Seven Habits of Highly Effective People*, pp. 32–35. Fireside Book, Simon and Schuster.
4 Gordon Training International was founded by Dr. Thomas Gordon. He is widely recognized as a pioneer in teaching communication skills and conflict resolution methods (P.E.T.) to parents, teachers, youth, organization managers and employees. He was the founder of Gordon Training International in 1962. His Gordon Model concepts are now known and used in over 50 countries.
5 James M. Kouzes, Barry Posner (2012). *The Leadership Challenge: How to Make Extraordinary Things Happen in Organizations*, 5th edition. Jossey-Bass.
6 K. Anders Ericsson, Ralf Th. Krampe and Clemons Tesch-Römer (1993). The Role of Deliberate Practice in the Acquisition of Expert Performance. *Psychological Review* **100**(3): 362–406.
7 Understanding Circle of Competence and Knowing the Edge of Your Competency. *Forbes*, Guru Focus, January 2, 2015.
8 Dental Economics – Future of Dentistry.
9 Ibid.

10 Ibid.

11 Ibid.

12 ada.org. *Dentists: Doctors of Oral Health*

13 Robert Greenleaf (1991). *The Servant as Leader*. Robert K. Greenleaf Center.

14 Geoff Colvin (2015). *Humans are Underrated*, p. 4. New York, NY: Portfolio/Penguin.

15 Marshall Goldsmith (2007). *What Got You Here Won't Get You There*. Hatchett Books.

16 Steven Pinker (2003). *The Blank Slate: The Modern Denial of Human Nature*. Penguin Press Science.

17 Donald Brown.

4

The Ultimate Losers In the End

"In the end, it's not the years in your life that count. It's the life in your years."

Abraham Lincoln

"If you look for truth, you may find comfort in the end; if you look for comfort you will not get either comfort or truth only soft soap and wishful thinking to begin, and in the end despair."

C.S. Lewis

"In the end, you're measured not by how much you undertake but by what you finally accomplish."

Donald Trump

Earlier, I asked the question, "What is dentistry?" Now I ask you the very self-evident question: "*Why* dentistry?"

Why did you choose dentistry? Was your choice influenced by a recent ranking in US News and World Report, as the number one job in healthcare? Was it that, according to the Bureau of Labor Statistics, there will be employment growth of 16% between 2012 and 2022, with more than 23 000 openings? Was it the low unemployment rate and agreeable work-life balance that made dentistry your choice? Dentistry has always been considered an admirable profession, yet if you diligently research the profession, you will find the truth about its darker side.

Although almost everything the business magazines tell us about the profession is true, dentistry is a high-stress and a high-risk profession. The stress that dentists encounter begins in dental school, from the competitive environment, to the pressures of completing requirements for graduation. As I mentioned in the Prologue, most dentists go into dentistry for their own reasons, including work-life balance, without realizing that a big part of the job is to motivate and influence people. Managing and leading other people is the most difficult requirement of any job. Health care and education require motivational skills and, the higher up on the ownership scale, the more leaderships skills are needed. Dentists soon find out that managing other people is difficult, and requires skills that they never realized they needed.

In Chapter 2, I discussed the importance of reconciling the paradox of duty and desire. The downside of not solving this problem is the possibility of burnout. Dentists are prone to professional burnout, anxiety disorders and clinical depression. According to the publication *Psychology Today*, burnout is a state of chronic stress that leads to physical and emotional

The Complete Dentist: Positive Leadership and Communication Skills for Success, First Edition. Barry Polansky.
© 2018 John Wiley & Sons, Inc. Published 2018 by John Wiley & Sons, Inc.

exhaustion, cynicism and detachment with feelings of ineffectiveness and lack of accomplishment. Occupational burnout is typically and particularly found within human service professions partly due to the high-stress work environment and emotional demands of the job.

Burnout is not recognized as a distinct disorder in the DSM-5; however, it can be found under problems related to life-management difficulty. Christina Maslach, author of *The Truth About Burnout* [1], calls burnout the antithesis of engagement. Engagement is characterized by energy, involvement and efficacy, the opposites of exhaustion, cynicism and inefficacy. As you will see, the latest research in positive psychology reveals that engagement in work is a key component to our well-being. The ultimate results of burnout can lead to any number of conditions, including cardiovascular disease, ulcers, colitis, hypertension, lower back pain, eye strain, marital disharmony, alcoholism, drug addiction, depression and suicide.

According to the blog oralhealthgroup.com [2], current research shows:

- Suicide associated with dentists is not a myth. Dentists commit suicide at more than twice the rate of the general population, and almost three times the rate of other white collar workers.
- Emotional illness ranks third in the order of frequency of health problems amongst dentists.
- Dentists suffer from coronary heart disease and high blood pressure at a 25% higher rate than the general public.
- Dentists suffer from 2.5 times more psycho-neurotic disorders than physicians.
- The #1 killer of dentists is stress-related cardiovascular disease.
- The dental profession loses the numerical equivalent of one large dental school class each year.

The dark side of dentistry can lead to serious consequences. Burnout is rarely discussed. I hate to sound like a cynic or a critic of what I feel is a wonderful profession but, as you will see in the next section, I have had my own personal history of burnout. One of the reasons I wrote this book was to help dentists to avoid any shadow of this serious condition. Another sequelae of burnout is that unhappy dentists do not do good work, and that affects patient care as well. Hence, the two biggest losers: dentists and patients.

There is a lot of information about occupational burnout. When I searched the Internet for the term "stress in dentistry," I came up with an article written in *Dental Economics* [3], the popular magazine for the dental community on all things related to business and practice management, about a dentist who was burned out and was offering his version of a cure. According to the author of the article, "the problem for many dentists is that the financial reward is much less than the risks encountered daily. In fact, the lack of financial reward actually becomes an added risk and stress, on top of everything else."

That sounds good, and many dentists who find themselves in that situation are susceptible to that type of thinking. Earlier, I discussed reductionist thinking. This is another good example of finding a *simple* cure for a complex problem. Burnout is a complex problem, and one cannot simply apply a multitude of practice management tips to cure a demanding psychological issue.

The author of the article continues his reductionist thinking by telling us he: "decided to sell my practice and work for the new owner as an associate. This way I would lower my risks, responsibilities, and stress by not having to own and run a business. I could just do the dentistry and go home." Through a series of circumstances, the dentist was able to buy the practice he went to work for when the existing owner died (murdered – but, that's another story!). The article then concludes by telling us that his new practice started to grow to over $7 million annually. He simplifies the whole process by asking us to ask ourselves two questions:

1) Do you see yourself as a practicing dentist that has to run a business?
   Or
2) Do you see yourself leveraging your skills into the business of dentistry?

I tell you about this article because, in a nutshell, this is how the dental industry tries to help dentists to answer some very difficult and serious questions we all have. They treat burnout in the same way they treat any other technical problem we face – "Just do this," and all of your problems will go away, or money will cure all ills. That is just not true, and actually has contributed to even more problems. The burnout usually gets worse, and it makes things worse for another group of people who tend to reduce complexity: patients.

Another lesson to learn from the article is that so many dentists today are doing just what that dentist did when the money issues get tight. They retreat from ownership and give the management, administrative and leadership issues to others. However, the retreat from private practice and ownership is leading to the trends we are seeing in dentistry today. Ownership and leadership are linked to one another. By abdicating the responsibility, for whatever reasons, we are losing the profession to those who are willing to take it on. In Part II, I will come back to why leadership and all that it entails is the true solution to all that ails this profession.

So why is dentistry so stressful? Is it just that, as the author of the *Dental Economics* article tells us, just a matter of the risks not equaling the reward? Just what are those risks? And will there ever be enough reward to justify them?

- *We live in a cave (I).* Every day, the dentist enters his or her practice by coming through the front door, only to enter the 10 ft × 10 ft operatory where they spend the majority of their days. But that's not the end. Their field of vision continues to be reduced by putting on loupes (the power increases as we age) and entering the oral cavity to perform highly intricate and demanding work. The work is physically and mentally challenging, and can lead to numerous problems, such as strain, back problems, vision problems, and fatigue.
- *We live in a cave (II).* Most dentists practice alone. Many of us, because of the psychographics and the personality traits of dentists, are very competitive with one another. We generally don't like to talk about our problems, personal or professional, with colleagues. Dental school can be quite competitive, and can be a contributing factor. When we have technical issues, we will call a specialist or a lab technician for answers. When we have business or emotional issues … well, we have consultants, and magazines, as I have already said, just don't do it.
- *Perfectionism.* Possibly another psychographic characteristic of dentists is their striving for flawlessness and setting excessively high performance standards, not only with their technical work but with their practice standards as well. When I graduated from dental school, the ideal was to strive for a $100,000 practice. The dentist I referred to above suggested a $7 million practice. Perfectionism leads to a life like an endless report card on accomplishments and achievements – a fast track to unhappiness. As I will show in Part II, our well-being is determined by more than what we accomplish, although it does play a role. Perfectionism is rooted in the avoidance of failure, and is nurtured by our current culture. It may even be in contrast to good leadership, which encourages failing forward.
- *Survival issues.* Ahh, but for the sake of survival, there is no greater trap than *the trap of the viable excuse.* Who could argue when you tell yourself you did something to "put food on the table?" Everyone, at some point in their career, has survival issues. My own survival issues pale compared to today's young dentists facing big school and practice loans. The constant worry over how to produce enough to make payroll and pay expenses can contribute to dentists making choices that can effect them for a long time to come. Maturing as a professional requires facing these obstacles and growing from them, ultimately to reach higher levels of responsibility and mastery. Young dentists, as well as many older dentists, make compromises, from working long hours and weekends, to working on people they resent for a variety of reasons, to accepting severely discounted fees, all for the sake of economic survival. This is probably the most obvious source of stress, because of how plausible it is.

- *Daily Murphy's Law.* Predictability at every level comes into play. From our work to our daily schedule, we can always count on something going wrong. Striving for some level of predictability is the dream of every dentist. Time pressure to do a job well is always on the mind of the dentist. Getting control of the daily schedule can go a long way to relieve stress.

- *Compromising dental treatment.* This was always my favorite, because it strikes right into the heart of doing meaningful work. Of all of the reasons for my burnout, this took center stage. I have already written about the subliminal need that exists in all of us to do meaningful work. Maybe for me it surfaced sooner rather than later, and I became more conscious of my unwillingness to do meaningless work that turns into sheer drudgery. We cannot change the realities of dental practice. Patients will always resist our ideal treatment plans because of time, money and fear issues. Yet we can, and must, find a way to overcome the resistance. This book will show you how.

- *The toll of fear.* We all knew this before we filled out our application for dental school. It comes as no surprise that many, even most, people have some anxiety about going to the dentist. What we don't realize (and there is now evidence) is that dentists experience patterns of physiological stress responses like increased heart rate, high blood pressure, and sweating, that parallel patient's responses when they are feeling fear and anxiety. This can't be good for the health of the dentist.

- *The secret lives of dentists.* Look, each of us have our own individual personality. We are not shocked when we hear of a colleague suffering from some health, financial, emotional, or marriage issue. Studies are beginning to show that many personality traits that make us good dentists are also detrimental to our lives. Those traits include: compulsive attention to details; extreme conscientiousness; careful emotional control; unrealistic expectations of ourselves and others; impatience; and a marked dependence on individual performance and prestige.

- *We're couch potatoes.* I admit that at one time I didn't exercise and I over-ate. In today's world, that is probably the exception rather than the rule, but I feel compelled to write about the idea that taking care of ourselves physically and mentally will help ward off burnout. My first cure for the stress of burnout was to start running. My thoughts became clearer, my energy was boosted, and I became more optimistic about my practice and my life. Hopefully this one tip will help you start on your road to leadership, unlike my dental friend, who believes that creating the $7 million practice is the answer. The Pankey Institute evaluated the health of 2400 dentists and found that their lives were characterized by DDS – dormancy, degeneration and stress.

In a way, managing stress is the point of this book. Living the life worth living has always been a theme driving my life. Invoking Carl Rogers once again: "Whatever is most personal is most universal." Let's take a look at my personal story and what some important research tells us about the ultimate price we pay when work doesn't satisfy our intrinsic and true needs.

Dentists and Stress

My first office in Medford Lakes, New Jersey was 600 square feet (confinement). It had two treatment rooms, a waiting room, a reception area, a dark room, a small laboratory, a private office, and a bathroom. It was tight in there. It was so tight that I had to keep my compressor in a small outdoor shed. I kept the shed heated during the winter with two portable electric heaters. During the winter, I would have to check the heaters frequently, to make sure the compressor didn't freeze. One day I came in and the compressor was frozen. I climbed through a window in my private office to see if I could fix the problem. I became so frustrated at the situation that I kicked the compressor and broke my toe.

That was the only time I was ever injured on the job. When I was in the Army, I worked with a dentist who was viciously bitten by a patient. I remember a friend of mine who sliced his finger with a Bard Parker blade. I also contracted Hepatitis B from a patient, but that was in the days before OSHA, and wearing gloves wasn't required. It is interesting to note that the United Nations' International Labor Organization estimates that approximately two million workers lose their lives annually due to occupational injuries and illnesses, with accidents causing at least 350,000 deaths per year. That is just the physical risks.

After I had my bout with hepatitis, I began to wear gloves routinely, and that was long before OSHA required it. Most of us seem to learn the hard way. We go along eating our cheese steaks and Twinkies until the doctor tells us that we have high cholesterol. Then we go to the gym for a few months, and it's back to our old habits. Maybe we need bypass surgery to finally learn the lesson. For me, as mentioned in my first book, *The Art of the Examination*, my life changed when I was diagnosed with Type 2 diabetes in 1990.

The biggest issue we all face is chronic stress.

It is my belief that, although I had a genetic predisposition for adult-onset diabetes, it was I who triggered my genetic capability through the chronic stress of daily practice. I believe that genetics is the gun, but the environment is the trigger. We may have no control over our genetic potential, but we have a lot of control over what we can do to prevent chronic disease like heart disease, diabetes, and some forms of cancer. There is much discussion these days about the rising costs of health care, and many are in the camp that believes we will never get a good handle on the costs until we can make behavioral changes.

In *The Heartmath Solution* [4], a book that attempts to show the connection between emotional stress and physical symptoms, authors Doc Childre and Howard Martin give this definition of stress:

> "Stress is the body and mind's response to any pressure that disrupts their normal balance. It occurs when our perception of events doesn't meet our expectations and we don't manage our reaction to the disappointment. Stress – that unmanaged reaction – expresses itself as resistance, tension, strain, or frustration, throwing off our physiological and psychological equilibrium and keeping us out of sync. If our equilibrium is disturbed for long, the stress becomes disabling. We fade from overload, feel emotionally shut down, and eventually get sick."

In other words, the chemical reactions of emotional stress occur at an organ or cellular level. This can be the Chinese version of a death by a thousand cuts. The biggest issue we face is chronic stress which leads to America's greatest scourge: chronic illness.

In a study found in the *American Journal of Epidemiology* (1997), Penninx *et al.* found that, of 2,829 people between the ages of 55 and 85, the individuals who reported the highest levels of personal "mastery" – feelings of control over life events – had a nearly 60% lower risk of death, compared with those who felt relatively helpless in the face of life's challenges.

In Childre and Martin's definition of stress, I think it is important to understand that stress is not about events so much as it is about a person's perception of circumstances. A person's stress has to do with what one believes, and one's expectations. It's about our perception of control and predictability in our lives and our work. It is ironic how many dentists blame TMJ disorders on emotional stress, leaving patients with the belief that there is nothing that can be done – that they will have to live with the circumstances. That seems to be the one area that I have found can be explained through biomechanics. True, there may be an emotional component in some cases, but the majority of cases have a functional cause. Yet, so many physicians dismiss the importance of mind-body diseases or psychosomatic ailments.

According to Don Colbert, M.D., author of the book *Deadly Emotions* [5], there are many psychiatric diseases that have been linked to long-term stress, including: general anxiety disorder; panic attacks; post-traumatic stress disorder; depression; phobias; obsessive-compulsive disorder – as well as other more rare psychiatric diseases. Colbert says that unmediated chronic stress can lead to a long list of physical problems, some of which I have dealt with:

- Heart and vascular problems
  - hypertension
  - palpitations
  - arrhythmia
  - dizziness and lightheadedness
  - mitral valve prolapse
  - premature ventricular or atrial contractions
- Gastrointestinal problems
  - gastro-esophogeal reflux disease
  - ulcers
  - gastritis
  - heartburn
  - indigestion
  - constipation
  - diarrhea and bowel irregularities
  - irritable bowel syndrome
  - inflammatory bowel disease
- Headaches
  - migraine headaches
  - tension headaches
- Skin conditions
  - psoriasis
  - eczema
  - hives
  - acne
- Genitourinary tract
  - chronic prostatitis
  - Chronic and recurrent yeast infections
  - frequent urination
  - loss of sex drive and impotence
  - frequent urinary tract infections
  - lower progesterone and testosterone levels
- Pain and inflammation
  - chronic back pain
  - fibromyalgia
  - chronic pain syndrome
  - tendonitis
  - carpal tunnel syndrome
- TMJ problems (note my comment above)
  - Lung and breathing problems
  - chronic or recurrent colds, sinus infections, sore throats, ear infections
  - chronic or recurrent bronchitis, pneumonia
  - asthma
  - bronchial spasms

- – shortness of breath
- – hyperventilation
- Immune impairment
  - – chronic fatigue
  - – chronic and recurring infections of all types.

As health care professionals, don't we really know how true this is? The American Institute of Stress claims that between 75–90% of all visits to primary care physicians result from stress-related disorders. As I have implied, the treatment for stress is usually very superficial. It is very easy to become addicted to stress. Many feel it's normal to work hard and stay overly busy, as if the constant flooding of adrenaline is good for us.

In my own case, I suffered from some of the things that appeared on the above list. Some of my ailments included: tension headaches; heartburn; irritable bowel syndrome; chronic fatigue; dizziness; lightheadedness; muscle soreness; panic attacks; and compulsive gambling – just to name a few. Most of us know dentists who have suffered similar fates from chronic ailments, to marital problems to suicide.

The idea that dentists commit suicide more than any other profession is real. However, the mortality rate in dentistry is also very high. For me, the turning point came when I was diagnosed with Type 2 diabetes. I took to heart what Mark Twain once said, "Get a small disease and really take care of it." After years of suffering from chronic stress, diabetes was my wake-up call. For me, diabetes was both a blessing and a curse, because I finally found the cause to many of my problems.

Many of you are probably thinking that diabetes is a disease caused by overeating in people, with a genetic background. There is some truth to that, but all of the facts are not in. Diabetes in America is reaching epidemic proportions. You don't need to have a relative with diabetes, or to be overweight, to get Type 2 diabetes. Seventeen million Americans have been diagnosed with Type 2 diabetes. Diabetes researchers are still coming up with new reasons for the disease, including chronic inflammation and viruses that affect liver function. I believe another possible cause of diabetes could be long-term chronic stress.

Years and years of frustration, hostility, or generalized stress can trigger the hormones that are responsible for the "fight or flight" syndrome. The hormones in question, adrenaline and cortisol, can have very damaging effects on the body. Elevated levels of adrenaline over time can also cause an elevation in triglycerides and blood sugar. Elevated levels of cortisol can raise blood sugar, insulin, and cholesterol, as well as the following, according to Don Colbert:

- Impair immune function.
- Reduce glucose utilization.
- Increase bone loss.
- Reduce muscle mass.
- Increase fat accumulation.
- Impair memory and destroy brain cells.

> "The sole reason for constructing my solo practice was to give me more life. If that's not your reason – it will suck up the life you have [6]."

My experience with Type 2 diabetes truly made me a believer in that last quote. Prior to that, I just tried to cope with the stress. The party line is, "If you can't take the heat; get out of the kitchen," or "That's just the way it is; deal with it." I remember a patient telling me one day while listening to me complain about dentistry, "It comes with the territory. If you didn't want the stress, you should have become a mailman." That was before the term "going postal" became popular.

It was shortly after I was diagnosed that I decided to take the bull by the horns and I resolved to take the concept of "vision" very seriously. I began to ask myself serious questions like, "What do I want?", "How do I want to spend my days? Who do I want to work with? Is my work making me ill, or is it my perception?", "Is my work keeping me from living the life I wanted?" These questions led me to rebuild my practice by starting with rebuilding myself.

I had to discover what a successful practice was. Was it someone else's idea, or one that I created?

Occupational stress is becoming more of a problem as we go into the future. A study by the American Psychological Association shows that about a third of the population feel isolated, and almost as many say their stress level has effected their physical and mental health [7]. Dentists today want control over their work. They are searching for meaning and autonomy. These are their intrinsic motivators and, when they are not acknowledged, stress happens, which leads to consequences that eventually affect the people we serve – the patients.

Dental Health Today

One Thursday evening in 2002, after teaching all day at the Pankey Institute, I gathered with a Continuum I class in "the condos" [8] to watch the premier of a new television show on ABC: *Extreme Makeover*. The show featured ordinary men and women who volunteered for extensive, extreme makeovers by a select group of Hollywood cosmetic surgeons and dentists. The show was an instant hit, and 55 episodes were broadcast through 2007. The show helped spawn other popular reality "makeover" shows like *The Swan, Extreme Makeover Weight Loss,* and *The Biggest Loser.* The dentists who were in that room that night believed the show was the greatest thing that ever happened for dentistry's public relations.

Although it can be argued that the cosmetic dentistry revolution began in 1994, when Dr. William Dickerson opened his Las Vegas Institute, the popularity of *Extreme Makeover* changed the way the public viewed dentistry, and changed the way dentists viewed themselves. Overnight, we wanted to do more cosmetic procedures. From porcelain laminates to sophisticated implant procedures, the whole profession was changing. With the acceptance of dental advertising, the promotion of cosmetic dentistry on a major television network and the growing popularity of organizations like the American Academy of Cosmetic Dentistry and others, committed to the advancement of cosmetic dentistry, the profession was changing rapidly.

Today, with the internet in full bloom, we can find a massive number of websites, blogs and social media posts that exhibit beautiful examples of cosmetic dentistry by some very talented dentists and laboratory technicians. But does this tell the real story of dentistry today? Has this image of dentistry become reality? I don't think so. The more things have changed, the more they have stayed the same.

Many people still see dentistry the way they viewed it 50 years ago. Although they acknowledge that dentists have better methods for controlling pain, better tools and technology, and much better materials that provide more beautiful results, they still have the same objections to dentistry: fear, finances, and trust issues. I will have a lot more to say about trust in Parts III and IV but, for now, let's take a look at how trust is on the decline in our culture.

Trust is central to human existence. As social animals, human beings have an instinctive need to cooperate and rely on one another. In other words, trust is a form of social capital, like love. According to Robert F. Hurley, the author of the book, *The Decision to Trust* [9], "Trusting means feeling comfortable with how a party will act in a situation in which you could be hurt. In terms of one-on-one relationships, it's been described as a willingness to make yourself vulnerable to someone else, based on positive expectations that the other person will either serve your best interests or at least not hinder them."

So why is trust even more important now, in the 21st century, than it was 50 years ago?

A 2012 Gallup survey showed trust has been on the decline. Actually, findings show a disturbing trend in declining trust since the 1960s, and the lack of trust in businesses has been a real issue for the last decade. In 2001, only 44% of people trusted business. In 2012, 45% trusted business in the US. In the UK, France and Germany it was worse in 2012 – 31%. There are many barometers of trust studies. One study found in Uslaner's, *Moral Foundations of Trust*, shows a disturbing trend of declining trust in major social institutions, including government and the media.

The public relations firm, Edelman, tracks people's level of trust in everything from the media to financial institutions. The 2009 Edelman Trust Barometer reported that three out of four Americans trust businesses less than they had done the year before. To make things worse, the same report said that Americans trust the media even less than business and government. The 2013 Edelman Trust Barometer found businesses were trusted by 58% of survey respondents globally, up from 53% in 2012. Despite trust being up, what this means is that, for every ten new patients, four do not trust you. Trust matters.

In other words, for various reasons, we now have become quite skeptical about messages coming from all institutions. Some have referred to 2008 as the year trust died in America, and say we are living in the post-trust era (PTE). There are many reasons for the breakdown in trust: the poor economy, corporate malfeasance, access to too much information, confusing advertising, and blogs. The world used to be a much smaller place.

Robert Hurley, in his book, *The Decision to Trust*, points to one reason for the erosion of trust as living in an age of extreme capitalism and an age of opportunism. He points to increased competition as having contributed to the evolution of a more economically driven, and less social and humanistic, model of capitalism. He claims, "More competition, more stress, and less slack in the system increase risk and make trust more difficult." The public has become acutely aware of a general lack of integration of ethics and morals in business models and organizations, which contributes to what Hurley refers to as *extreme capitalism*. We hear from many on the lecture circuit, and from within the profession itself, that "dentistry is a business." This extreme viewpoint might be one of the factors in the decline of trust.

More important than what the statistics tell us about trust levels is what most dentists see in their practices on a daily basis. In spite of what we see on Facebook, or in the glamour magazines, patients come into our practices with greater needs than ever before. It seems that fewer and fewer people can afford the advanced dentistry that technology allows us to do. Most new patients enter our practices with very poor oral conditions and even worse existing dentistry. People are staying away from dental offices for longer periods of time because of the rising costs of dentistry.

In addition to the trust factor, the financial factor is even more significant. The oral health landscape has changed over the past decade. The percentage of Americans with private dental benefits declined from 2000 through 2012. For working-age adults, this trend has been accompanied by a significant decrease in dental care utilization. While dental care utilization is at its highest level ever among children, utilization among adults is in steady decline, with only 35.4% of working-age adults visiting the dentist in 2012.

There are various reasons why adults do not visit a dentist. The most apparent reason is financial barriers, with one study finding that one out of five individuals are unable to afford needed dental care. At the same time, "supply-side" barriers are falling, with fewer individuals reporting problems with dentist office hours or the distance to a dental office being too far. While finding a dentist remains a challenge in some settings, in recent years, financial barriers to dental care have been declining. Moreover, various surveys and research methodologies measure barriers to dental care in different ways. Clearly, the available evidence does not provide a complete picture, which leads to renewed questions of the true underlying reasons why adults continue to forgo visiting a dentist.

On June 26, 2012, the television show *Frontline* broadcast a documentary called *Dollars and Dentists* [10] on the PBS network. The show was hosted by investigative journalist Miles O'Brien, who concluded that America was in a dental crisis. The general theme of the program was that patients were going to the dentist less because of the high out-of-pocket costs associated with dentistry. Frontline does not have the power of ABC-TV, but still many people were exposed to this problem, which was both an industry issue as well as an economic issue. In either case, it was dentistry's reputation that was being called into question.

Most of the show was concerned with welfare dentistry and access to care issues. The show highlighted the fact that government and Medicaid reimbursement is too low for most dentists to accept. The result is that corporate dental practices have come in to fill the void, making a big profit in welfare dentistry. O'Brien raised many ethical questions, like who should make dental decisions for patients? Dentists, or businessmen with profit motivations? What about dentists who are strictly driven by profit? He also exposed the numerous lawsuits against some of the for-profit corporate dental practice chains that are appearing all across America.

So, as dentistry has tried to enhance the message of what we can do for people, the same conditions that have kept people away from the dentist are still at work. The high cost of dentistry, patient anxiety, and the trust levels of all businesses and government programs, have made dentistry less accessible to many people. If there is a dental crisis in America, who should a manage the crisis? Government? Corporate? Non-Profit? Or can it be a grass roots issue? Can individual dentists contribute to get a handle on this crisis, or will we continue to watch the profession transform itself into something other than what its architects meant it to be?

During my own career, I have seen many examples of critical publicity aimed at dentistry. The year I graduated from dental school I was given a gift of a newly published book, *Dentistry and Its Victims*, by Paul Revere D.D.S. The dental community did not like reading about its darker side. In 1987, the *Reader's Digest* published an article titled, *How Your Dentist is Ripping You Off* [11]. Once again, the dental community was up in arms about how this bad press would affect the reputation of dentistry. Online, we see not only the beautiful work dentists have done, but we also see biting critical reviews of dental practices. All of these examples are not true versions of the character of most dentists, but they all contribute to a reputation that has hurt the profession for years.

The sad truth is that we do have a dental crisis in America. In 2000, the Surgeon General's Report on Oral Health addressed the inequities and disparities that affect those least able to muster the resources to achieve optimal oral health. The common theme that emerged from this extensive study "is that across all ages, income levels, and health insurance statuses, cost is a major factor. This is consistent with previous studies showing cost is the main barrier preventing adults from obtaining needed dental care." The report goes on to say, "the major message of the report is that oral health is essential to the general health and well-being of all Americans and can be achieved by all Americans. However, not all Americans are achieving the same degree of oral health."

I witness this in my practice everyday. Although I do my fair share of complete dentistry, and have had a fulfilling career, in every way, over the last 40 years, I would be blind to deny that we have a growing crisis in dentistry. There are many reasons for the crisis and the disparities in the oral health of Americans. It is a complex problem that cannot be reduced to simple reasons, as the media has portrayed. Mostly, the reasons are socio-economic. Other reasons include everything from inadequate public programs, poor distribution of dental facilities in remote places, an over-reliance on inadequate insurance programs, a lack of third party funding, and a lack of public understanding of dental health and prevention, among others. There is one problem that is rarely mentioned, and it is evidenced by the harsh criticism of the media and even some dental professionals – a lack of leadership within the profession.

I have been aware of our profession's reputation throughout my career. I understand what dentists must overcome to get our best dentistry off the shelf. I am not sure what control I could have over the numerous contributing factors to today's issues that I have discussed in this part of the book. I have little control over the general economy, the extreme capitalism that Hurley writes about, or the mainstream levels of trust that exist in these present times. I feel the same about our current healthcare crisis. There is no simple answer; it's just too complex.

Some economists are turning to psychology to explain why our health care system does not function optimally. The growing field of behavioral economics studies the effects of psychological, cognitive, social, and emotional factors on an individual's economic decisions. When we make decisions, we unwittingly allow our emotions, prejudices and biases guide us. In other words, we are not as rational as we would like to believe. This is why perceptions and reputation is so important. The late John Wooden, who many consider the doyen of coaching, had a fondness for aphorisms, and used to teach others to "Be more concerned with your character than your reputation, because your character is what you really are, while your reputation is merely what others think you are."

Who you are is a question that is at the heart of leadership. As a leader, it is your duty to be aware of this and to use leadership skills to your advantage. Through over 40 years of dentistry, I have faced the same professional and personal issues that dentists still speak about currently. I have found that the one discipline that holds the key comes under the general heading of leadership. I wrote this book to help dentists and the dental community take a deeper look into leadership and communication. When it becomes part of our dental education maybe, collectively, we will cure what ails American dentistry.

References and Notes

1 Christina Maslach (2001). *The Truth About Burnout: How Organizations Cause Personal Stress and What to Do About It.* Josses-Bass.

2 Randy Lang (2007). *Stress in Dentistry – It Could Kill You.* DDS Oralhrealthgroup.com.

3 Michael Kesner (2003). Burnout in Dentistry: The Cause and The Cure. *Dental Economics* **101**(9).

4 Doc Lew Childre and Howard Martin (2000). *The HeartMath Solution: The Institute of HeartMath's Revolutionary Program for Engaging the Power of the Heart's Intelligence.* New York, NY: Harper One.

5 Don Colbert (2006). *Deadly Emotions: Understand the Mind-Body-Spirit Connection That Can Heal or Destroy You.* Paperback.

6 Barry Polansky (2003). *The Art of the Examination.* Word of Mouth Enterprises.

7 American Psychological Association (2015). *Stress in America: Paying With Our Health.*

8 The condos are the housing facilities for students and faculty for The Pankey Institute in Key Biscayne Florida.

9 Robert Hurley (2011). *Decision to Trust: The Decision to Trust: How Leaders Create.* High-Trust Organizations Hardcover.

10 *Dollars and Dentists* (June 26, 2012). www.pbs.org/wgbh/frontline/film/dollars-and-dentists/(still available for viewing online).

11 www.dentistat.com/ReaderDigestArticle.pdf

Part II

The Solution

"There is nothing so powerful as an idea whose time has come."

Victor Hugo

"Visionary people face the same problems everyone else faces; but rather than get paralyzed by their problems, visionaries immediately commit themselves to finding a solution."

Bill Hybels

"With violence, as with so many other concerns, human nature is the problem, but human nature is also the solution."

Steven Pinker

"The solution often turns out more beautiful than the puzzle."

Richard Dawkins

Leadership and communication is the solution. How's that for some good, old-fashioned reductionist thinking? But I hear it all the time. In business, the word *leadership* has become so trendy that it has lost all meaning. One of the best ways to understand what leadership is, is by looking at an exemplar. I began my quest to learn about leadership many years ago, while studying the Pankey philosophy. I found many outstanding technical dentists who were not leaders, yet I never met a dental leader who was not an excellent technical dentist. Becoming a true dental leader is a long and involved process and, possibly, that is why I don't see many. Leadership development is the answer; and, if it is the answer, then the dental community must acknowledge that and provide a leadership development curriculum.

Motivational speaker Earl Nightingale, who was also an acquaintance of Dr. Pankey's, tells about a response given by Henry Ford when asked the question, "What's the problem with men these days?" His response according to Nightingale was that men just don't think, and he went on to say, "Thinking is the hardest work there is, which is probably the reason so few engage in it."

All leadership begins in the mind. We must become high quality thinkers before we can execute high quality work. I believe Henry Ford, after observing today's digital tools, would say that most men are either still not thinking, or are thinking at a shallow or superficial level. Leadership is deep work. In chapter 6, I will discuss the reasons why broadening and building a knowledge base through deep work will not only enhance leadership skills, but will also benefit our general well being.

L.D. Pankey was a role model for thinking dentists. He was challenged by similar problems dentists face today. Sure, times were different, but most of the problems we face, as Steven Pinker tells us in the quote above, are problems of human nature. I never met Dr. Pankey; much

The Complete Dentist: Positive Leadership and Communication Skills for Success, First Edition. Barry Polansky.
© 2018 John Wiley & Sons, Inc. Published 2018 by John Wiley & Sons, Inc.

of what I know about him comes from the teachers who knew him, and books and articles written about him [1]. I imagined him to be a man like any other, who had to grapple with the same problems we all face. I set out to learn his story because I was sure that, if he could become one of dentistry's most revered leaders, then so could I. In retrospect, I have concluded that Pankey, like all of us, travelled his own Hero's Journey, faced his own demons and, in the process, matured into the wise leader he became.

The Hero's Journey was first described by Joseph Campbell in his bestselling book, *The Hero With a Thousand Faces* [2]. Campbell described the journey as:

> "A hero ventures forth from the world of common day into a region of supernatural wonder: fabulous forces are there encountered and a decisive victory is won: the hero comes back from this mysterious adventure with the power to bestow boons on his fellow man."

L.D. Pankey's early life was committed to being the best dentist he could become. On a trip to Europe in the summer of 1932 for the European Dental Conference, his life changed course after meeting his mentor, Dr. Daniel Hally-Smith. Hally-Smith had a dental practice at the fashionable Place Vendomme in Paris. Pankey left Europe with two important pieces of advice: first, learn as much as you can about examination, diagnosis, treatment planning and communication. He told him there was a three-month course given at Northwestern University that taught just those things. The second piece of advice came in the form of a letter that L.D. kept under a glass plate on his desk for the rest of his career. The letter, essentially, was a verse from the famous book, *As a Man Thinketh* by James Allen [3], "thoughts are things, and as you think so you become."

Oh, there was one more thing: L.D. was told to learn about the science of occlusion. So, he contacted the most renown expert at the time – Clyde Schuyler.

During his sabbatical, he developed his "philosophy of practice."

Those two pieces of advice made an impression on my own leadership studies. Pankey was advised to put a premium on the skills of communication, and he was also advised to "think." He didn't take the thinking part lightly. His philosophy begins with taking an inner journey to know himself better. In other words, he committed to an inside-out approach to leadership, rather than the shallow approach most people take these days – outside-in. The last thing I noted was what I mentioned earlier, that in order to be a leader, we must take technical dentistry very seriously.

In Part II of this book, I will discuss the foundational principles of leadership. I will go over many of the reasons why leadership is the solution and, as leadership expert Dr. John Maxwell claims, that "everything rises and falls on leadership [4]." I will show that no matter how skilled one becomes, ultimately success, happiness and a meaningful life depends on the ability to lead.

Parts III–V will show you strategies on how to become a leader through three fundamental elements: the inner journey of self-management and self-development; the outer journey of developing relationships by mastering communication skills; and the third element of how to become a master technical dentist.

References and Notes

1 William J. Davis and Lindsey D. Pankey (1985). *A Philosophy of the Practice of Dentistry*, Medical College of Ohio.
2 Joseph Campbell (1972). *The Hero With a Thousand Faces*, 2nd edition. Princeton University Press.
3 James Allen (1903). *As a Man Thinketh*.
4 John Maxwell (2007). *The 21 Irrefutable Laws of Leadership*, p. 267. Nashville, Tennessee: Thomas Nelson Publishers.

5

The Fundamental Value of Leadership

"Everything rises and falls with leadership."

Dr. John Maxwell

"The empires of the future are empires of the mind."

Winston Churchill

"He who has a why to live for can bear almost any how."

Friedrich Nietzsche

Leadership development is important – more important than we give it credit for. Do you remember what ex-president George H.W. Bush once said about not getting "the vision thing?" In 1987, George Herbert Walker Bush, then vice-president to the outgoing Ronald Reagan, asked a friend to help him identify some cutting issues for his coming presidential campaign. The friend suggested he go up to Camp David for a few days to figure out where he wanted to take the country. A *Time* Magazine article quoted Bush's response, "Oh," said Bush in clear exasperation, "the vision thing." Since then, "that vision thing" has become part of our culture and has been associated with people who don't quite get the leadership thing.

After writing *The Art of the Examination*, I sent copies to those whom I considered my mentors. One of them, Dr. Peter Dawson, who is still one of dentistry's preeminent leaders, reciprocated my gift to him with another book. Dr. Dawson is the author of one of dentistry's bestselling technical books, *Evaluation, Diagnosis, And Treatment Of Occlusal Problems* [1].

Through the years, I have received gifts from many dentists with titles that would help me to become a better technical dentist – '*How to*'s about every procedure to make me more successful. The book was a signed copy of John Maxwell's *Becoming a Person of Influence: How to Positively Impact the Lives of Others* [2]. That gift, in one way or another, revealed to me that the genuine leaders in dentistry saw leadership as a discipline or something that needed to be studied, in addition to technical dentistry.

Some years later, after being honored by speaking at a Dawson Alumni Meeting, I was Dr. Dawson's dinner guest. At dinner, the discussion turned to L.D. Pankey, one of his mentors. I will never forget what he said that night about Dr. Pankey. Very simply, he said, "L.D. was no fluke." I took that to mean that L.D. Pankey was different from the other great dentists of his era, because he loved dentistry and the profession of dentistry, and understood what leadership meant to the profession.

So what is this thing called leadership, anyway – and how do we become leaders?

The Complete Dentist: Positive Leadership and Communication Skills for Success, First Edition. Barry Polansky.
© 2018 John Wiley & Sons, Inc. Published 2018 by John Wiley & Sons, Inc.

One requirement of leadership is that the leader must have followers. That simply means that the dental leader must have certain qualities that would cause patients and staff to be influenced by them. That is the simple definition of leadership. Unfortunately, leadership is a bit more complex, and is defined differently by different people. We all have our own ideas about what it means to be a good leader. While the definitions may vary, the general guidelines remain the same: leaders are people who know how to achieve goals and inspire and influence people along the way. Leadership is about success.

Type in "leadership" at Amazon.com, and you will get back an astonishing 180,000+ matches. Typing in "communication" will return over 300,000 matches, and "success" brings back 275,000 matches. That's a lot of opinions and theories. Leadership, communication and success are very robust categories on the business book shelf. It can get pretty confusing. My own library is filled with over 750 books on leadership, success, and communication, and I have read most of them. Many of the books are redundant and, truthfully, are filled with an abundant amount of self-evident information. Yet, as discussed, this information is indispensable for success. I wanted to write a book that makes this information accessible to the dental community.

For many, the idea of leadership is reduced to just common sense. That is the opinion of many within our profession, and may be the reason why it is not taught in dental school. There are times when I read these books that I feel the information "should" be self-evident. Yet, I say to myself, if it is common sense, then why is it so uncommon these days. As mentioned earlier, maybe reductionist and superficial thinking is at play. There is no doubt that the dental profession needs to develop more leaders for the sake of the individual dentist, as well as the entire profession.

Essentially, there are no shortcuts to leadership. Leadership development is a process. In all of my studies throughout the years, I have found that there is an underlying process and structure to everything – including leadership development. You will read more about process later on, when I discuss technical dentistry as well.

For now, I want you to understand that developing leadership skills, mastery and effectiveness is a process that takes time, growth and change. You will find that leadership development is more than just theoretical. It is practical and, although it begins in the mind, such as the idea that "thoughts are things," it takes action, emotional courage, and vulnerability to make the changes necessary to grow into the role of leader. After all, essentially, leadership is about behavior change.

In the introduction to this Part I, mentioned the Hero's Journey. My own life changed when I was introduced to the work of the mythologist Joseph Campbell. You will not find his books in the business or self-help section of the library. Mostly, his books are found in the literature, mythology or psychology sections. A mythologist is, at the most fundamental level, a storyteller. Storytelling is becoming very popular these days. You will recall that "story" and "leadership" are two of the elements included in the human universals. Stories help us to understand complex concepts by helping us to visualize the emotional issues better. Stories help us create meaning. Stories can help us sift through the complicated theories of leadership that fill those thousands of books on Amazon. That is why people read biographies, and it is also the reason why working with role models and mentors is so effective. A story can reduce the learning curve significantly, because there are no shortcuts. As T.S. Eliot once said about learning something difficult like leadership, it will "cost not less than everything." But it will be worth it.

I honestly believe it will be worth your while to read about Campbell's Hero's Journey [3]. The journey, as described by Campbell, is also known as the "monomyth." George Lucas, the creator of *Star Wars*, admitted that he rewrote the original screenplay to portray the monomyth. When I go to the movies I can see the monomyth structure that many writers use to develop their stories. I saw the monomyth structure when I read about L.D. Pankey. When I look back on my own life and career, then yes, I see the monomyth.

One of the best business books I have ever read was Walter Isaacson's *Steve Jobs* [4]. Jobs is both a good and bad example of leadership. In reading his book, I learned a lot more about the hero's journey. Jobs [5] gave a famous commencement speech to the graduating class at Stanford University in 2005, after his terminal cancer diagnosis. In it, he reviewed his life, and listening to it today sounds very much like the monomyth. One piece of advice he gave that day was: "You can't connect the dots looking forward; you can only connect them looking backwards. So you have to trust that the dots will somehow connect in your future. You have to trust in something – your gut, destiny, life, karma, whatever. This approach has never let me down, and it has made all the difference in my life."

Structure and process is like a template. The monomyth has stages. The mythic structure has twelve stages that can be identified easily in the movie *Star Wars*. The key stages include:

- *Your Ordinary World.* This is the beginning of the story, when our hero is in a safe place, before the adventure begins. The adventure begins by understanding the true nature of ourselves – our outlooks, our beliefs and our values. Above all, we are all human. Prior to my burnout, my everyday world was what many would consider ordinary. I remember complaining to an elderly patient about the stress I was experiencing, and his response was something I considered par for the course: "If you didn't want pressure, you should have become a teacher." That's just the way is was.
- *The Call to Adventure.* This is *the* early stage when we realize something is wrong in the world. It may come to us in he form of a message (think about R2D2 and C3PO giving Luke Skywalker the bad news after an ordinary day of work). Any threat to our safety and security and well-being would be considered a call to adventure. My diagnosis of adult-onset diabetes was my wake-up call. Sometimes life whispers; sometimes it screams. High blood sugar was my R2D2.
- *Refusal of the Call.* For the first time, fear is realized. This is the emotional courage I eluded to earlier. For dental *leaders*, this refusal is common. We feel the fear and stay put in our ordinary world. This is a moment of truth if our roles and lives will change. Change is emotional – it is scary.
- *Meeting the Mentor.* Although this has become a cliché in modern times, another important stage that is reduced to the simple advice of "find a good mentor," it really means finding your Obi-Wan Kenobi. Someone who realizes that it will take more that teaching you how to place an implant or extract a third molar to find success. This mentor understands the true nature of your journey – that it is an inner journey, of finding yourself. For that, you will need more than simple advice. It may be insight into the dilemma the hero faces, wise advice, practical training or even self-confidence. Whatever the mentor provides, it serves to dispel his doubts and fears and give him the strength and courage to go on.
- *Crossing the Threshold.* For me, the threshold was the Pankey Institute. When I first went down to Key Biscayne, I wasn't fully committed. I met people whom I thought were my mentors but, looking back, they were strictly helpers. I wasn't fully committed. I became more committed after Continuum III. At that point, after studying Pankey's story, I met Dr. Bill Lockard from Oklahoma City. He was retiring from dentistry that very same week. I listened to his "story," and I was convinced and committed that week. I was ready to cross the threshold. Bill showed me the difference between a true dental leader and many of the "gurus" of the day. I will explain those differences later, but most had to do with taking the inner journey.
- *Tests, Allies and Enemies.* Now I was officially out of my comfort zone. I was not only committed to get my very best dentistry off the shelf, but I had to bring it home to my practice and explain it all to family, staff and patients. I needed tools, and a light saber wouldn't do it (neither will lasers or digital radiographs). I went home to practice in a new way. My patients had not changed, my staff had not changed. I knew if I was to succeed, I would have to be the

leader. They would have to follow me. I was tested every day by patients and staff. At this point, I need allies, and my wife was very understanding and provided the support I needed. There were family members who believed I was crazy to spend so much money and effort to practice in a way that would bring me happiness which was my idea of success. Within the dental community, there were local dentists who didn't share my views of comprehensive relationship-based dentistry, and who let their opinions be known. On a national level, there were dentists who ridiculed the Pankey philosophies of restorative dentistry. Completing and actually practicing the Pankey way was the true test.

- *Approach To The Inmost Cave.* Throughout the journey, definite themes will continue to emerge. For me and, as I have come to find out for many in leadership positions, the theme of low self-esteem would come up. Joseph Campbell used the analogy of the inmost cave to describe what we still had to conquer was our own selves. When a difficult task came up, whether technical or behavioral, I would feel the discomfort that went along with the question of whether I was good enough. For many, these feelings have been with us since childhood. In 1978, psychologists named this feeling as the *Imposter Syndrome* [6]. It was first described as an issue for women but, today, the leadership industry has recognized it as a common theme among all business leaders. There are many causes, and most begin in childhood with expectations of success. I remember writing down a quote by Marianne Williamson that I kept in my wallet: "Our deepest fear is that we are powerful beyond measure. It is our light, not our darkness that most frightens us. We ask ourselves, 'Who am I to brilliant, gorgeous, talented, and fabulous?' Actually, who are you not to be?"

- *Ordeal.* This is your supreme test if you continue along the hero's journey. For many, it may be to become accredited in one of dentistry's esteemed organizations. It may be to go back to school to become more specialized, or to learn a new technology that wasn't available when they graduated. For me, my supreme test was writing my first book, *The Art of the Examination* – not only writing the book as a physical and mental task, but something that changed my direction in dentistry. I now became committed to teaching and writing about leadership and the soft skills needed to help dentists become successful.

- *Reward (Seizing the Sword).* This is the point of total transformation. The dragons have been slain, the enemies defeated. The rewards await you. The interesting part of the journey is that we never know the extent of the rewards. For me, I found a new passion in writing which led to a second career. I also met new people whom I never would have met if I had never accepted the challenges. My ordinary world has totally changed in every way, and I have changed in so many ways.

- *The Road Back.* At this stage, the anxiety of the original call to adventure is gone. There is a greater sense of self-confidence. Self-esteem is at its highest levels, and there is an immunity to feeling incapable of most anything. Some may claim this is a natural outgrowth of maturity and aging, but I disagree. I see so many people, not only dentists, who advance in age and never reach the equivalent levels of success – I believe it is because they refused the call.

- *Resurrection.* This is considered the climax of the journey – the point in the story where the hero has his most dangerous encounter. As I write this, I am laughing, because maybe this book is my resurrection. As I already explained, this book is taking on some of dentistry's biggest issues. The demons I challenged earlier in my career pale compared to what younger dentists face currently. Yet, I feel this will be my final expression to do something for the profession. When I opened Niche Dental Studio with my son in 2010, I thought that was a new pinnacle that would be my last, but Josh, my son has carved his own path. Hopefully I had something to do with that.

- *Return With The Elixir.* According to Chris Vogler, the author of *The Writer's Journey*, which explains the monomyth as a template for storytellers, "the final reward that he obtains may be literal or metaphoric. It could be a cause for celebration, self-realization or an end to strife, but whatever it is it represents three things: change, success and proof of his journey. The return home also signals the need for resolution for the story's other key players. The Hero's doubters will be ostracized, his enemies punished and his allies rewarded. Ultimately the Hero will return to where he started, but things will clearly never be the same again." My own journey hasn't ended yet, but I can see the future – I have always seen the future in one way or another.

As you can tell, the hero's journey is a process of growth and maturity. Joseph Campbell developed his thinking from the ideas of the psychologist Carl Jung, so you can see this isn't just the work of a storyteller. It has deep philosophical and psychological roots, and they have been described by many others, like the renowned psychologists Erik Ericsson and Abraham Maslow. Erikson is famous for mapping out the developmental stages of life and defining identity through the stages. Maslow, who I discussed in Chapter 2, defined his stages in his famous Hierarchy of Needs. Each stage evolved as defined by one's needs: physiologic and survival needs,; security and safety needs; love and belonging needs; esteem needs; and, eventually, self-actualization needs – this last one being that one fulfills one's potential. In Campbell's version, the idea of self-transformation is present throughout – the idea of self-actualizing and becoming what we are meant to become.

That would be success.

What *is* success? Success is personal. Each of us has our own version of what success means. TED is a non-profit organization devoted to spreading ideas, usually in the form of short, powerful talks of 18 minutes or less. It began in 1984, as a conference where Technology, Entertainment and Design converged, and today it covers almost all topics – from science to business to global issues – in more than 100 languages. When I searched for TED talks on the question, "what is the definition of success?", eleven presentations came back. Many definitions included the accumulation of material wealth, power and prestige. On reaching this point of the book, you can guess that I would argue.

One of the TED talks was of John Wooden, the legendary coach of the UCLA basketball team who won ten national championships in 12 seasons. Coach Wooden considered himself primarily a teacher before being a coach. Coaching basketball was another way of teaching life lessons to students. In his TED talk [7], he eloquently defined success as "peace of mind attained only through self-satisfaction and knowing you made the effort to do the best of which you are capable." In so doing, we become better people. When you listen to Wooden's ex-players, you constantly hear the theme of what better people they became, and they won the prize as well.

My own definition of success is "the accomplishment of a worthy goal." I will have more to say about well-being, happiness and success in the next chapter.

Becoming a leader ensures the pathway to success, no matter how one defines it. Most dental courses I attend focus on the end-product, rather on the process of getting there and how we evolve as true leaders. The focus is on beautiful dentistry, or closing the sale to get patients to accept dentistry. This is the usual and customary way dentistry has always been taught. I love the term "usual and customary," as it so implies mediocrity. Leaders are never satisfied with mediocrity. Leaders understand that the most desirable future is one of excellence – virtuous, worthy and valuable. These are the terms leaders speak about – not mediocrity.

As I wrote about earlier, one of the problems we have is reductionist thinking. Thinking wholistically takes effort. We all want to reduce complex ideas to simple ideas. I am reminded of the fabled scene in the movie *City Slickers*, This was a 1991 comedy with Billy Crystal playing Mitch, the city slicker who goes to a dude ranch to reconcile his life crises, and Jack Palance, the stoic cowboy who plays his advisor, Curly. The scene which has become known as "the one thing" scene captures both of them in a deep conversation about life.

Mitch is at fault for causing a stampede and, as his punishment, Curly chooses the fearful Mitch to accompany him to find the stray cows. They spend the night alone and slowly begin to bond. Mitch discovers that, despite Curly's tough exterior, he is a very wise man. Curly advises him how to face his problems, by singling out the "one thing" that is most important in life. And so it is with leadership. We all want to know the one thing about leadership that will provide us with the answers to all of our life and professional problems.

Although there is no one thing, there are fundamental components to be mastered. Personally, I agree with author Marcus Buckingham, who wrote a book titled *The One Thing You Need To Know: ... About Great Managing, Great Leading, and Sustained Individual Success* [8]. His "one thing" (and he admits there is no one right answer) is that what sets leaders apart is their ability to turn people's legitimate anxiety about the future into confidence. They do that by showing people vividly what the future is going to look like.

Leaders do that through various skills and traits that can be learned. One of those is "the vision thing." Vision and future focus are fundamental to leadership, so let's start there.

That Vision Thing

In Chapter 1, I told the story of the three stonecutters. The moral of the story is that the third stonecutter was most happy because he saw himself as building a cathedral, rather than as just doing a job. Although he was working on an incomplete project, in his mind he saw something else. He saw a bigger picture; he saw the future. Beyond just the project, he also saw his own future and his own legacy – that the cathedral, and he, would live on forever. Some might call this purpose. I call it vision, and I believe it is the "one thing" all leaders possess. More important, I believe, is that it is the starting point for all leadership. All leaders are forward-looking. All leaders have to be able to imagine a positive future. *That* is the "one thing."

Everything starts in our minds. Visioning is simply the ability to see and feel the possibility of a future that doesn't yet exist. We all do it at some point in our lives. An author of children's books, Antoine de Saint-Exupery, once said, "If you want to build a ship, don't drum up people to collect wood and don't assign them tasks and work, but rather teach them to long for the endless immensity of the sea." The endless immensity of the sea is a powerful image that compels the pursuit of a worthy goal that I described at the start of this chapter. Our forefathers guaranteed our right to pursue happiness. They guaranteed the pursuit, but left the definition of happiness up to each of us. That happiness may lie in a better future that compels us to follow. Children love to follow their dreams. All leaders are dreamers and possibility thinkers.

It is the compelling vision that unleashes the energy that is necessary to move toward that vision. It is what calls out when work is more than a job. It is the voice behind the calling. I believe this is what Albert Einstein meant when he said, "Imagination is more important than knowledge." Creating a vision, for most of us, is the easy part – as I said, we all have the ability to dream. The difficulty lies not in creating the vision, or what Stephen Covey recommends, "to begin with the end in mind." The dilemma is to make that vision crystal clear and prominent every day. Joel Osteen, the televangelist, author and extraordinary leader, writes about leadership for his followers. His favorite topics are vision, imagination and dreaming. One piece of advice that is repeated in many of his books is, "Always keep your vision in front of you."

Let's explore the ideas of creating the vision and then how to keep it out in front of us for active pursuit.

Fifteen years into my practice, I closely identified my life with the opening line of Dante's poetic magnum opus. *The Divine Comedy* opens with the line, "In the middle of our life's journey, I found myself in a dark wood." For the first 15 years, I was living a life that others offered up to me. I was the furthest thing from being a creation of my own destiny. I remember thinking to myself when I left my ex-business partner that I wanted to be the master of my own destiny. Up until that point, I was living the scripts handed to me by my parents, teachers, the education system, and other people's agendas.

I had not heard Steve Jobs's Stanford commencement speech yet. In that speech, he told the young graduates, "Knowing your time in life is limited, think carefully about how to spend it. Don't waste it living someone else's life. Don't be trapped by dogma – which is living with the results of other people's thinking. Don't let the noise of others' opinions drown out your own inner voice. And most important, have the courage to follow your heart and intuition. They somehow already know what you truly want to become. Everything else is secondary." Re-reading that today sounds a lot like Joseph Campbell's "follow your bliss" advice.

My very first action was to physically move my practice. That was my first attempt at becoming the master of my own destiny. We have all used that expression to reveal what we sincerely want to do with our lives. Who doesn't want to be the master of their own destiny? But destiny implies a destination. A destination is a landing place, a goal, a target; even an aim, a purpose or a mission. Most people just wish for their destiny, and most people never take the time to create that place and make a plan to get there. My first step was to build a new practice.

I would drive around looking for potential sites. I only had a vague idea of what I wanted; I only knew that things had to change. One day, I saw a For Sale sign on the main road that ran from my existing practice to my home. I stopped to look. A minister had recently died and had left his wife with overwhelming debt and in bankruptcy. The house was in disrepair. It was weathered and small. My first impression was that it would be a major renovation; too expensive, and saddled with unpaid back taxes that the new owner would have to take care of.

I parked my car and stood outside for a while. I closed my eyes and began to imagine what my new practice would look like. As I write this, I keep thinking of the line from the movie *Field of Dreams*: "If you build, it they will come." The children's book author I quoted earlier, Antoine de Saint-Exupery once said, "A rock pile ceases to be a rock pile the moment a single man contemplates it, bearing within him the image of a cathedral." The rock pile was in front of me and the cathedral was in my mind.

This was my starting point. The dark woods were getting a bit brighter. The vision, if not the actual building, was inspiring. The vision itself provided the inspiration and the energy to begin the project. As you will see, one of the attributes of a compelling vision is inspiration. At this point, all I had done was drive my car, stand outside an old house and use my mental capacity to imagine what could be. This clear picture would be the starting-point for the next 25 years of my life and practice. But, like all visions, it was just a starting-point.

In 1964, songwriters Burt Bacharach and Hal David wrote the song *A House is Not a Home* for a movie by the same name. The song was recorded by the singer Dionne Warwick, but never reached any level of popularity. In 1981, R & B singer Luther Vandross included the song on his debut album. The seven-minute version became Vandross's signature song for many years to come. The lyrics imply an apropos lesson:

> "A house is not a home,
> A chair is still a chair,
> Even when there's no one sittin' there
> But a chair is not a house
> And a house is not a home
> When there's no one there to hold you tight
> And no one there you can kiss goodnight."

Inanimate objects are brought to life through context. Relationships create context. The energy, the inspiration, the power and the spirit needs to be created. But it all starts with a vision. Regardless of whether your vision is a personal vision, a practice vision, a family vision, or a vision for parenting your children, it all starts in the mind. As Stephen Covey reminds us, "All things are created twice; first mentally; then physically. The key to creativity is to begin with the end in mind, with a vision and a blueprint of the desired result." This is leadership job number one.

In the business world, the idea of creating a vision has become a cliché. What I have come to find out is there is much more truth in the biblical axiom, "man plans, God laughs." It has been said that most businesses, at one time or another, have referred to the Wayne Gretsky philosophical doctrine about the future: "Skate to where the puck is going, not where it has been." I have discovered that my original vision acted more as a map than a template. As a map, it afforded me the chance to chart a course, rather than to copy a model. I was more of a navigator, making sure we were going in the right direction. But what direction was I going? Toward what destination?

How do we choose a destination? An end? Can we really see that far into the future? Does it really matter what the physical properties of a practice look like in terms of how it will function, 10, 15, 25 years later? The real questions that need to asked are the questions of philosophy, such as how we treat people, and how to bring those principles to life within the practice. That is why philosophy is important. To set the direction. As leaders, we have the responsibility to look into the future. We get paid to be dreamers.

How do we create the vision? I did it by looking at the past. I knew what I did not want. I realized, because of my burnout, that I wasn't satisfied with what my work was bringing to my life. I craved meaning. I hated the repetitive, monotonous, routine that became drudgery. I needed change, so I set out on my journey by creating a picture of my ideal practice based on what I did not want. My new practice started with people – people who trusted me, people who appreciated the level of care and skill that I was trained to do. I was capable and ready to do whatever it took to make my dream come true. Mostly, the changes required other people. That is when I realized that leadership and communication skills would be most valuable in manifesting my destiny.

Frequently, people ask the question, "What is the difference between leadership and management?" The simple answer is *effectiveness*. Leaders are effective, and managers are efficient. I want to make this distinction because many people think I write about practice management. Practice management is about doing things right. Although I do write about doing things right at times, I am mostly writing about doing the right things. I believe that doing the right things comes first. Being effective precedes being efficient.

There is a story that is told by many business writers, including Stephen Covey, Warren Bennis and Peter Drucker, that describes management as efficiency in climbing the ladder of success, while leadership determines whether the ladder is leaning against the right wall [9]. I have seen my whole career change when I focused on leadership and communication. It was difficult to change. Maybe that is why so many dentists I meet take the path of least resistance. They focus on *things* – shiny new things like products and equipment. They focus on management. They attempt to gain more and more control by practice management techniques like time management and people management, neither of which lend themselves to being controlled. Instead of managing themselves, their attention and focus, and their energy levels, they manage things that are outside of their locus of control. Leaders focus on their internal locus of control.

Creating a vision for your own life and practice is important. Creating a vision for your children's lives is also important. Creating a vision for the health of your patients is also important, because it defines a standard of practice. Your vision is the starting point for your intentions. If I haven't convinced you of just how important creating a vision is to your life, consider this: Joseph Campbell's biographers [10], Robin and Stephen Larsen, wrote that one of Campbell's favorite questions was, "Do you know what depression is?" Then he said, responding to his own question: "It's when you have spent your life climbing the corporate or whatever kind of ladder and you finally reach the top and it's against the wrong wall."

How important is vision? Make sure you're climbing the right wall.

Climbing The Right Wall

My vision wasn't cast in stone. I was very flexible and open to new ideas. I recall how insecure I was, compared to many of my colleagues. I always found myself around extremely confident people, who seemed to know so much more than I did. It was intimidating, but I didn't mind, because I was committed to making changes. When I went to the Pankey Institute, I would hear so many conflicting stories from dentists bragging about their practices. Later on, I found out that my insecurities are what kept me open to better ideas and thinking. I discovered that the insecure path was truly the secure path – in the end.

It took time to clarify my vision. One day, during lunch, I was listening to Wayne Dyer, the self-help guru and motivational speaker. On the tape, Dyer suggested to his audience to sit down in a quiet place and write a letter to yourself … from the future … from your future self. I did it. I was searching for guidance from anywhere. It was a good exercise – maybe even my first attempt at journaling. I learned a lot about myself from that exercise. Then I changed it a bit. I wrote a letter to myself from the future from Dr. L.D. Pankey.

If you remember, I did not know Dr. Pankey but, at the time, he represented all that was ideal about dental practice to me. I remember that it was a long, detailed letter. That exercise did more to clarify my vision than anything I had done to date.

Another exercise I did back then was the Tombstone Test. It has been called various names, but essentially it is very straightforward. It asks you to look in the mirror and ask yourself: "If I died tomorrow, would I want, whatever it is that I am pursuing today, engraved on my tombstone as my epitaph?" Covey, in *7 Habits of Highly Effective People* [9], described the Tombstone Test by asking readers to imagine their own funeral. All of these exercises involve using your imagination to communicate with your future. Ever since I did these thought experiments, I came to find out that the social psychologists have a lot to say about our future selves.

In his seminal bestseller, *Stumbling on Happiness* [11], Harvard social psychologist Dan Gilbert writes about his research in the field of affective forecasting (also known as hedonic forecasting), which is the prediction of one's emotional state in the future. Affective forecasting is studied by psychologists and economists in order to decide what present choices can be made, based on how we will feel in the future.

Gilbert writes at the outset that, "the human being is the only animal that thinks about the future." This trait is especially prominent in leaders. Gilbert has given three very popular TED talks, including one of the most-viewed talks of all time. After reading and watching him speak, I have concluded that creating an accurate vision of our future selves is a tricky business. He describes a concept known as synthetic happiness, which explains why, when we don't quite reach our dreams, we are happy anyway. We synthesize our happiness and settle for something we never planned. Why is that? Because of time. We all live in the now, and we all make choices that will eventually effect and affect our future selves. That's why this vision thing is so important, because our future selves must live with the choices we make right now.

I know so many dentists who never think about their future and end up settling. When you ask them, they're happy. That's how our psychological immune system works. As Shakespeare said, "Nothing either good or bad, but thinking makes it so." At any point along our personal or practice journey, we tend to believe that who we are at that moment is the final destination of our becoming. This is not only wrong, because we live dynamically changing lives, but it is also the source of much of our unhappiness. Although humans are the only animals who can use imagination to think about the future, imagination is still difficult. It is difficult because of time. Our values and personalities change over time.

Another social psychologist, Hal Hershfield, a Professor of Marketing at New York University's Stern School of Business, also studies affective forecasting. Hershfield's research focuses on judgment and decision-making and behavioral economics, with a specific interest in how thinking about time can strongly impact decision-making and emotional experience. If this research sounds esoteric, it's not. It has very common application. Our present selves behave on a daily basis in ways that are detrimental to our future selves. Just think about obesity, drugs and the entire retirement industry. We do things today that our future selves do not thank us for.

Hershfield's research used virtual reality to help participants to vividly imagine their own old age. They were given virtual reality goggles and sent into a room where they encountered a kind of mirror that made them look 68 or 70 years old. Half of the people in the study saw versions of their future, older selves, and the other half saw images of their current selves. Then the participants were taken to another room, and asked questions about their retirement. Those who had seen images of their future selves were willing to put twice as much money into long-term savings accounts than those who had seen images of their current selves.

In other words, they were able to close the gap between their current selves and their future selves. Instead of seeing the future as something that only happens to others, or strangers, they started to behave as if their current decisions meant so much more. In a way, they had a vision.

So how can leaders apply this research to their work? It starts with vision. We must learn to close the gap between our current and future selves. Just starting a conversation, like I did by writing a letter from my future self to my current self, is one way. They have actually found that letter writing of that sort helps in making better ethical decisions now. As Dan Gilbert's research reveals, we can't just depend on our imaginations and dreams, as I first read about with the Tombstone Test. Hirshfield adds credence to the age-progressive images by getting us closer to realty to close the gap.

There is another that is suggested by Dan Gilbert, that is to find a surrogate, or people you admire who have faced the challenges you are facing. My letter from L.D. Pankey was a variation on that theme. I then used that letter and asked people who knew him, "What would L.D. do?" Creating a vision cannot be reduced to dreaming … and as I have come to find out if you *just* build it … they will come.

My Pledge to You

Now that we have some idea of what we want to create, it's time to figure out why. The answers to *"why?"* for leaders come in the form of self-reflection on purpose and are then expressed in written form, as a promise to their followers in the shape of a mission statement. The vision is an aspirational description of what an organization would like to achieve or accomplish in the long-term future. It is intended to serve as a clear guide for choosing current and future courses of action.

Now that you see how creating a vision is not as easy as closing your eyes and dreaming, purpose is just as daunting. Both take a considerable amount of time for self-reflection and introspection. Purpose may be more discovered than created. Generally, we think about our purpose when a crisis appears. My burnout was my crisis. Sometimes, a crisis can be a blessing and a curse. It seems that I have always used my crises, whether financial, health, or relations, to make positive changes.

Even before I entered dental school, I had visions of what kind of dentist I would be. I don't mean what I would do every day in terms of choosing a specialty, but more of how I would relate to my patients. I daydreamed about my role in their lives. I saw myself as an advisor, a trusted friend. I genuinely believed in the importance of what I was going to do. I saw myself as the head of a clinic where patients and others came to me for advice. I felt special because I was choosing a profession that afforded me the chance to work with people and make a difference in their lives. Making a difference in people's lives, I discovered, has always been a theme in my life. Maybe it is for you, as well. I believe it is with most people.

When I graduated from dental school, I was hit with a big dose of reality. The value that I had placed on my services wasn't matched by what others wanted from me. My role was being diminished by what most of the public (not all) wanted from dentistry. I think, in the end, this is what actually caused my burnout, and I will have more to say about this in the next chapter, on what the positive psychologists have taught us about well-being. Many years ago, I heard a famous lecturer describe the situation as going from a "doctor" to a "mechanic" in a blink of an eye.

This went on for many years, as I described earlier. The human brain can only focus on only so much information at one time, and with the Internet and so many other distractions today, it's so much more difficult to live in the gap between stimulus and response [9]. I think that is why we tend to react, rather than respond, to our daily trials that test our resolve to become all we are capable of becoming. Self-awareness is great, but it has become another bromide that popular psychologists and self-help speakers throw at us.

Self-awareness is also easier said than done. It wasn't until I was diagnosed with type 2 diabetes that I began my introspective years. I reassessed what I really wanted for my life, my family, and my patients and my staff. I realized I had drifted unconsciously from my original vision of making a difference. I had lost my way. I had lost sight of my purpose, and was I was paying a price that was unacceptable.

Recall the story of the three stonecutters from Chapter 1. I believe the third stonecutter was the one who saw his work in relation to other people. He saw his work in a much wider context. I also believe that the results in the Gallup study mentioned previously, that only 13% of workers are actively engaged in their work, is a result of taking too narrow a view of work. The context of all work is other people. We only exist in relation to other people. I believe very simply that it is our obligation to be the best we can become, so that we can make other people better: our children, our spouses, our friends and family and, at work, our patients and our staffs. By keeping that purpose in front of me, just like my vision, I was able to stay on track. That is why discovering purpose lies at the heart of every leader.

The dictionary defines purpose as: an aim or a goal, the object toward which one strives, or for which something exists, an intention, the result or desire that is intended. Purpose is the reason why something is done. The result is your destination; actually, as I will discuss in the next chapter, it may very well be your destiny. Your purpose provides the energy to continue to drive toward that end.

In one of the most highly recommended books for dentists, *The E-Myth* [12], author Michael Gerber begins his description of small business development with an explanation of what he calls a *primary aim.* He describes the primary aim as a starting point which includes *a vision*, *a purpose* which provides the *energy*, and it answers the following questions:

- What do I value most?
- What kind of life do I want?
- What do I want my life to look or feel like?
- Who do I wish to be?

Your practice ultimately has to provide the resources to accomplish your primary aim.

I realize this is a book about leadership. As I have come to find out through my years of practice, leadership doesn't exist in a vacuum. It is a blend of many branches of knowledge. My own research has led me to articles and books in such diverse fields as business, sales and marketing, cognitive psychology, positive psychology, social psychology, personal growth and development, management, behavioral economics, and decision-making, not to mention leadership and communication. For me, leadership is an all-inclusive term that covers so many disciplines. At some point, the reader may be asking, what does all this talk of "purpose" have to do with leadership?

The answer is everything. The dentist must be the beacon that his or her followers look toward. The beacon is the source of energy. It is the light that must never burn out. Over and above that, the dentist works to provide a good life for himself and his family. That energy comes from vision and purpose.

Everyone needs a reason to get out of bed in the morning. Richard Leider, the author of one of the more impactful books on the topic of purpose, *The Power of Purpose* [13], has made that single question the focus of his whole career: *What is your reason for getting up in the morning?* Leider uses a formula to describe how to find your core sense of purpose: $G + P + V = C$. His formula suggests, and most would agree, that we must first have a clear understanding of the things we most cherish in life, our core values. The V in the formula is for values, the G stands for our gifts (others refer to gifts as our strengths), and the P stands for our passions. Fundamentally, the formula is asking another deeper question: "Are you using your gifts (strengths) on something you feel passionate about in an environment that values you?" If so, says Leider, "You're on purpose. You have a reason to get up in the morning."

I will have more to say about passion and strengths in Chapter 7. For now, I want to convey the idea that our individual purposes are derived mostly from our core values. Most leadership books include a section on clarifying values. Like finding our purpose, this involves deep intro-spection. If purpose provides the energy for the trip, then our values provide the direction. Leaders are driven by principles and values. As noted in Chapter 3, principles are rules or laws that hold up over time. Principles are like guidelines that our best leaders use as boundaries for ethical behavior. They are the human universals that exist in all cultures across all time – like empathy, leadership and reciprocity. My favorite principle is the Golden Rule.

Dr. Peter Dawson always lectured about his version of the Golden Rule. He called it his WIDIOM rule. It was a guideline for ethics in his practice. It translated to *Would I Do It On Me?* That is a principle that simply states treat others as you would like to be treated. It's fundamental to all service industries. Covey calls principles the territory, while values are the maps within the territory. Principles are not values. Of course, "when we value natural laws and principles we have truth – a knowledge of things as they truly are." Once again, the principle of WIDIOM implies that our purpose somehow should center around other people.

Values are who we are as individuals. Elvis Presley once said, "Values are like fingerprints. Nobody's are the same, but you leave 'em all over everything you do." They act as your daily guide. Your behavior, like it or not, is centered around what is most important to you. As the leader of your practice, it is up to you to clarify and communicate those values to the members of your practice. Once those values are communicated and shared, they have a major influence on the day-to-day behaviors and attitudes of the practice.

The opposite of not clarifying values can lead to much confusion. I have seen many dental practices that do not reach their potential because of mixed messages around what is truly important and the core beliefs of the dentist. Simply put, when the dentist puts profit over people, it shows up with less compliance, high turnover and possibly legal issues.

In the next section, I will explain the various processes in creating a vision, defining your purpose and clarifying your values. I want to end this section with a discussion of the most conventional way to communicate your vision, purpose and values. It is called your mission, and it is expressed through a mission statement.

According to Wikipedia, "a mission statement is a statement which is used as a way of communicating the purpose of the organization. Although most of the time it will remain the same for a long period of time, it is not uncommon for organizations to update their mission statement and generally happens when an organization evolves. Mission statements are normally short and simple statements which outline what the organization's purpose is and are related to the specific sector an organization operates in."

For me, the mission statement is my promise to my patients. After much self-analysis, and getting to "know myself" better, the mission statement is the distillation of what I want to simply communicate. Dr. L.D. Pankey brought his philosophy of practice to dentistry by codifying very complex ideas into simple tools that can be remembered very easily. One of those tools is his Cross of Dentistry. The Cross has four arms: Know Yourself; Know Your Patient; Know Your Work; and Apply Your Knowledge. At a very fundamental level, this book is an analysis of the Cross of Dentistry.

In teaching the Pankey philosophy through the years, I have encountered many dentists who do not understand what "know yourself" actually means. Pankey was a student of the Greek philosophers – the original wholism thinkers. Socrates was famous for saying "the unexamined life is not worth living" and, although I do not agree with the "not worth living" part, I have seen too many people not examining their own lives to the degree I am recommending. Maybe the unexamined dental practice is not worth starting. Maybe L.D. was referring to another philosopher, George Santayana, who observed, "He who does not remember the past is condemned to repeat it." By examining our lives and getting to know ourselves better, we have a chance for growth and change, otherwise we will continue the same patterns of behavior that took us only so far in life. Another way of saying it is, and I can't resist using the oft-quoted Albert Einstein, "the definition of insanity is doing something over and over again and expecting a different result."

At the end of the self-analysis is a mission statement, both personal and professional. The mission statement is less about what the destination looks like – the vision – and more about how my practice will achieve the defined results. It makes the values and purposes come alive. The mission statement speaks more to the core values of the practice and the patients, rather than being a description of what the practice will look like in the future. Mission statements are also flexible because, over time, circumstances change, people change, and values change. The mission statement should reflect the purpose and the core values of the practice. It should be brief, simple, and clear enough for the constituents to understand and apply. It needs to be the basis of all strategies that guide the day-to-day activities of the practice. It should live.

Yes, mission statements should come alive. I have seen too many mission statements hung up on the walls of businesses, that are there for decoration only. The leader played a major role in developing the mission statement and should be the one who lives it daily. It is those traits, behaviors and qualities that everyone will look toward. It will define your leadership. Leadership experts James Kouzes and Barry Posner, in their book, *The Leadership Challenge*, advise leaders, as one of their five practices, to model the way [14].

Some years ago, when I first learned about writing a mission statement, I struggled to find the right language. As time went by, my practice was developing into a practice that I created through Pankey's philosophy. I had developed the values of clinical excellence, honesty, education, and empathy, among others, into my practice. I adopted Dr. Pankey's original mission statement:

> "The goal for my practice is to help people keep their teeth for their lifetime, in proper health, comfort, function, and esthetics. And to do it appropriately according to their circumstance, objectives and temperament."

Throughout this book, I will refer back to this mission as an expression of values that I have applied in my dental practice. In time, the statement was lived by not only myself, but my staff and my patients.

If you think that many of the ideas or concepts I have presented so far in this book are too abstract, too philosophical and too difficult to apply, then take heart, because I, too, once thought that these principles were hard to apply. In the following chapters, I will bring these principles to life so that they come alive in a practical way. I live in the same world as you do. I believe, as John Maxwell claims, "everything rises and falls on leadership." But those are just the words of a philosopher, and what good is philosophy if it can't be useful? Thoreau once said of the best philosophies, that they "solve the problems of life, not only theoretically, but practically." The next section will explain how to discover your vision, values and mission.

Creating Your Vision Statement

1) Your vision statement should be short and memorable. I like the words "brief", "simple" and "clear". Use descriptive word pictures that suggest where you are going to be in the future.
2) The language should be very specific to dental outcomes. Dental leaders think in terms of long-term value.
3) Use very specific language. Don't use language or terms that are open for interpretation. For example, "optimal care" means different things to different people. Use specific time frames.
4) Make sure it can be understood by others outside of dentistry. Don't use jargon.
5) Make sure the vision is realistic and achievable, yet audacious enough so the practice must stretch to reach the vision.
6) Make sure the vision is aligned with your values.
7) Bring your staff in to brainstorm. Take a long-term view. Imagine that your practice was going to be featured on the cover of a prominent dental magazine. What would the headline read?

References and Notes

1 Peter E. Dawson (1989). *DDS, Evaluation, Diagnosis, And Treatment Of Occlusal Problems*, 2nd Edition. Mosby.
2 John Maxwell (2006). *Becoming a Person of Influence: How to Positively Impact the Lives of Others*. Nashville, Tennessee: Thomas Nelson Publishers.
3 There are many sources that describe the Hero's Journey. My favorite is the discussion in the book *The Power of Myth* – and interview by Bill Moyers and Joseph Campbell.
4 Walter Isaacson (2011). *Steve Jobs*. New York, NY: Simon and Schuster.
5 Steve Jobs (2005). You've Got to Find What You Love. *Stanford News*, June 14, 2005.
6 Pauline Rose Clance and Suzanne Imes (1978). The impostor phenomenon in high achieving women: Dynamics and Therapeutic interventions. *Psychotherapy Theory, Research and Practice* 15(3): 241–247.
7 www.ted.com/playlists/77/11_must_see_ted_talks.
8 Marcus Buckingham (2005). *The One Thing You Need to Know About Great Managing, Great Leading, and Sustained Individual Success*. Free Press.
9 Stephen R. Covey (2013). *The Seven Habits of Highly Effective People*, 25th Anniversary Edition, p. 108. New York: Simon and Schuster. Covey suggested in Habit 1 to be proactive by finding the gap between stimulus and response.

10 Stephen and Robin Larsen (2002). *Joseph Campbell: A Fire in the Mind*. Inner Traditions.

11 Dan Gilbert (2006). *Stumbling on Happiness*, pp. 5–6. New York: Knopf.

12 Michael Gerber (2004). *The E-Myth Revisited: Why Most Small Businesses Don't Work and What to Do About It*. New York: Harper Collins.

13 Richard J. Leider (2015). *The Power of Purpose: Find Meaning, Live Longer, Better,* 3rd Edition, p. vii. Oakland, CA: Barrett-Koehler Publishers Inc.

14 James Kouzes and Barry Posner (2012). *The Leadership Challenge: How to Make Extraordinary Things Happen in Organizations*, 5th edition. Jossey-Bass.

6

Positive Psychology and Leadership

"The purpose of life is not to be happy. It is to be useful, to be honorable, to be compassionate, to have it make some difference that you have lived and lived well."

Ralph Waldo Emerson

"Well-being cannot exist just in your own head. Well-being is a combination of feeling good as well as actually having meaning, good relationships and accomplishment."

Martin Seligman

"The only prerequisites to leadership are that you remain positive, calm, and open-minded."

Alexis Hunter

The late positive psychologist Chris Peterson said, "Positive institutions facilitate the development and display of positive traits, which in turn facilitate positive subjective experiences." Creating positive cultures in our profession may be just the solution our profession needs. Too many people inside and outside of dentistry only see the negative side. The fear, the costs and the distrust have helped to paint a dismal picture. This is not only true of dentistry, but of the entire field of psychology as well. Throughout its history, the science of psychology has mostly focused on what is wrong with people – the bad, not the good. Positive psychology may be the answer, and the science is what makes it different from the history that preceded it.

Positive psychology is a relatively new field. Actually, psychology itself is a relatively new field; many like to say psychology has a long past, but only a short history. The history of psychology as a scholarly study of the mind and behavior dates back to the Ancient Greeks. The psychologists of that period were known as philosophers. Psychology, as a self-conscious field of experimental study, began in 1879, when Wilhelm Wundt founded the first laboratory dedicated exclusively to psychological research in Leipzig, Germany. Many of the philosophers and psychologists concerned themselves with finding the meaning of life, or what makes life worth living. Many fell back on one word ... happiness. The reductionists have concluded that finding or pursuing happiness is the single focus of positive psychology. The true scientists have recently shown this to be erroneous. The science of positive psychology is complex, learnable, and not simply just a matter of the genetics of feeling good. It takes some work, as you will see.

As you can probably tell by now, my professional life has been a search for finding happiness, but I was never able to find it. I didn't know what it was. I would see images of a song from my youth, *The Elusive Butterfly* [1], whenever I thought of happiness. That was my view, that of a songwriter. To some people, it is the Peanuts comic strip's view, "Happiness is a warm blanket,"

The Complete Dentist: Positive Leadership and Communication Skills for Success, First Edition. Barry Polansky.
© 2018 John Wiley & Sons, Inc. Published 2018 by John Wiley & Sons, Inc.

or John Lennon's cynical view, "Happiness is a warm gun." In any case, I was never satisfied with the answers. They were way too reductionistic for me.

The Pankey Philosophy appealed to me because it was the first time I heard anyone in dentistry address the concept of happiness. Dr. Irwin Becker's philosophy class was the highlight of my first week at the Institute. Dr. Pankey's philosophy was focused on balance around a center which was the reward of happiness – both material and spiritual. Pankey developed his philosophy from studying Aristotle's explanation of achieving "the good life." In Aristotle's view, all human action is for the purpose of achieving happiness, and Pankey's philosophy depended on that view. But I wasn't satisfied, because it was too vague and not easily translated to the technical part of his philosophy.

I don't blame Dr. Pankey for not explaining happiness any better than the likes of Aristotle, or Freud for that matter. We do know that "work" is an important component of the "good life." Most psychologists had a difficult time going into detail about such an amorphous subject. Freud, too, referred to a balance when he said, "Work and love, love and work – that's all there is." Bookstores and libraries are filled with books on self-help and psychology, for people who are searching for that elusive butterfly. One psychologist, Dr. Martin Seligman, has spent his entire career searching for a workable theory on happiness. He claims he detests the word *happiness* because it is overused and has become meaningless. Since he is commonly known as the founder of Positive Psychology and the Director of the University of Pennsylvania Positive Psychology Center, he is quite the authority on the subject. Since 1997, when he was the president-elect of the American Psychological Association, he has been developing his theories.

Seligman's first theory was published in his best-selling book, *Authentic Happiness* [2]. In that book, the first description of positive psychology, Seligman defined happiness as being composed of three different elements: positive emotion, engagement and meaning. Finally, someone was describing terms that I could relate to, rather than the virtues and values that Thomas Jefferson said we had the right to pursue. I knew these elements were important, but I also knew that I was pursuing success, regardless of how one defines it. For many people, success includes some degree of external and material rewards and feelings of contentment. What I had already realized was that happiness precedes success, so I needed a working model. Seligman's next book, *Flourish* [3], filled that need.

In *Flourish*, Seligman updates his original theory by stating that the goal of positive psychology is to increase life satisfaction. According to his new theory, "the topic of positive psychology is *well-being*, that the gold standard of measuring well-being is flourishing, and that the goal of positive psychology is to increase flourishing [4]." He also states in the book that the goal of positive psychology is to increase the amount of life satisfaction on the planet. Talk about a worthy goal. Think about what that would do for the dental profession.

I am not a psychologist. Through my years in practice, I have met many dental lecturers who have claimed to know how to find peace and happiness in a profession that is known not only for its material successes, but also for its morbidity. By morbidity, I am referring not only to suicide rates, but to any other conditions that effect the quality of dentist's lives, like divorce, drug usage, depression, chronic and other psycho-immune illnesses. This is the elephant in the room of most continuing education courses. In my studies of positive psychology, I found ways, in actuality, to create conditions and circumstance that will lead to what many have called the good life. To create these conditions and circumstances is the work of leadership, which is why I have included this discussion of positive psychology in a book about leadership.

In the last chapter, I cited Dan Gilbert's advice about finding a surrogate to visualize your future. I enjoy reading books that mine for the wisdom and advice of the elderly, such as Mitch Albom's *Tuesday's With Morrie*, about a man, Morrie Schwartz, a 78-year-old sociology professor who was dying of the last stages of ALS. It became a bestseller because it gave readers a perspective on how to live their lives. Albom wrote the book as a series of conversations that covered acceptance, communication, love, values, openness, and happiness. He emphasized the importance of forging a culture of one's own, to transcend the tyranny of popular culture, suggesting that the media are preoccupied with death, hatred, violence and depression. As you will see, leaders forge cultures; they build empires of the mind and positive workplaces that go beyond surviving (negative) to thriving (positive).

In another book, *30 Lessons for Living, Tried and True Advice from the Wisest Americans* [5], Karl Pillemer, PhD, asked more than 1000 Americans over the age of 65 to share their advice for living. From lessons on creating a happy marriage and living like an expert, to lessons on getting up everyday for a good reason, and being excited to work, these interviews led to 30 lessons, which Pillemer distilled down to the five most important:

- Control over one's time (Autonomy).
- Being happier (Positive emotions).
- Working with their strengths or gifts (Competence).
- Doing less.
- Having faith that everything will work out (Optimism).

Are you beginning to sense a theme with what is important in life?

A nurse, Bronnie Ware, made a practice of asking all of her patients, before they died, if they had any regrets. Her book, *The Top Five Regrets of the Dying: A Life Transformed by the Dearly Departing* [6], offers the following five regrets:

- Being true to oneself. Not being authentic was the number one regret. Most people did not honor their dreams.
- Wishing they did not work so hard. This was especially true of the male patients, that they didn't honor their own time. This will be discussed later under the heading of autonomy.
- Having the courage to express their true feelings (Relationships).
- Staying in touch with old friends and family (Relationships).
- Not letting themselves be happier (Positive emotions).

This material is important. It not only can be life-changing but, if taught properly, it can change the profession. It needs to be part of a leadership curriculum, so that dentists will have access to a much bigger – a whole, if you will, picture of the dental profession. L.D. Pankey did not have access to the science of positive psychology during his career. I know he studied Maslow and Carl Rogers, both humanistic psychologists who believed in a client-centered approach to dentistry. It has been debated about who first developed the term *positive psychology*. Maslow and Seligman both used similar language. Maslow used the term a bit differently – more in the human potential sense – while Seligman describes it more descriptively as a course of study. Although I still believe the work of the humanists can be very helpful with motivating people to become the best version of themselves, positive psychology offers leaders an approach for leaders to create better lives for themselves and their followers.

The science of positive psychology is growing rapidly. As recent trends of physician and professional burnout increase, this issue can no longer be ignored. As I mentioned in Chapter 4, the consequences of burnout are quite pressing. Christina Maslach has developed the Maslach Burnout Inventory, which is now recognized as the leading measure of burnout. The MBI incorporates the science that has been conducted over the past 25 years since professional burnout was considered a problem. The inventory addresses three separate scales:

- Emotional exhaustion – measures feelings of being emotionally overextended and exhausted by one's work.

- Depersonalization – measures an unfeeling and impersonal response toward recipients of one's service (patients and staff), care, treatment or instruction.
- Personal accomplishment – measures feelings of competence and successful achievement in one's work.

Maslach defines burnout as "the index of the dislocation between what people are and what they have to do. It represents erosion in value, dignity, spirit, and will – an erosion of the human soul. It is a malady that spreads gradually and continuously over time, putting people into a downward spiral from which it's hard to recover [7]."

Kapoor, Puranik and Uma, in a recent article addressing burnout in dentistry, concluded that dentists are particularly prone to burnout as measured by the Maslach Burnout Inventory [8]. Dentists, they point out, are not alone in trying to cope with the chronic emotional strain of dealing extensively with other human beings. As mentioned earlier, positive psychology deals with what is good in life. There may be some controversy in some circles about what is "positive" and what is "negative". When it comes to burnout, it can easily be seen how negative it is when compared to its metaphorical polar opposite condition … passion. If passion is the fire, the fuel and source of energy we need to sustain our work and careers, then burnout is a hollow, vacuous, depleted state that can ruin or end a career. As Maslach's definition states, it is the erosion of the human soul. The cure is passion, and I will discuss that in Chapter 7.

Specific to dentistry, there are some factors which would potentiate occupational burnout in the daily work lives of dentists: confinement, patient anxiety, compromised treatment, perfectionism, economic pressures, low self-esteem [9], time and scheduling pressures, pay-related stressors, patients' unfavorable perception of dentistry and dentists, technical problems, patient management issues, patient relationships, posture and chronic pain problems, and unhappy marriages [10]. Reviewing my own career, I can see some, if not many, of these circumstances in my own burnout. As I reversed my condition through developing passion, I realized how much it was dependent on learning skills that I could not classify without using words like leadership, communication and connection [11].

Burnout in all of the health professions is a serious issue, causing "both a threat to the workforce and a tragedy to the individual dentist and thus could be considered a public health issue [12]." Most physicians and dentists who suffer from burnout do not seek help, because of the expectations of health professional in society as being strong individuals who generally are in control.

Of course, if a dentist is in the throes of burnout, leadership skills may be too late to the party; psychiatric help may be the alternative. If, like me, the dentist is highly sensitive to his or her working conditions, then the lessons in this book and what we can learn from positive psychology will go a long way. It takes work, but it is worth it.

In summary, positive psychology is a science, but many would argue that it is just common sense, because it seems to have been around forever. Psychologists from William James to Maslow, and philosophers from Aristotle to Thales, have been theorizing about happiness since someone realized there even was such a state of being. The word *happiness* actually comes from the Old Norse *happ*, meaning "chance" or "luck. [13]" But the science of happiness, positive psychology, has come a long way since then. It is also much more than the scores of pop psychology trade books that get published every year to fill the desires of those searching for that elusive butterfly. Positive psychology today is backed by reams of data and evidence, and that has resulted in many conclusions that can help us to be better leaders and to create our own version of the good life.

The following is a list of some of the recent findings that have been backed by the science [14]:

- Most people are happy.
- Happiness is a cause of good things in life, and not simply along for the happy ride. Happiness leads to desirable outcomes at school and at work, to fulfilling social relationships, and even to good health and long life.

- Most people are resilient.
- Happiness, strengths of character, and good social relationships are buffers against the damaging effects of disappointments and setbacks.
- Crisis reveals character.
- Other people matter mightily if we want to understand what makes life most worth living.
- Religion matters.
- Work matters as well, if it engages the worker and provides meaning and purpose.
- Money makes an ever-diminishing contribution to well-being, but money can buy happiness if it is spent on other people.
- As a route to a satisfying life, eudemonia trumps hedonism.
- The "heart" matters more than the "head." Schools explicitly teach critical thinking; they should teach unconditional caring.
- Good days have common features, such as feeling autonomous, competent, and connected to others.
- The good life can be taught.

This book is about applying many of these tenets. It should be noted that science has shown that these results show causes and correlations, but none are 100% effective. During my career, I have found that some are most important. The last two are of particular importance: that these skills can be learned and, as I will reveal in Chapter 7, that autonomy, competence and connection may be the keys to a fulfilling career.

The next section will discuss some of the more prominent features of Martin Seligman's Well-Being Theory.

The Well-Being Theory

My father drove a taxicab for a living. He owned his own cab. Every night, when he came home, my mother would ask him the same question: "How was your day?" I assumed that she meant how much money he made that day. When I went into my own dental practice years later, my wife would ask me the same question. It was then that I realized that it was more than production that contributed to the making of a good day or a bad day. Looking back, it was the accumulation of those days, good and bad, that contributed to my overall well-being. It is true as author Annie Dillard says, "How we spend our days is, of course, how we spend our lives."

I remember, when I was in the middle of my burnout, that I would take a vacation or a long weekend just to get away. There was no getting away from burnout though. It would follow me around like a dark cloud. I realize now that well-being is like the weather – it is a construct composed of many elements. That is how Martin Seligman describes life satisfaction in his most recent theory on well-being – as a construct. Our days are constructed or built with elements that make up our subjective well-being. Happiness then, is a thing, the result of the well-being that we can construct or actually design. With this view, the idea of "you build it and they will come," made sense. Instead of viewing happiness as something we all deserved in a "just world," Seligman's new theory could actually be pursued. The only change is that, instead of building something outside of ourselves, we build it inside, by working on the elements or nutriments of well-being.

The major difference between Seligman's original theory of happiness, as explained in his first book, *Authentic Happiness* [15], is that the newer well-being theory defines each nutriment or growth factor as a measurable component, rather than just a subjective feeling. When we view the components as nutriments or agents of growth and development, we see that leadership skills can be learned and that growth is possible. As a construct, no single component can be responsible for happiness. That means that high production alone will not result in happiness. Production and money is just a piece of the well-being and life satisfaction picture.

Semantics is the branch of linguistics and logic concerned with meaning. The word nutriment, as stated earlier, is any agent of growth and development. I am a big believer in the concept of labeling your emotions. I believe that if you name it, you can tame it. Any feeling that will help us to grow and sustain is worth developing.

When I was dealing with my own issues, the three things I did were:

- First, get into physical fitness. That enabled me to have a clear head.
- The second thing I did was to read. Leaders, as you will learn, read. Reading helped me to explain my feelings to myself. Only by making small distinctions was I able to tame the negative and convert them to the positivity of well-being.
- The third thing I did was to find other leaders and view them through a prism. I would see them as possessing some, if not all, of the elements of a good leader.

Throughout this book, you will read about the various nutriments that contribute to well-being. Seligman's theory contained five elements. Remember, there is no such thing as the perfect leader.

Dr. Pankey's philosophy was more aligned with Aristotle's original ideas. Happiness was hazy and ill-defined. I believe that is one area that needs to be further clarified for dentists to be able to apply in the real world of dentistry. According to Seligman, each component has definite parameters. Each one would be chosen as something anyone would choose for its own sake. In addition, "each nutriment had to have three properties to count as an element [16]:"

1) It must contribute to well-being.
2) Many people pursue it for its own sake, not merely to get any of the other elements.
3) It is defined and measured independently of the other elements.

Seligman's five elements are positive emotion, engagement, positive relationships, meaning, and accomplishment. He calls these elements by the mnemonic PERMA. I will look at each of these nutriments through the lens of a dentist trying to pursue happiness by becoming a more effective leader. Marty Seligman added a sixth module to his theory. It is now known as PERMA-V. The V stands for vitality, and includes items that add or renew levels of energy which add to our well-being.

Figure 6.1 Martin Seligman's Well-Being Theory PERMA-V.

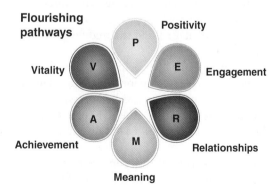

Positive Emotions

How can we talk about well-being, positive psychology, and life satisfaction, without talking about the pleasant life, or positive emotions? I know what you're thinking – are you kidding? In a dental practice? Well, there seems to be a lot of confusion around this topic. Most would agree that they would like to spend their lives in eternal bliss. Here is the obvious bad news. It's just not possible. Our days are filled with both positive and negative emotions. In this section, I will try to explain why being more positive will lead to greater effectiveness and make you a better leader.

Barbara Fredrickson is a Kenan Distinguished Professor of Psychology and principal investigator of the Positive Emotions and Psychophysiology Laboratory (a.k.a. PEP Lab) at the University of North Carolina at Chapel Hill. Her research reveals how positive emotions, fleeting as they are, can tip the scales toward a life of flourishing. She is the author of the bestselling book, *Positivity* [17]. In her foundational research with mathematician Marciel Losada, she developed a theory on positive emotions called the Broaden and Build Theory. They discovered that experiencing positive emotions broadens people's minds and builds their resourcefulness in ways that help them become more resilient to adversity, and to effortlessly achieve what they once could only imagine. With positive emotions at a ratio of 3 : 1 to negative emotions, you'll learn to see new possibilities, bounce back from setbacks (resilience), connect with others, and become the best flourishing version of yourself.

Losada's mathematics has come under fire in recent years, but the general theory of positive emotions over negative emotions still substantiates the Broaden and Build Theory. The original theory was based on working with high-performance teams. They built a laboratory especially designed to capture the behavior of teams in action. Through one-way mirrors, Losada's assistants videotaped, recorded and captured all interactions on specially programmed computers. Every single word and gesture was analyzed. Losada tracked three dimensions: whether people's statements were:

1) positive or negative;
2) self-focused or other focused; or
3) based on inquiry (asking questions) or advocacy (defending a point of view).

The results were amazing. After analyzing over 60 teams, he found three groups: the high performers (25%), who scored the highest in profitability, customer service and evaluations by superiors; the "flounderers" (30%), who were not making money and left dissatisfaction in their wake; and the rest (45%), who had a mixed profile of some good and some bad, but nothing consistent.

Losada quantified the trait of influence and called it *connectivity*. As he studied the groups more, he found that, according to the three dimensions, the high performers stood out, with an unusually high positivity ratio, at about 6 : 1 positive to negative statements, compared to the lowest group at 1 : 1 and the middle group at 2 : 1. Losada called the 3 : 1 ratio or higher the Losada Line.

The groups that fell below the Losada Line showed behavior that was not conducive to success, or to leadership for that matter. They lost their good cheer, their flexibility, their ability to question, and they languished in an endless loop in which people defended their own position and became critical of others. Keeping our positive to negative statements above the Losada Line, or 3 : 1, involves asking questions instead of defending a position, and always staying other-focused.

As if Losada's work isn't convincing enough, John Gottman, the world's leading expert on the science of marriage, and the author of the book *The Science of Trust*, confirms a similar ratio in married couples that Losada found in working groups. Gottman's work was done in what he calls his "love lab," at the University of California at Berkeley. Gottman used very sophisticated methods to measure not only the language of married couples interacting, but also their heart rate, sweat gland activity and other physiological changes, during conversation. He captured all verbal and non-verbal communication. What he found was amazing. He followed the couples for years and predicted, based on those early initial conversations, which couples would stay together and which would divorce. Gottman confirmed that married couples had a positivity ratio of 5 : 1. Any way you slice it, being positive during group or couple interaction pays off in big dividends.

So what are these positive emotions that act as nutriments for our growth and development? Positive emotions all have something in common. They are all *reactions* to our current circumstances. During the course of our days, these feelings come and go. They are fleeting – even more so than negative feelings. The thing about positive feelings is they are what Fredrickson calls "wantable" feelings. They not only feel good, but we want them. People actually pursue positive feelings (happiness?).

There is a distinction between positive feelings and pleasure. As Barbara Fredrickson explains, "Positive emotions are triggered by our interpretations of our current circumstances, whereas pleasure is what we get when we give the body what it needs right now. If you're thirsty, water tastes really good; if you're cold, it feels good to wrap your coat around you. Pleasures tell us what the body needs. Positive emotions tell us not just what the body needs but what we need mentally and emotionally and what our future selves might need. They help us broaden our minds and our outlook and build our resources down the road. I call it the 'broaden-and-build' effect."

As I mentioned earlier, a friend once told me that dentists are either crying or lying. That may be a gross exaggeration, but I have found that, in general, many dentists fight off negative emotions on a daily basis. Although I do encounter happy dentists, mostly at social events and meetings, mostly I hear a lot of complaining about their day-to-day frustrations. I hear from staff members how anxiety ridden and insecure their bosses are – that they worry for their health. I have already discussed the morbidity issues, but I want to mention the effect of negative emotions on attitude and demeanor, because that grimly effects leadership issues.

We live in a country where we tend to equate stress with success – busyness, rather than being positively effective and productive, is valued. Emma Seppälä, the science director of Stanford's Center for Compassion and Altruism Research [18], says that our culture values persevering to attain our goals, and fighting to outperform others – all of which involve some form of stress. Success is popularly equated with busyness, high stress and aggressiveness. Leadership is equated with low-intensity positive emotions like calmness. Low-intensity positive emotions make us more influential, a trait common among leaders. Even high-intensity positive emotions must be monitored, because of their effect on our stress levels and, hence, our leadership effectiveness.

A calm, low-stress, highly productive practice is a worthy goal. Leaders can build that first internally, and then through building a positive culture. I will have more to say about building positive cultures in Part III but, for now, realize that building a positive environment is enabling the dentist, the staff and the patients to work easily and fruitfully.

Psychologists regard emotions as more than just subjective feelings. The word "emotion" has the same root as "motion", conveying that emotions move through us and, perhaps, drive us. They drive our thoughts, arousal patterns and, eventually, our behavior. Let's look at the emotion of fear. Fear is constant in a dental practice. We always talk about the patient's fear of the dentist. What are the staff's fears? What about the doctor's fears? Are doctors fearful of the responses of their patients or their staff? Can fear actually drive the behaviors and attitudes of a dental practice? When someone experiences fear, the natural reaction is avoidance. Fear is the number one emotion for patient's avoidance of dentists. It is also the number one reason why dentists do not do, or present, comprehensive dentistry. I can think of many reasons why focusing on positive psychology is important for leaders, but this may be the most obvious and the best.

As stated at the beginning of this chapter, positive psychology focuses on the bright side of life. So why do so many of us focus on the negative? Wikipedia, the online encyclopedia, describes a *negative bias* as "the notion that, even when of equal intensity, things of a more negative nature (e.g., unpleasant thoughts, emotions, or social interactions; harmful/traumatic events) have a greater effect on one's psychological state and processes than do neutral or positive things. In other words, something very positive will generally have less of an impact on a person's behavior and cognition than something equally emotional but negative." Or, to put it another way, "life is difficult." It was first documented by psychologists Roy Baumister, Ellen Bratslavsky, Kathleen Vohs, and Catrin Finkenauer in an article titled *"Bad is Stronger than Good.* [19]"

As leaders, how do we get more control?

This is where positive psychology meets behavioral economics meets neuroscience. Leadership is hard work. Becoming a leader is not just about putting on a happy face. Leaders spend most of their time overcoming resistance. Negativity bias is another form of resistance. That resistance comes from patients, staff and mostly their biggest adversary: themselves. Lao Tzu, in his classic book, Tao Te Ching [20], wrote, "Knowing others is intelligence; knowing yourself is true wisdom. Mastering others is strength; mastering yourself is true power." Of all the nutriments that promote growth toward leadership, knowing yourself and building a positive mindset may be the most difficult. There are things we can do to build the positive mindset.

For a dentist, here are some ways negativity bias manifests itself:

- We remember insults more than we remember praise. "The squeaky wheel gets oiled" is another way to look at it. Most dentists look at their schedule and make positive and negative assessments.
- Negative experiences tend to be more memorable than positive ones. "How was your day, honey?"
- The brain has a tendency to be vigilant and wary.
- For positive experiences to resonate, they have to occur much more frequently than negative ones (3 : 1)
- The brain reacts more strongly to negative stimuli than to positive stimuli. Watch out for dooming and glooming your patients – it just may backfire.
- When your mind wanders, it's more likely to recall something that made you angry or upset, instead of recalling something that made you happy and filled you with pride.

On that last point, as an example, I recall the advice from Clayton Christensen, the author of *How Will You Measure Your Life* [21]. In finding fulfillment in your life, we will not please everyone, and we will not succeed with everyone, but we can measure our success by the number of people we have helped in our lives. That's good advice to use when that negative bias creeps in. There are many other ways to look on the bright side of life. The first one is just being aware. Remember: if you name it, you can tame it.

First, let's look at a few things we should know about how the brain works and what makes leadership hard work. As leaders, we must be aware of how others will look for the cracks in our armor – and we all have cracks. Every day we are reminded by the media of one leader or another who falls from grace. I am writing this just after watching the 2015 Super Bowl, won by the Denver Broncos over the Carolina Panthers. During the week preceding the game, both quarterbacks were highly scrutinized: Peyton Manning, the Broncos quarterback, for a rumor circulating about his supposed use of human growth hormone; and Cam Newton, for his "conduct unbecoming of a leaders", because of his excessive demonstrating and showing off. The evening before the game, Cam Newton, was voted as the NFL's most valuable player.

What happened after the game was a lesson in leadership. Newton was labeled as a sore loser. He stormed out of a press conference without answering questions. His behavior was truly unbecoming of a leader. Those who study leadership should not have been surprised. He, like all NFL players, was coached on how to lose with dignity. His whole career was on display for the public and the press to see yet, in this one moment to shine even after defeat, he looked bad to the press, to the public, and even to his own teammates. Cam Newton, in that moment, was emotionally hijacked. It happens all the time. If leaders like Bill Clinton, Eliot Spitzer, and my favorite football player, Odell Beckham Jr., are susceptible, we all are open to what Daniel Goleman [22] termed the "emotional hijack."

In our world, a four-second outburst can tarnish anyone's career and reputation. It is what becomes chiseled in other's minds about you. Goleman originally called it the amygdala hijack for the emotional part of the brain, which regulates the fight or flight response. When threatened, it can respond irrationally. A rush of stress hormones floods the body before the prefrontal lobes (regulating executive function) can mediate this reaction.

Every discussion on leadership falls back on our level of control. There are moments when we seem to lose control. The emotional hijack is one of a multitude of ways we lose control, and all of them fall back on our brains. That is why we see so much written these days on the human brain; it is the new frontier. From avoiding debilitating chronic conditions like dementia and Alzheimer's disease, to leading better lives and helping to lead others, it all starts with the brain. Having influence over others begins with having influence over ourselves. I guess, at a scientific level, this is what Lao Tzu and Socrates meant by knowing ourselves.

Let's take a look at three principles of neuroscience that can help to understand just what we are up against during the course of our day-to-day lives.

From Plato and Aristotle to today's cognitive psychologists and neuroscientists, there is agreement on the two-system brain theory. Plato described the brain as a wild horse and a rider. Nobel Prize-winning behavioral economist Daniel Kahneman, in his best-selling book, *Thinking, Fast and Slow* [23], describes intellect as two separate systems: System 1, the deliberate rational system; and System 2, the automatic system, which operates automatically, intuitively, involuntary, and effortlessly. In all cases, the metaphors refer to the anatomic components of the brain, which continue to be mapped out. Those two areas are known as the prefrontal cortex and the aforementioned amygdala.

The two-system brain requires vigilance and care. No one can have a perpetually rational mind; we could not live our lives without releasing most of our daily functions to our automatic or fast-thinking minds. There are two reasons for this: first, the prefrontal cortex is very small compared to the emotional mind (hence Plato's metaphor of the wild horse in relationship to the small rider); and, second, the prefrontal cortex is an energy-sucking organ. It requires more fuel, oxygen, and glucose to function at its highest levels. The "slow" System 1 is responsible for *reasoning, self-control and forward thinking*, which are instrumental in serving the moral obligations of a leader. System 1 is accountable for the "duty" element I wrote about in Chapter 2, reconciling the paradox of duty and desire.

For the dentist/leader, reasoning and logic is used throughout our day to solve problems in a rational manner. L.D. Pankey would say that a good dentist is endowed with "care, skill and judgment." The second function of the rational brain is self-control. This is the element that gets hijacked when we do not exhibit self-control. We use it when we resist temptation. Dentists face self-control issues all the time when dealing with patients who demand being treated in a way that counters better treatment. Working with people of so many different temperaments requires the dentist to maintain a level of emotional regulation. The last function of the prefrontal cortex is the ability to be forward-thinking. In creating a vision and focusing on long-term values, the dentist uses his or her rational mind to imagine the best possible future for all concerned.

So why is it that we are so susceptible to the emotional hijack?

As mentioned earlier, the pre-frontal cortex is small and requires lots of energy. It can only deal with so much at one time. We are granted only a limited amount of *working memory*, and this restricts the number of things we can concentrate on at one time. That is a good reason why dentists should limit the number of things they are working on at the same time. Science has made it known that multi-tasking is ineffective, because of the overload it places on working memory. In Part V, when I write about how to do an examination, I will describe why and how building "sacred time" into our most pivotal daily moments can make the most out of our System 1 thinking.

The other side of the paradox – desire – is managed by System 2, Dan Kahneman's fast-thinking system. That system takes care of all of our automatic needs, like breathing and digestion, so we can get through each day and we can preserve energy to use System 1. This subconscious system is also capable of some multitasking if we can create good habits. What it cannot do is allow someone to answer emails or take messages or a phone call in the middle of a procedure that requires more concentration. The emotional brain is also responsible for giving people what they need in the moment, rather than allowing the rational mind to make sense and interpret the real circumstances. The automatic brain can actually distort our sense of reality by altering our selective attention. Hence, we become hijacked.

Attention is a key component. Slowing down and paying attention not only allows us to see more clearly but also to preserve the energy that is required for the rational mind to work. I wish this were more within our control. What is in our control are the conditions and circumstances we create in our work environment that are brain friendly.

Reading Stephen Covey's *7 Habits of Highly Effective People* had a profound impact on me many years ago. I was so impressed with his first habit: *Be Proactive*. The problem I encountered was that just knowing wasn't good enough. How could I slow down and stay within that gap between stimulus and response? I totally understood the quote mentioned by Covey by the psychologist, R.D. Laing:

> "The range of what we think and do is limited by what we fail to notice. And because we fail to notice that we fail to notice, there is little we can do to change; until we notice how failing to notice shapes our thoughts and deeds."

The Harvard Business Review [24] (2003) reminds us of importance of self-awareness: "Executives who fail to develop self-awareness risk falling into an emotionally deadening routine that threatens their true selves. Indeed a reluctance to explore your inner landscape not only weakens your own motivation but can also corrode your ability to inspire others."

My problem was slowing down, creating conditions and preserving the energy to make me more effective. The number one job of all leaders, Peter Drucker tells us, is self-management [25]. Self-management begins with self-awareness and that begins in the brain. As the Broaden and Build Theory promises, by accumulating more positive emotions (3 : 1), becoming other-focused and living in the question, we can build a great career in dentistry.

Another brain attribute that leaves us susceptible to being hijacked is what author Carolyn Webb calls the Discover-Defend Axis [26]. This may be the true essence of the emotional hijack. Every day our brains maintain a level of vigilance by determining pleasant vs. unpleasant things in our environment. We evaluate whether something or someone is a threat or a reward. Is it friend or foe? This constant evaluation process has allowed our species to survive. It can be the trigger to the fight or flight response that provides for our survival. The problem is that it makes mistakes in modern times, because the actual threats are mostly in our minds, and we don't get to encounter too many saber-toothed tigers in our practice.

The amygdala is in the privileged position as the emotional sentinel. It is the first responder. The stimuli come from anywhere at any time, and go straight to the amygdala without consulting the prefrontal cortex. This survival mechanism lets us react to things before the rational brain has time to mull things over. It has a hair trigger. Neuroscientists tell us the reaction time could be as little as twelve thousands of a second. Any strong emotion, anxiety, anger, joy, or betrayal trips off the amygdala, and impairs the prefrontal cortex's working memory. The power of emotions overwhelms rationality. That is why, when we are emotionally upset or stressed, we can't think straight.

Matthew Lieberman [27], a neuroscientist from UCLA, has found an inverse relationship between the amygdala and the prefrontal cortex, the brain's executive function where rational thought and judgment sit. When the amygdala is active with blood and oxygen, there is less activation in the prefrontal cortex. Our thinking power is disrupted, and there are deficits in our problem solving, because the blood and oxygen are in the amygdala versus the prefrontal cortex. It is like losing 10–15 IQ points temporarily, which explains "what was I thinking?" So we *are* thinking, but with less capacity and brain power.

Few dental practices are stress free. In today's economy, more dentists than ever, as already noted, are suffering from burnout and stress. If we could slow down and gain control over our daily emotional hijacks, that would go a long way in relieving stress. It doesn't take much for a person to get hijacked and, before you know it, the entire practice is hijacked and working in a dumbed-down mode. I have always said that stress makes us stupid. High stress is an emotional contagion, and that is why leadership is so important.

The leaders' ability to manage their emotions then, is fundamental to the practice performance as they are the "emotional thermostat" and can influence the practice mood and productivity. The global management Hay Group has found that the leader has 50% to 70% influence over the climate of the team. Freedman and Everett (2008) state that 70% of the top issues in the workplace are tied to leadership. Thus, the leader and their emotional intelligence have an enormous influence on the team.

A leader's role, then, as stated earlier, is to keep calm in spite of our own brain's survival instincts. When the "defend" mode acts up, all we want to do is provide what we need most, rather than take the time to interpret the circumstances and go into what Carolyn Webb calls the discovery mode. Our emotional brain, like that raging horse, wants to go into fight or flight – or, in other word, we want to "eat it, kill it or make love to it", as the popular social media advice goes. When we gain that level of control, our positive emotions, as fleeting as they are, help us to create a more positive, stress-free practice.

Webb advises us to try to get into the discovery mode by focusing and engaging the brain's reward system. It is interesting to note that our brains love many of the ideas that the leadership lessons in this book attract. Building relationships delivers the reward of belonging and social recognition. The dental leader focuses on a sense of autonomy, competence, and purpose, as well as continual learning. All of these things are rewarding for their own sake, and counter the daily slings and arrows of dental practice. Research by Edward Deci and Richard Ryan, at the University of Rochester, has shown that having a sense of autonomy and personal competence is profoundly motivating [28]. As you will discover in the next chapter, dental education fails to develop leaders, because they fail to nurture what really matters for leadership development – passion, mastery, autonomy, competence and relationships.

Throughout my entire career, I have been hijacked. I believe that, until I became more aware of how to combat the emotional ups and downs of practice, I was doomed to more of the same – poor working conditions, poor health and poor results. It took time, and I will explain how I did it and what the experts recommend before I close out this section. It seems that every day I speak with and coach dentists who are having issues that just get more out of control, because of negative emotional responses, like: misreading people's true intentions or moods; blaming people for not listening to them or not accepting their recommendations; and frustrations with patient's lack of compliance and poor behavior. I can never give advice that will fix the patient, only advice to fix the dentist – and it's always a leadership issue.

Let's take a look at the third brain attribute that either helps or hinders leaders. This is the one we have the most control over – the mind-body loop.

I breed and raise dogs. At any one time, I could have eight dogs living in my kennels. In addition to the joy they bring to my life, I have to take responsibility for managing their "emotions." Animals do not possess the same brains as humans. Their behavior is mostly determined by hormones. That means I have to be very vigilant when mixing and matching play times. Puppies seem to get along with everyone. At approximately eighteen months, things change, especially when there is an intact male in the house and a bitch in season.

I have broken up my share of dogfights in my time. One interesting observation that I made many years ago was that it was rare for the dog to get injured, but I always walked away battered and bruised. One time, two of the girls really got into it. Gracie snuck her way into Ellie's kennel and, in an instant, began to have a free-for-all that looked like it would be a fight to the death. After what seemed to be an eternity, I separated them, and lay down in a sea of blood. My flight-or-fight mechanism was fully charged. Adrenaline was furiously pumping, my heart was pounding, I was sweating and I was gasping for air. It felt like it took me 30 minutes to recover. When I looked into Gracie's kennel, she had cut on her ear, but her tail was wagging. She was back to normal in minutes. That is what is known as resilience; the ability to bounce back quickly.

As noted earlier in this chapter, science tells us that most people are naturally resilient. That episode showed me the difference between the levels of resistance we can exhibit. My early burnout was most likely helped along by shorter, less acute episodes, that set off my flight or flight reaction. Enough of those will effect our ability to bounce back, and it is an example of the mind-body loop that we humans must cope with. As an aside, it's a good time to point out that our patients don't recover from dental stress as quickly as we would like.

So, if we are naturally resilient, how do we lose it? Why do we carry our fears and anxieties around longer than we need to? Why does our stress linger until it becomes chronic? The answer, as I alluded to earlier, is in the brain. Our brains tend to focus on the negative emotions; toughing it out, or thinking it away, or putting on a happy face, just doesn't work in most cases. We can't talk our way out of chronic stress. Actually, toughing it out by suppressing emotions can make things worse, by increasing the ratio of negative emotions to positive emotions. This will lead to lower self-esteem, optimism, and well-being, and even higher rates of depression, as well as impaired memory [29]. We need to build our resilience by understanding the physiology of the brain and the way the body can help make the mind stronger. What many of us do is just the opposite. We drink, smoke, and use drugs to make us feel better.

We need to restore the balance in our bodies to strengthen our resilience. If you recall, one of the first things I did after my personal burnout was to exercise. I still believe that getting into shape was the best possible thing I could do for my career – and my life. Science shows us that we can do many things that will improve our emotional state, outlook and well-being by focusing on the body. Let's take a look at a few.

- **Sleep**: Dentists today are really getting into the physiology of sleep, mostly as a profit center, rather than taking their own medicine. A tired brain devotes less blood to the prefrontal cortex. We need between seven and nine hours of sleep to operate efficiently. Sleep deprivation makes us dull. It also cuts down on our optimism or, in other words, our ability to nurture positive emotions.
- **Exercise**: Exercise increases blood flow to the brain. I have heard many people say that "sitting is the new smoking." The antidote to sitting is moving. Famed Harvard psychiatrist John Ratey has taken up the call for revealing the scientific evidence on the link between exercise and mental function [30]. Exercise will increase mood, motivation and ability to deal with stress.
- **Meditation**: Remember when I was lying on the floor, after breaking up the dogfight? Well, slow as it was, the thing that brought me back into calm and balance was slowing down my

breathing. Yes, that was a natural response to the circumstance, but making a practice of concentrating on the breath as a habit goes a long way toward calming the mind and making our prefrontal cortex more functional. I began meditating long after my burnout. These days I do hot Yoga three days per week. The Yoga includes a session of deep breathing exercises, physical exercise, and it fatigues me just enough to get a good night's sleep every night.

In summary, this section has dealt with the P in PERMA-V: positive emotions. Obviously, this discussion was more than just putting on a happy face, as the happiologists would have us believe. Positive emotions, it turns out, is a fairly complex discussion. Intuitively, my journey led me to read about my own mental and emotional health, to look for examples to follow with exemplary role models, and to take better care of myself through diet and exercise, meditation, by becoming more aware and naming my emotions and, mostly, to realize that most of my positive emotions had more to do with other people than myself.

Now let's take a look another element of well-being: engagement.

Engagement

Do you love dentistry? There was a time when I did not love it. I would dread coming into the office. Luckily, I had a dental assistant who was forthright enough to tell me the truth. And I was fortunate enough to listen to her feedback. Ken Blanchard, author of many books, including *The One Minute Manager*, is known for saying, "Feedback is the breakfast of champions." When Micki told me that it seemed I wasn't interested in my work or my patients, that was a turning point for me. Of course, I was ready to hear it, because I was suffering inside. I guess another way of saying it is, "when the student is ready, the teacher will appear."

Sure, as you know, I was burned out. I needed to turn things around, so I began to take lots of continuing education courses. It was soon after, at a Dawson Seminar, that my desire for dentistry was rekindled. Dr. Dawson, a master teacher and presenter, had a way of making the very same complex ideas we learned in dental school about occlusion come alive. I was excited about going back to my practice to apply my newly understood knowledge. I am still excited about the things I learned so many years ago. In retrospect, I was experiencing the proof of Barbara Fredrickson's "broaden and build" theory that I wrote about in the last section. Once the dread of burnout lifted, I truly began to enjoy my work more. A fire was lit that still burns, and I believe, by becoming so engaged in dentistry – every component of dentistry – that my employees also became more engaged.

According to Dr. Arnold Bakker, a professor of Work and Organizational Psychology from Erasmus University in Rotterdam, work engagement is most often defined as "a positive, fulfilling, work-related state of mind that is characterized by *vigor, dedication, and absorption* [31]." In essence, work engagement captures how workers experience their work: as stimulating and energetic and something to which they really want to devote time and effort (vigor); as a significant and meaningful pursuit (dedication); and as engrossing, and something on which they are fully concentrated. In other words, work engagement is not just a fluffy way of saying someone likes their work, but that they are psychologically connected to the work.

Bakker's research also showed that engaged employees are most energetic, self-efficacious workers who exercise influence over events that affect their lives. Influence is a defining trait of leadership as we will see later. In addition to being more influential, engaged workers create their own positive feedback (Broaden and Build Theory), in terms of appreciation, recognition and success. Engagement creates renewal and a sense of increased energy. To engaged workers, the work is fun, not drudgery. Professor Bakker sums it up by saying, "Enthusiastic employees excel in their work because they maintain the balance between the energy they give and the energy they receive."

So what is the problem? Not only in dentistry, although that is my main focus in this book, but in a Gallup World Poll of 47,000 employees in 120 countries, only 11% reported engagement in their work (The State of the Global Workforce 2010, © 2010, Gallup, Inc.). That is down from the 17% reported in a similar poll in 2005. Among the 2010 interviewees, 62% reported they are not engaged – that is, they are emotionally detached and are likely to be doing little more than is necessary to keep their jobs. And 27% are actively disengaged, indicating they view their workplaces negatively, and are liable to spread that negativity to others. A very recent Gallup Well-Being Index was the subject of an online article by Elizabeth Mendes, *"America's Life Outlook Better Than in 2008, but Not Best,"* [32].The index indicates that life ratings for all age groups declined in October 2012, revealing that whatever issues are causing Americans to be less optimistic about their lives recently are affecting everyone, regardless of age. That's sad.

You may be asking yourself why engagement is a leadership issue. I want to make it clear that engagement not only is a component of the dentist's own well-being, which makes him or her a better leader but, without engagement, the dentist and the practice will eventually lack followers and fail to build a culture of trust and excellence. I constantly hear dentists complain about staff members who do not take interest in their work. I hear complaints about hygienists and assistants who don't promote or "sell" dentistry. My answer to those dentists is to take more ownership of that particular problem. Remember, I had that same issue as well – before I became more engaged in my work and took ownership.

There is no leadership issue that cannot be solved without looking in the mirror first. Engagement is an emotional contagion, the same as high stress in the negative sense.

Many years ago. the former CEO of the Pankey Institute asked me why Pankey dentists seemed so happy. That question stayed with me for a long time. The only reason I could ever attribute their apparent happiness to was complete emotional engagement in all aspects of their work. Studies have shown that engagement is still only one element of well-being yet, because our work is so important to our overall well-being, it is a big one.

Prominent happiness researcher Mihalyi Csiksentmihalyi, of the University of Chicago, has written extensively about a concept known as *flow*. Flow is defined as a state of consciousness where people become totally immersed in an activity and enjoy it intensely. Some have described the intense feeling as peak performance or peak experience. Researchers have found scientific evidence for flow during the performance of a large number of different activities, including sports, art and music. In the next chapter, I will continue this discussion in relation to the role that passion plays in sustaining a long and successful career. For now, let's understand the relationship of engagement, as a first step to creating passion, to leadership and culture building.

Csiksentmihalyi describes flow activities as "the more involved we become, and the more positive the experience. When the job presents clear goals, unambiguous feedback, a sense of control, challenges that match the worker's skills, and few distractions, the feelings it provides are not that different from what one experiences in a sport or artistic performance [33]." To spend our days in flow would be unrealistic; however, if you have experienced these feelings while performing dentistry, wouldn't it be nice to build a practice that provides more and more potential flow circumstances?

Dental practices that have high staff turnover are practices that do not engage employees or patients. As already stated, the symptom, for the dentist, is depression, burnout and chronic illness. For the practice, it is languishing, high stress and high turnover. Since I brought my passion back to my practice, I have had no turnover. No turnover, unless a staff member had to leave due to illness, or they were moving. My staff includes Geri, who has been with me for 38 years, Michele, my hygienist for 40 years, Carol, my other hygienist for 24 years, and Mo, my dental assistant for 12 years. I am as proud of that record as any dentistry I have ever done. It is, as Clay Christensen wrote, one way to describe how I will measure my career.

Flow is like a wave on the ocean, or an athlete being "in the zone." It can be described as pure elegance and effortlessness of movement and thought. It occurs when a person faces a clear set of goals, with clear rules and guidelines. The clarity of mission, based on values and purpose, is a leadership requirement. Flow experiences also provide immediate feedback. The feedback is possible because dental leaders plan every step through a systematized treatment planning process, which I will describe in Part VI.

The process ensures that every step is ordered for the best possible result, rather than just random procedures that have no apparent arrangement. The dentist and the staff get to say things like, "I love it when a plan comes together" a lot. That builds confidence, trust and certainty for everyone. For the dentist, it builds his or her sense of control and predictability. Every day is planned and organized around the mission, and the practice is more than focused on production. There are goals that directly relate to purpose. It makes a difference between a practice full of daily surprises, with everyone on roller-skates, instead of a calm, peaceful, positive practice where everyone has the time to focus.

Engagement and flow experiences help to accelerate the leader and his team's growth and education. In my early career, we used to use the term "amalgam jockey" for dentists who did the same thing every day for their whole careers. Through engaging work, the team enjoys their work more, because they grow with the challenges of new things. They get comfortable with expanding their skill sets, so that they are challenged rather than bored. The dentist who leads the charge in continuing education learns exactly what he or she is capable of doing, and never gets overwhelmed by what can't be done. The practice becomes defined by victory after victory, rather than by what the fee for a crown is, or how many crowns did we do this week? Great dental teams learn to love their work, and the production takes care of itself.

In his book, *Finding Flow* [34], Csiksentmihalyi writes, "When goals are clear, feedback relevant, and challenges and skills are in balance, attention becomes ordered and fully invested. Because of the total demand on psychic energy, a person in flow is completely focused. There is no space in consciousness for distracting thoughts, irrelevant feelings. Self-consciousness disappears, yet one feels stronger than usual. The sense of time is distorted; hours seem to pass by in minutes. When a person's entire being is stretched in the full functioning of body and mind, whatever one does becomes worth doing for its own sake; living becomes its own justification. In the harmonious focusing of physical and psychic energy, life fully comes into its own."

Maybe, then, it's physical and psychic energy, rather than happiness, that we are seeking. Maybe, more than fame or fortune, we want to feel better at a physical and emotional level. Maybe it's not the drink at the bar that the Miller Lite commercials tell us is what we want, but the work we did that day that gave us that moment of happiness and comfort.

Authors Jim Loehr and Tony Schwartz [35] might agree. Both, through their books and lectures, specialize in helping executives, professionals and athletes to achieve full engagement in high stress environments. Their mission is to ignite a fire in the hearts of organizations and their leaders. Most dental consultants focus on time management and money management as indicators for success. According to Loehr and Schwartz, truly effective leadership is more about managing and investing in your energy – physical and psychic.

Their book is based on four basic principles that show why energy is the most important thing leaders can manage. Energy, they say, not time, is the fundamental currency of high performance. Every one of our thoughts, emotions, and behaviors has an energy consequence, for better or for worse. The four principles are as follows:

- Principle 1: Full engagement requires drawing on four separate, but related, sources of energy: physical, emotional, mental and spiritual.
- Principle 2: Because energy diminishes both with overuse and with underuse, we must balance energy expenditure with intermittent energy renewal.

- Principle 3: To build capacity, we must push beyond our normal limits, training in the same systematic way that elite athletes do.
- Principle 4: Positive energy rituals – highly specific routines for managing energy – are the key to full engagement and sustained high performance [36]."

Early on in my career, I was taught by the practice management people that my success depended on getting "warm bodies" into my chair. I focused on production goals and ergonomics. I designed my entire practice around productivity. Although my production went up, my energy level went down, as previously described. When I learned to work smarter, I had the time and energy to enjoy the work and take care of my staff and patients in a much more meaningful way. Looking back, it was taking control of myself first – my health, both physical and mental, that gave me the energy to make the changes I needed to make. Working in a fatigued state didn't do much for production, time management or, most importantly, keeping people happy.

I found out the hard way that people are not machines. People need to stay relaxed and calm to do their best work. Today's working environments are not conducive to human values and needs, so it is the job of an effective leader to develop a work environment that provides conditions that do not put people at risk of burnout. We can't spend every minute of our workday producing dentistry as if that is the sole reason for our existence. In Part VI, I will discuss some of the ways to build in practical methods to work within the rhythms of the human body, while acknowledging the need to spend more time with patients.

Engaging work and finding flow is an element for good reasons. One of the observations I have made in my own journey is that nature itself has a pulse, a rhythmic, wavelike movement between activity and rest. As Cziksentmihaly says, it has a flow. We are all guided by rhythms, and one of the themes of this book is to help dental leaders find those rhythms through the use of what Loehr and Schwartz call rituals: consistent, congruous activities that help promote success and well-being.

In the next section, I will discuss the context in which we do all of our dentistry: other people.

Positive Relationships

We can learn a lot about leadership by reading the biographies of famous people who are in leadership roles. Coaches like John Wooden, military leaders like George Patton, spiritual leaders like Pope Francis and the Dalai Lama, business leaders like Steve Jobs, and political leaders like Ronald Reagan, can teach us a lot about leadership. Since leadership is my passion and it is ubiquitous in our daily lives, I look for examples of good and bad leadership continuously. I am a big fan of the National Football League. I believe that a team's success rises and falls on the leadership at the very highest level – the owners and the head coach.

Recently, a report came over the radio that the much-publicized head coach of the Philadelphia Eagles, Chip Kelly, was being fired. I had followed Chip's career since he left the University of Oregon Ducks to coach at the professional level. Kelly was the most highly sought-after coach coming out of the college ranks in 2012. In the four years at Oregon, he led the program to four consecutive BCS (Bowl Championship Series) bowl game appearances, including the 2011 BCS National Championship Game. Kelly's record at Oregon during the four years he was there contributed to his reputation as an offensive genius, who truly knew the 'X's and 'O's of football. I took a particular interest in Kelly because my team, the New York Giants, are the Eagles' main rivals.

Kelly led the Philadelphia Eagles to two consecutive winning seasons. He went to the playoffs in his first year and just missed in his second year. However, the third year was a disaster.

Numerous off-field incidents led, ultimately, to him being fired. Most of those incidents centered around bad leadership, rather than an inability to put together a system that could win. Ultimately, Chip Kelly was fired because he failed to communicate with players, fans and the press. Two days before he was fired, he failed to take responsibility for letting some of his key players go to other teams. As the head coach and general manager, he shifted the account-ability for his behavior to others in the organization. In other words, he broke the first rule of leadership by not taking ownership of his results. Those who watch NFL football know that every Sunday, at least 16 head coaches and quarterbacks say, "the blame belongs right here with me." But even that is not what got him fired.

The next day, at a press conference, owner Jeffrey Lurie admitted that the real reason Chip was being let go was "he wanted the next coach of the Philadelphia Eagles to value "emotional intelligence." Chip Kelly, in other words, lacked people skills and the ability to create positive relationships.

At its core, football, like dentistry, is a people business, and being able to maximize the personnel on hand has as much to do with massaging their egos as their muscles. In the following days, many players came forth and repeated the same feeling, with stories that painted a picture of Chip not being the most likable coach around. In college, Chip never had "people" issues, because he was a coach who ruled college students through his position. In the pros, the context changed. These players were adult men, not students. Context matters.

In dental school we focus on the 'X's and 'O's of dentistry. After graduation, context matters, and the context is other people.

Leadership is a funny subject. It is open to various styles and methods of working with people. Leaders, as we will discuss further, are mission-based. They set goals and inspire others to help complete the mission, whether in sports, or at war, or in school. How that mission is accomplished is always with other people. All leaders, over time, must develop their own style. Some people have natural leadership ability, but most must learn through trial and error. One such leader is Tom Coughlin, the former head coach of the New York Giants.

Tom Coughlin's story is a tale of transformation that did not start out well. When Coughlin came to the Giants as their head coach, in 2004, he came with a reputation of being a strict disciplinarian. Some of his "rules" included being five minutes early for meetings, keeping both feet on the ground while sitting, wearing suits and black socks for road trips, and wearing high socks on the practice field. These strict rules rankled some of the star players, like Tiki Barber and Michael Strahan. The Giants finished that disastrous season with a losing 6-10 record. The following years were rocky for the coach and his team. After losing in the playoffs in 2006, owner John Mara took Coughlin aside and told him he would have to be more player-friendly. The ownership stuck with the coach, and they were rewarded the following years with a Super Bowl victory.

The championship season would not have been possible without the changes that took place in Coughlin's leadership. Offensive lineman Shaun O'Hara claimed that, in the first years, if a player walked by the coach and said, "Good morning, coach," he would reply by saying, "What's so good about it?" The following year, with the help of ownership and his wife, Tom Coughlin made the biggest change in his career – he focused on creating positive relationships. He admitted he looked at his players as people, rather than players with numbers on their uniforms. Stories have become legend about Coughlin's change in demeanor. At one point, running back Brandon Jacobs almost passed out when the old disciplinarian told his team he loved them. It was those moments that changed the players' perception of Coughlin forever.

I had my own personal experience with Coughlin. After the 2007 Super Bowl win, I wrote an article for the industry magazine, *Dental Economics.* It was based on the Giants' victory and Coughlin's leadership, and I referred to him as the master of the intangibles. I sent a copy of the article to the coach. Two weeks later I received a package in the mail from the offices of the NY Football Giants; it was a signed photograph of the coach accepting the Lombardi Trophy. He also included a short letter, which read:

Dear Barry,

Thank you for your letter and your article.
I really enjoyed your admission, "I am a die-hard, hard-core, blue-bleeding Giant's fan!"
<u>Realize</u> one thing.
Perhaps the biggest accomplishment was the Art of Communication –
And through the "Leadership Council" we improved communication –
But with that ownership, responsibility and the <u>veteran</u> players drew the <u>young</u> players into the Web of Accountability,
And the entire team "would not let the other guys down."

Sincerely,

Tom Coughlin

Tom Coughlin retired after the 2015 season. In his final press conference, he continued to express the love and admiration he had for his players and the Giants organization. It was an amazing turnaround from his early years. For me, it represented how leadership can be developed, and how important creating positive relationships are to the overall well-being and success of everyone. The language of the letter he sent to me is the language of a leader – relationships, communication, accountability and trust. One of his players was quoted in the newspaper the day after his retirement as saying, "He's one of the greatest men I've ever been around, for what he's done for me and my family and always believing in me, always putting me in a position to be great. The stuff he did for a lot of players that were going in the wrong direction and how he gravitated to us as players and men, he made an imprint on my life and the lives of others. Tom Coughlin should run for President."

Coughlin was always known as a "football guy." Someone who truly understood the nuances of the game. It was only after learning how to build positive relationships that he achieved the ultimate success. That's leadership, because other people matter.

Recently, I did a self-assessment of my own leadership strengths after reading Clay Christensen's book, *How Will You Measure Your Life?* I reviewed my career and made a list of things I could remember that placed me in a leadership role; things that worked out, and things that did not work out. My list included my practice life as well as my private life. The long list included many successful achievements and some disappointments. The good outweighed the disappointments. The biggest lesson for me was that every success was about working with other people, and I felt better about how I helped other people. America has become a very individualistic society, yet I believe the human brain is inherently a social brain, and that we have evolved to become more cooperative and helpful.

It has been said that the main purpose of the human brain is social. Part IV of this book is titled *Other People Matter.* In that part, I will discuss the specific skills of communication. I want to make the point here that so many dentists and professionals do not like to engage in conversation – it's just about the teeth for many of them. Through the years, I remember mostly the people and their stories, because I took the time to truly get to know them. Conversation is important, and studies show that, the more meaningful the conversations, the more they contribute to the happiness of both parties.

Leadership is about communication, and leadership is best understood from a relationship and communication perspective. One of my strengths is conversation. When I teach dentists about getting to know their patients during the preclinical examination, they seem confused about the conversation element. They tell me that they're okay with "small talk," but they would rather just get to the teeth. This is a problem, because small talk isn't very meaningful, and dentists use it only as a stepping stone to get on with their examination. A 2010 study by Matthias Mehl and colleagues defined small talk as "the banal and uninvolved exchange of trivial information," and substantive talk as "the involved exchange of meaningful information [37]."

The results were pretty important for dentists who just go through the motions of conversation. First, they found that happier participants spent more time talking to others, "an unsurprising finding given the social basis of happiness." The surprising thing was that the extent of small talk was *negatively* associated with happiness. The last finding was that the extent of substantive talk was *positively* associated with happiness. So, happy people are socially engaged with others, and this engagement entails matters of substance. That sounds a lot like the Tom Coughlin experience. I know it is what I have experienced. Getting to know our patients and their stories goes a long way in developing positive relationships that will last for years. It takes more than small talk. I will have more to say about the importance of conversation later in the book.

As we go into the future, we will see more and more emphasis on technical dentistry. We will pay the price of less human interaction. This is becoming more evident. For years, dentists would complain that the public was unable to distinguish between dentists. I would argue that the dentists who spent the time getting to know their patients would have a competitive advantage, but I acknowledged it was a tough road. Lately, I have been seeing patients who actually stop to ask, "whatever happened to doctors like me who sit down and talk with their patients, rather than being in a hurry to get on with their day?" I wondered why I was beginning to see this, and determined that, with the rise of corporate settings, large practices and overwhelming technology, dentists are spending less time with patients, and patients are seeing the difference.

Recall service expert Leonard Berry, whom I mentioned in Chapter 3, who said that the most important aspects of service are dependability, reliability, assuredness and empathy. All of these are built on the foundation of positive relationships – the softer components of relationships, rather than the hi-tech tangible components.

As I write this chapter, Americans are being entertained by the antics of the politicians who are vying for the next presidency. One candidate, Donald Trump, is getting the majority of the attention. To say his behavior is somewhat controversial would be an understatement. One of the biggest criticisms I hear is that he's just not nice. Like it or not, we are judged on our degree of niceness; it is part of our social brain to be nice and get along. One of the more popular reasons for patients changing dental practices, besides financial, is that the practice or the doctor wasn't nice. Being nice goes a long way in developing positive relationships.

I remember when my father was dying, and was in the last stages of acute myeloid leukemia. The physician in charge and the nurses treated my family as if we were annoyances that they had to deal with. Many times, I heard them say things that were just – well, not nice. On one particular occasion, the doctor, whose name I will never forget, spoke to my mother and I as if my father had already died and his presence was a burden on the nursing staff. Suffice it to say that it is years later, and I still remember that discussion. Just like Donald Trump's caustic remarks about his opponents will continue to be remembered long after the elections. It pays to be nice, and science backs it up.

Legendary baseball manager Leo Durocher is credited with the famous quote, "Nice guys finish last." There are many people who believe that this is true; however, taking the high road and building positive relationships will lead to more success. This isn't one of those either/or discussions; we know that building positive relationships is good for our well-being, but is being nice conducive to great leadership? In other words, what style of leadership should we choose – and is there a choice?

Sociologist Max Weber defined a type of leadership he called "charismatic authority", where the leadership is derived from the leader's charisma. He contrasted this type of leadership from two other types of authority: legal or positional authority, and traditional authority. Weber defined charismatic leadership as, "resting on devotion to the exceptional sanctity, heroism, or exemplary character of an individual person, and of the normative patterns or order revealed or ordained by him." By the term "charisma", Weber means a virtue which sets apart leaders from other men as being endowed with supernatural, superhuman or, at least, specifically exceptional powers or qualities. He called them a "gift." This begs the age-old question about whether leaders are born or made.

The ability to create and maintain positive relationships in the leadership role requires more work than most people realize. I believe it can be developed if we define it properly. Olivia Fox Cabane, in her book *The Charisma Myth* [38] explains charisma as consisting of three components blended together: power, warmth and presence. By power, she means that we have the ability and influence to help them. Warmth refers to the trait of intention – that you are willing to help them; and presence means you listen to them without distraction. Thus, there is a sense of presence in combination with – well, just being nice.

Cabane cites research that shows that our reaction to power and warmth is deeply wired. We rely on instinct to assess people we encounter, as a survival mechanism. We get a gut reaction that tells us whether to like and trust another. The combination of power and warmth – or charisma, she claims – plays powerfully on our instincts. "From lab experiments to neuro-imaging, research has consistently shown that they are the two dimensions we evaluate first and foremost in assessing other people [39]."

In numerous studies at the Yale University Infant Cognition Lab, researchers Paul Bloom, Karen Wynn and Kiley Hamlin [40] showed that infants prefer nice people. In one study, infants were shown puppet shows in which one character in the show assists another character by helping it climb a steep passage, open a box and retrieve a bouncing ball, as opposed to another character who impedes these actions by running away with the bouncing ball. Afterward, the puppets were set down in front of the infants. Each puppet was placed next to a pile of treats. At this point, the infant was asked to take a treat away from one puppet. Like most children in this situation, the infant took it from the pile of the *naughty* puppet. But this punishment wasn't enough – the infant leaned over and smacked the naughty puppet in the head.

So what can we surmise from these experiments about being nice and morality, and what do they have to do with positive relationships and leadership?

Firstly is that, just like the human universals that I noted earlier, we are endowed with certain innate qualities from an early age. Like empathy, fairness and reciprocity, a sense of good and bad is innate. In other words, there is a connection between niceness and morality. You will see later in this book that morality is fundamental to leadership. This growing body of evidence suggests that humans do have a rudimentary moral sense from the very start of life [41].

Another point is that we instinctively know when someone is *helping* or *hindering*. Did the babies teach us that helpful behavior is good behavior, and that hindering was bad? All that can be deduced is that the babies preferred the good puppet over the other. Everything was based on how the puppets treated "the other." The babies were responding to what the adults described as "nice" or mean." These very same conclusions have been found in the work of primatologist Franz DeWaal [42] with his work on bonobo apes on the evolution of ethics. What's really important is that the infants, wrong or right, made a judgment, and judging moral behavior is a survival instinct.

These instinctual qualities may be brain-based as well. Neurotransmitters and hormones, oxytocin and dopamine are released when we feel a desire to bond and develop positive relationships. Dr. John Gottman, mentioned earlier in this chapter on positive emotions, claims that we need a 5 : 1 ratio of positive to negative thoughts to build a positive relationship. In his latest book, *The Man's Guide to Women: Scientifically Proven Secrets from the "Love Lab" About What Women Really Want*, a scientific approach to building long-lasting relationships, he claims that what both parties are seeking is trustworthiness.

Hopefully, you are convinced that building positive relationships is very important, not only for your well-being, but also to your eventual success in becoming a dental leader. Unlike what Leo Durocher claims about nice guys finishing last, nice guys are winners before the game even starts. In order to build relationships though, things must truly matter. The next section describes the next element of PERMA – purpose.

Meaning

In 1984, John Scully had been the vice-president of PepsiCo, where he had successfully made Pepsi the number one brand in the Cola Wars. He was secure in his job and, by all measures, quite successful. There was no reason for him to join a young company that was making some noise in the computer industry. However, Apple lured Scully away from Pepsi through one pitch by founder and CEO of Apple, Steve Jobs. The pitch has become legendary: "Do you want to sell sugar water for the rest of your life, or do you want to come with me and change the world?"

Scully admitted later that those words helped him to reassess his life. He took the job at Apple. Jobs appealed to Scully at the level of meaning, the fourth element of PERMA. In 2011, upon hearing the news of Jobs' death, Scully issued the following statement: "Steve Jobs was intensely passionate at making an important difference in the lives of his fellow humans while he was on the planet. He never was into money or measured his life through owning stuff ... a world leader is dead, but the lessons his leadership taught us live on."

In Chapter 5, I discussed the concept of mission and the attainment of a worthy goal. In this section, I would like discuss the role of purpose and meaning toward our well-being, and what it means for leadership. Although I have always been goal-oriented and mission-based, I had always felt a void because I wanted, like Jobs, to make a difference in the world. I wanted my life to have meaning. In my early years, the dentistry I was doing lacked meaning for me.

Nothing matters. Those two words are very important, because what matters is only what is important to you. You define what truly matters. When I realized that nothing matters, only what truly matters to me, I became free to focus on my mission, my values, my goals – and, yes, my purpose. I came to realize why most self-management people say that "constancy of purpose is the first principle of success." It is not up to me to provide you with the meaning and purpose of your work. For me, comprehensive, relationship-based dentistry provided the meaning that was missing when I was spending my time "filling and drilling." There are many dentists who are content with this level of meaning. I also believe that most dentists don't take their thinking to another level and truly wonder about these things.

Creating meaning and purpose is a subjective experience. The purpose of this book is to help those who have decided that their purpose in dentistry is to take on a role that is bigger than themselves, to find a way to accomplish that purpose. Leadership requires the dentist to serve something bigger than self. I agree with Richard Leider [43], a clinical psychologist, author and the founder and CEO of the Inventure Group, who is committed to helping organizations to find more purpose and meaning in the workplace. He believes that the "process of unlocking your purpose and finding the courage to live it – the power of purpose – is the single most important developmental task we can undertake today."

Leider devoted his whole career to answering one question: "What is your reason for getting up in the morning?" He became obsessed with the work of Viktor Frankl and his seminal book, *Man's Search for Meaning*. He distilled Frankl's work into a common theme that runs through all of Frankl's work. That theme is that the last of human freedoms is the freedom of choice – the freedom to choose, not only in an existential sense, but in the very practical sense of living moment to moment on a daily basis. Science has shown, since Frankl's book, that people who exercise their freedom of choice to live more meaningfully live longer, healthier lives, and they are happier and more productive.

People who have exercised their freedom of choice to make meaningful decisions that are bigger than themselves make better leaders. Sometimes, I think people look too deeply into the existential meaning of finding purpose. It's quite simple. Like John Scully did, either you want to make a difference in the lives of others, or you want to focus on yourself. Scully made a choice. Most leaders make similar choices, and reap the reward of a longer, healthier life. Young dentists who are part of the Millennial generation are now being asked to make these very same choices that have existed for generations. For these Millennials, filling this existential vacuum will be critical. The longer someone decides to live with purpose, the more energy they will have to sustain their career.

Purpose and meaning provide the energy and resilience to keep on going when obstacles appear. That energy is what I was missing during my burnout. In another, less-known, book by Viktor Frankl, *The Doctor and the Soul*, he devotes a lot of the discussion to the meaning of work. He acknowledges, like his mentor Freud, the importance of work, where we spend considerable time and our self-worth is on the line. He distinguishes the social status, fame and fortune that we derive from work and the degree of meaning a job offers. This is the paradox of duty and desire, as well another dissection of Pankey's Cross of Dentistry. Because of his familiarity with medicine, he uses being a doctor as an example. He claims that all health care professionals are not saved from this paradox, and that "the meaning lies beyond making the right diagnosis and incisions (preps and impressions), or drawing blood and cleaning wounds [44]." These tasks, while important, won't satisfy the human soul.

Frankl says in his book that "to practice all of the arts of medicine is not to practice the art of medicine." The art of medicine is to find the right words to say to a patient. The art of medicine (and dentistry) is to live in the world of purpose, meaning, language, communication and story. In today's professional world, we have reached an impasse, because the true art of dentistry is not being taught. The practical application of the "knowledge" that L.D. Pankey talked about can be summed up in one word: leadership.

One of the skills leaders use is storytelling. In later chapters, I go over the whys and hows of storytelling. Story is linked to purpose and meaning, because it provides the context for our work and lives. Story is the emotional connection that provides the energy that drives us to get out of bed in the morning to go to work. Humans are meaning-making organisms, who are wired for storytelling. One of our objectives is to discover our purpose by telling our story. Ask yourself a few questions. Take notes in your journal.

1) Why did you choose dentistry?
2) What does your dental practice represent? To you? To your patients? To your family?
3) What are you passionate about at work?
4) Who are your favorite patients, and why?
5) What makes your heart sing [45]?

After answering these questions, see if a story emerges. Within that story, you will find the purpose and meaning of your life in dentistry. That story is the building block for every piece of communication in your practice. The story will reveal your values, which essentially drives all behavior as well.

My simple definition of a leader is someone who achieves a worthy goal and inspires others along the way. Your story will unlock what is worth striving for – the worthy goal – and the story will help inspire others to join you in your mission. Recall the story about the stonecutter. The biggest difference between him and his fellow workers was the story he told himself about how he viewed his work, and that made all the difference.

As a dentist-leader goes through his day, people see his purpose in his eyes. He looks alive, as if he came to work for an intention higher than himself. I see so many dentists who work with what I call zombie-eyes. I had them once. I couldn't wait till my hours were over. Indifference was written all over my face. Then I came alive. People see that. Ralph Waldo Emerson said, "What lies behind you and what lies in front of you, pales in comparison to what lies inside of you." Purpose and meaning are the two elements that light up what lies within you. Living everyday with purpose, meaning, and intention provides leaders with inspiring reasons to go on in the face of adversity.

One question to ask yourself is, "Is dentistry important?" In other words, does it matter? When a dentist gives up and becomes apathetic about his or her work and the people, dentistry becomes very mechanistic. Our roles change. I have already written quite a bit about the importance of roles, or how we see ourselves, and how we define ourselves. I first entered dentistry in 1973. The theme of dental education back then was a mechanical view of dentistry. I have written about how dentists complained that their work was similar to a car mechanic [46]. The motif in dental schools was more of a glorified and dignified technical school, focused on tasks, duties, and technology. Biology and science is what differentiated the young dentist, but mostly we were mechanics of the mouth.

In the years following my graduation, things began to change. Bonding was invented in 1955 by Michael Buonocore but, by 1977, dentists were becoming very proficient at creating beautiful smiles with the rapidly growing dental product industry. However, dentists were still mechanics, with some leaning toward being more cosmetic. That revolution was beginning to change the role of dentists. Even more important during the 1970s was a much greater emphasis on the role of periodontal disease in changing what the dental community meant to patients.

It is true that periodontists have always understood the importance of periodontal disease, and practiced prevention and surgical techniques (soft tissue mechanics) but, during the 70s, men like Dr. Robert Barkley and Dr. Paul Keyes and others were beginning to change the way that dentists saw themselves in playing a new, more important role in helping people to keep their teeth. Dentists and hygienists would become more involved in prevention, care and hygiene. For the first time, dentists would do more than scaling and surgery to save teeth. They now realized the importance of spending time with patients to motivate, educate and inspire people to keep their teeth.

Bob Barkley, a student of L.D. Pankey, understood the people skills that were necessary to help people. He knew that he could do more for patients. There are many stories (there's that word again) about Barkley and what inspired him to change the way he treated patients [47]. Barkley studied the psychologist Carl Rogers, who developed the concept of client-centered therapy. To apply Roger's concepts in dentistry required the dentist to become more than a mechanic. It required the dentist to operate out of a sense of purpose. It required committing oneself to examination and diagnostic procedures that required skills beyond the technical – people skills.

Barkley's own epiphany is a well-documented story that is often told by many of his disciples [48]. He practiced in the small town of Macomb, Illinois during the 60s and 70s. During his early years, he practiced like many of us: examine, diagnose and present a fee. One day, a young girl came in for an examination. She had rampant caries, but they were treatable. Barkley quoted a fee, as many of us do, but the father could not afford the fee. He lost track of the patient until a few years later, when he saw her in a local Dairy Queen pageant. He asked what had happened to her. To his utter shock and surprise, she told him that it was too expensive, so she went and had all her teeth extracted. She now had full upper and lower dentures – she was barely 20 years old! He was so disheartened that he vowed never to quote a fee that was more than it would cost for dentures, if money was a barrier.

This story revealed meaning and purpose to Barkley. It inspired his practice until the day he died in a plane crash in 1977. L.D. Pankey, his mentor, tells another story of his own mother having all of her teeth extracted after he moved to Coral Gables from his hometown in Kentucky. I have had similar stories in my own practice, and in my personal life, that shook me to the core and brought me right up to the meaning of dentistry for myself and others. To many people, dentistry is more than just a photograph that we can put on Facebook. It can make the biggest difference between a life of health vs. disease, comfort vs. pain, function vs. dysfunction and self-esteem vs. embarrassment. In other words, we must always keep our purpose in front of us, and not get distracted by the everyday routine of our work.

Barkley went on to develop the American Society for Preventive Dentistry. He wrote a book titled *Successful Dental Practices*, which was eventually translated into Japanese, and he is considered the father of the preventive dentistry movement of the 70s. In 1977, one month before his fatal plane crash, Barkley prophetically told a room full of dentists, if he died tomorrow he would want the following written on his tombstone: "The man most responsible for humanizing dentistry." For a moment in time, Bob Barkley did his part, like L.D. Pankey, to redefine the role of dentists. But it didn't last long.

Dr. William Brown, in an essay commenting on Barkley's article, "On Becoming a Humanistic Dentist," noted how Barkley observed dentists misunderstanding his core message by converting his philosophy into business and more technique [49]. Dr. Brown personally knew Bob Barkley. In 1971, at the first Prevention Convention at the Hilton Hotel in Chicago, Barkley commented that the atmosphere was carnival-like. "There were rows upon rows of commercial booths hawking floss, polished-bristle toothbrushes, Floxite mirrors, and any manner of tools to use for plaque control." The energy was high, as the dental community was beginning to embrace this new movement in the most commercial way. A new market was born.

But Dr. Brown reported that Barkley had seen a problem that was based upon the fact that many "disciples" went home to their practices and found that the "5-Day Plaque Control Program" wasn't as easy to integrate into a traditional dental practice as it had seemed when they heard Dr. Barkley. In other words, the dental community was commercializing the idea, rather than humanizing the concept.

The business of dentistry acts as a lens that clouds how dentists see themselves and define their roles. It did in the 70s, and it has been steamrolling since dental technology and corporate dentistry have taken a firm position in the dental community.

During the eighties and nineties came the cosmetic revolution. As the 20th century turned to the 21st, implants and social media contributed to how dentists defined their role. We became cosmetic dentists and bondodontists. The public was obsessed with health and beauty. We share our conquests on Facebook. Lost in all of this is the message of humanistic dentistry and the changing role of dentists. To review, we went from mechanics of the mouth, to gardeners of the mouth, to beauticians of the mouth.

In 1990, I heard Dr. Peter Dawson use the term "physician of the oral cavity." I liked that term, because it made me feel as if my work was more important – that is, it had more meaning. I bought into the concept and used it in my practice, because Dr. Dawson was teaching a comprehensive view of dentistry. Mostly, that comprehensive view was more about occlusion, rather than the relationship between the mouth and the rest of the body. Since that time, we have learned a lot about the role oral health plays in the general health of our patients, and Dr. Dawson's term has taken on a much more significant meaning. Most recently, the dental community is embracing the importance of sleep dentistry and its relationship to the oral cavity. Is this another attempt at making us see ourselves as "physicians of the oral cavity?" Or is it another profit center, just as Bob Barkley noted at the 1971 Prevention Convention?

Are you beginning to get the sense that the more things change, the more the more they stay the same? That is one of the driving forces for me writing this book. I understand that purpose is the starting point for everything. It is the driver. It provides the energy and the fire.

Many people have advised me not to retire from clinical dentistry. Through 42 years, I have painfully developed meaning and purpose for clinical dentistry. I have had my difficulties and disappointments through trial and revelation. I have also been rewarded, spiritually and materialistically. I probably would have stayed on (I don't play golf), but I have developed a new purpose – that is, to carry on the work of Pankey and Barkley through writing and teaching. To make a real difference. Everything, as author Simon Sinek says, "starts with why [50]." We spend the majority of our working lives focused on the "how."

Earlier I wrote that "nothing matters" until you make it matter – until you give it meaning. Most dentists go to courses and watch how others practice, then go home and copy the presenter. I chose my role models carefully, but one thing I have found is that, when it comes to purpose and meaning, we must discover that from within ourselves. We can't just make purpose up. During my early years, I would go home after a weekend course and try to copy the presenter's style. I would memorize their scripts. I never succeeded in that endeavor. It sounded good when they taught it, but there was a disconnect.

This lesson was driven home for me after I wrote *The Art of the Examination*. Dentists would visit my practice to observe how I did the exam and case presentation, They were looking for some magic words, just like I had done earlier in my career. Some thought I was getting better results because I had strong conversation skills, and I was a good storyteller. This was discouraging for me, because I knew that copying wasn't the answer. At this point, I came to realize that leadership development was the answer. Teaching dentists to become authentic leaders started with purpose. Bob Barkley himself used to tell his audiences, "If you try to copy me or anyone else, the best you will be is oleo margarine! You gotta be you." It is this very nuance in Dr. Pankey's philosophy about "knowing yourself" that results in authentic leadership.

In a 2014 *Harvard Business Review* article [51], authors Nick Craig and Scott Snook said that, "clarity in purpose is the key to accelerating growth and deepening impact in both professional and personal lives." They concluded their article by saying that less that 20% of leaders know their personal purpose. Leaders who lack a clear purpose risk struggling with health issues, and show a lack of consistency in leadership style. In other words, clarifying your purpose is essential to developing your leadership.

Your relationship with yourself is probably the most important relationship you can develop. Copying others is unsustainable, as I have found out. Ralph Waldo Emerson once said, "To be yourself in a world that is constantly trying to make you something else is the greatest accomplishment." It's the ultimate act of congruency to have one's thoughts and actions in perfect harmony, all driven by purpose and meaning.

The most popular practice management courses teach wonderful scripts and role-playing that mimic patient situations and circumstances. Dentists love this type of learning; a manual for every scenario, like a cookbook. But it's not authentic.

Finding meaning and purpose takes work. In the coming chapters, I will have more to say about how to discover purpose. Let me tell you how I discovered my purpose. You already know much of my story, the burnout years, etc. Early on, after listening to Dr. Dawson and Dr. Becker at the Pankey Institute, I was bitten by the desire to learn more, so I read and I read. I couldn't get enough of everything to do with dentistry. One thing led to another, and I found that I would spend much of my spare time doing two things – reading and physical fitness.

Reading was about educating myself, and fitness was about self-improvement. I loved every minute of it. Finally, I realized that reading, writing, and teaching others how to become their best selves was my purpose. That same purpose drove my practice. That same purpose is driving me right now as I write this book, or write my blog, or speak to an audience of eager dental students. Purpose and meaning are sustainable over time.

In Chapter 5, I wrote about Joseph Campbell and the Hero's Journey. There is this thought that the journey is only for special or extraordinary people. However, Bill Moyers, in the PBS Special [52] for television, asked Campbell about the significance of the myths: "so myths are stories of the search by men and women through the ages for meaning, for significance – to make life significant – to find out who we are?" Campbell answered that he thought most people search for a meaning of life. He went on to say, "most people are really looking for an experience of being alive – so that we feel the rapture of being alive." Moyers then asked if these myths were meaningful in contemporary life. Campbell responded that the myths provide the clues about how to live life at any time – it's up to each of us to answer the call.

For me, indifference and apathy was my call to adventure. I became convinced, as Campbell says, that all of us – not just extraordinary people – have the opportunity to answer the call. No one is born with a single purpose in life. When the fire goes out, we must ignite ourselves with purpose. Indifference kills. In a dental practice it can potentially kill patients, staff, relationships, and careers. On the other hand, purpose inspires and can breathe life into work, life, practice, and all existence.

In July 2011, the United Nations passed Resolution 65/309, which was adopted unanimously by the General Assembly, placing "happiness" on the global development agenda. March 20th was declared as International Day of Happiness. It was inspired by the tiny republic of Bhutan, which measures prosperity by gauging its citizens' happiness levels, not the GDP. Instead they use a GHP, a gross happiness product. I questioned why the UN thought this to be important enough to commemorate as a special day. Their reasoning was to make people aware to the fact "that the pursuit of happiness is a fundamental human goal."

It is ironic that so many of us need this constant reminder. Today's healthcare landscape continues to place obstacles in the way of that pursuit. This hasn't gone unnoticed by the Millennials. Numerous Gallup polls show that lack of engagement in the workplace leads to a lack of meaningful work. One way to change this is for leaders to become meaning makers. A DeVry University study showed that 71% of Millennials said meaningful work was the top career factor defining success [53]. In other words, today's younger dentists are willing to trade money for meaning. They understand the long-term benefits of meaningful work.

There are many benefits of living with purpose and creating meaningful work, both personally and professionally. Since this chapter is about well-being, it may be time to acknowledge the connection between well-being, leadership and success. Many studies have shown that happiness precedes success, therefore happy leaders are successful leaders. Let's start with the personal benefits of finding purpose.

Some of the healthiest people in the world live on the islands of Okinawa. The islands are part of one of five regions in the world that author Dan Buettner, in his best-selling book *The Blue Zones*, has identified where people live longer and lead healthier lives. One of the factors that contribute to health and longevity is living a purposeful life. The Okinawans actually have a word for it: *ikigai*, which literally means, "the reason you wake up in the morning."

In a 2008 Japanese study, Toshimasa Sone [54] and his colleagues sought to find out how *ikigai* led to longer life. They studied over 49,000 Japanese men and women over seven years, to see if there was a correlation to mortality. What the researchers found was encouraging for those who had clarity of purpose. Those lacking clarity in intentional living had a higher incidence of cardiovascular disease and other life-threatening diseases. Ninety-five percent of those participants with *ikigai* lived seven years longer than the 83% of the study's participants without a sense of meaning and purpose in their lives. The study presents a strong case for the value of knowing your purpose and the potential positive impacts on your well-being. In other words, purpose can inform the choices we make and the behaviors we intentionally demonstrate as leaders.

A Google search for the benefits of living with purpose will lead to more than I can write about in this book. The point is that living with purpose has proven to be essential in living a long, happy and healthy life – certainly the qualities we look for in a leader.

Some of those benefits can be used in day-to-day practice. Purpose keeps us focused and ready to guide us through personal relationships. It grants us permission to do what is right over what is expedient, by keeping us on track. Here is a short list of some practical examples for anyone in a leadership position:

- It helps maintain a sense of calm and positivity during the day.
- It increases your ability to stay motivated and learn from negative experience.
- It helps to keep priorities and "what really matters" in proper perspective. To develop a better balance with work-life issues.
- It maintains mental and emotional clarity during stressful, demanding times.
- It increases your ability to take time with people.
- It works on your intrinsic motivation to experience lasting enjoyment.
- It enables a quicker recovery time from emotional upsets.
- It allows greater awareness of and control over emotional responses to demanding and life situations [55]

So, besides all of the positive benefits that bring well-being and joy to our lives, including: the ability to have stronger and happier relationships; more and better creativity; earning more money; and having better health and a longer life, a life of purpose gives us the power and strength to bounce back quickly from the day to day stress of life. Purpose builds resilience.

Andrew Zolli, author of *Resilience* [56], describes these people as being able to "cognitively reappraise situations, and regulate emotions, turning life's proverbial lemons into lemonade." According to positive psychologist Barbara Fredrickson, this kind of long-term resilience can lead to better cardiovascular health, less worry, and greater happiness over time [57]. With dentists being such perfectionists, it seems that resilience would be a good trait to develop, and it starts with purpose.

Resilience increases with a strong sense of purpose. Together with the overall life improvements of *ikigai*, and the strength of resilience, the dentist can flourish and can better relate to people to put their practice in a position for long-term success.

There is a painting hanging in the offices of The Pankey Institute. It is from *Alice in Wonderland*. Alice is standing at a fork in the road, wondering which road to take. The Cheshire cat is in a tree, and they have the following conversation:

> "Which road do I take?" she asked.
> "Where do you want to go?" was his response.
> "I don't know," Alice answered.
> "Then," said the cat, "it doesn't matter."

None other than the father of modern Yoga, Patañjali, said it all:

> "When you are inspired by some great purpose, some extraordinary project, all your thoughts break their bonds: Your mind transcends limitations, your consciousness expands in every direction, and you find yourself in a new, great and wonderful world. Dormant forces, faculties and talents become alive, and you discover yourself to be a greater person by far than you ever dreamed yourself to be."

Now let's take a look at the final element of well-being. The one that get the most attention: accomplishment.

Accomplishments

Then there is the classic parable of the Mexican fisherman. The story was originally told by German author Heinrich Böll, about an encounter between an enterprising tourist and a small fisherman on a European coast, in which the tourist suggests how the fisherman can improve his life. The story may actually have originated with the Chinese philosopher Chang Tzu. It's been told, retold and adapted to modern life. The following is the most current version that can be found on the internet:

"A vacationing American businessman standing on the pier of a quaint coastal fishing village in southern Mexico watched as a small boat with just one young Mexican fisherman pulled into the dock. Inside the small boat were several large yellowfin tuna. Enjoying the warmth of the early afternoon sun, the American complimented the Mexican on the quality of his fish.

"How long did it take you to catch them?" the American casually asked.

"Oh, a few hours," the Mexican fisherman replied.

"Why don't you stay out longer and catch more fish?" the American businessman then asked.

The Mexican warmly replied, "With this I have more than enough to meet my family's needs."

The businessman then became serious, "But what do you do with the rest of your time?"

Responding with a smile, the Mexican fisherman answered, "I sleep late, play with my children, watch ball games, and take siesta with my wife. Sometimes in the evenings I take a stroll into the village to see my friends, play the guitar, sing a few songs …"

The American businessman impatiently interrupted, "Look, I have an MBA from Harvard, and I can help you to be more profitable. You can start by fishing several hours longer every day. You can then sell the extra fish you catch. With the extra money, you can buy a bigger boat. With the additional income that larger boat will bring, before long you can buy a second boat, then a third one, and so on, until you have an entire fleet of fishing boats."

Proud of his own sharp thinking, he excitedly elaborated a grand scheme which could bring even bigger profits, "Then, instead of selling your catch to a middleman, you'll be able to sell your fish directly to the processor, or even open your own cannery. Eventually, you could control the product, processing and distribution. You could leave this tiny coastal village and move to Mexico City, or possibly even Los Angeles or New York City, where you could even further expand your enterprise."

Having never thought of such things, the Mexican fisherman asked, "But how long will all this take?"

After a rapid mental calculation, the Harvard MBA pronounced, "Probably about 15–20 years, maybe less if you work really hard."

"And then what, señor?" asked the fisherman.

"Why, that's the best part!" answered the businessman with a laugh. "When the time is right, you would sell your company stock to the public and become very rich. You would make millions."

"Millions? Really? What would I do with it all?" asked the young fisherman in disbelief.

The businessman boasted, "Then you could happily retire with all the money you've made. You could move to a quaint coastal fishing village where you could sleep late, play with your grandchildren, watch ball games, and take siesta with your wife. You could stroll to the village in the evenings where you could play the guitar and sing with your friends all you want."

There are many lessons that can be drawn from this story. For me, the big lesson is knowing what really matters in life, and realizing that it is already much closer than we think. There are other lessons that support Seligman's Well-Being Theory as well, like: spending time with your friends; you can't put a price on a happy life; small is beautiful, less is more; appreciate the information and knowledge, but realize that wisdom is more useful; and one that affects all of us when we enter into this profession: advice is nice, but intuition is better.

The American businessman was full of advice and sounded quite persuasive, but at some point we all have to sit back and reflect on what truly matters and realize it's okay to want what is truly important to each of us, that will contribute to what will become your best life. It takes time, but if you're always too busy to sit back and smell the coffee because you have been pursuing the siren of achievement, the pursuit of happiness becomes a pursuit of material wealth.

It's more complicated than that, I know. The first step is to get out of survival, in order to find the time. In reality though, things have not changed in years.

Accomplishment is important – a very important component to our well-being. When I graduated from dental school, the goal for a successful practice was "The $100,000 Dental Practice." Don't laugh – it's just a number. Everything is relative. As a matter of fact, there is still a book in print, titled, *Building the $100,000 Dental Practice* [58]. It was written in 1981. Today, we see articles online and in the dental magazines on how to grow your monthly production by $100,000, or how to build your million-dollar, or even multi-million dollar, practice. One thing is for sure; in the history of dentistry, there has never been a shortage of advice. And most of the advice has centered around achievement and accomplishment of goals. But whose goals are they?

In developing the Well-Being Theory, Martin Seligman faced the same dilemma. The point is that we devote so much of our lives toward success, and we mostly define success materially, because it is measurable and tangible. I have always been fond of the Albert Einstein quote: "Not everything that can be counted counts, and not everything that counts can be counted." If you have read this far, I am sure you realize that I believe there is more to the life well-lived than how much money we can accumulate. Yet, because we are so susceptible to that, most of the advice is related to that one particular problem.

If you recall, in the description of the Well-Being Theory, one of the criteria for becoming an element of well-being was that it had to be done *for its own sake.* There is no doubt that people do pursue "success, accomplishment, winning, achievement, and mastery for their own sakes [59]". Winning at all costs has become a sport in our culture. Football coaching legend Vince Lombardi is often quoted by those who have made winning at all costs their personal mantra, when he said, "Winning isn't everything, it's the only thing." Lombardi and others had much more to say about how to go about winning, yet this quote stands out as being a battle cry for our times. It's a slippery slope because of the measurability and tangibility of accomplishments. Earlier, I referred to coach Tom Coughlin as a "master of intangibles." I felt it was his ability to focus on the positive emotions and relationships that were responsible for his ultimate successes. As dental leaders, we must learn to master the intangibles.

But people are people, and the accomplishment of goals will always be a major piece of the agenda. It is human nature to want to win. Donald Trump has created his entire presidential campaign on winning, and he is appealing to the masses. Every day, all over the world, dental practices start off with a morning huddle that includes a discussion of daily production goals. I practiced for 40 years with daily targets. We all feel good when we hit our goals. It's when hitting the goals at all costs seeps into the practice culture that our influence and well-being diminish. I will have more to say about this in Part III, Leadership Ethos. Winning only for winning's sake may just be a mask for the pursuit of wealth.

The accumulation of wealth and major achievements do not preclude happiness and well-being. People can certainly spend their attention and efforts on balancing achievement with the other elements – positive emotion, engagement, meaning and great relationships. Maybe this is what inspired the Biblical quote, "Again I tell you, it is easier for a camel to go through the eye of a needle than for a rich person to enter the kingdom of God." I know many successful dentists who have accumulated wealth, practiced many years producing the finest, highest quality dentistry on people they would call their patients and friends, and couldn't wait to get back into their highly energetic, optimistic practice everyday. Those are the ones I would say had the qualities I am writing about in this book. They are dental leaders.

I have also seen the dark side of the "winning is everything" culture. I have attended courses where dentists are taught to close cases at all costs. How to manipulate people into buying dentistry by pressuring them into unaffordable loans. How to increase the practice volume so that dentists spend as little time with patients, for the sake of production. Being a lab owner as well, I have seen cases in the lab that show no signs of planning or thought, for the sake of just getting it done. I have heard one too many lab technicians and dental assistants question the doctors' morals as well as skills. And, as insurance companies and corporate dentistry have become more of a presence, these issues just get worse.

So, just like in the last section on purpose we asked, "*why?*", in this section I am suggesting we ask ourselves, *what?* What does success mean? In Chapter 2, I wrote about reconciling the paradox of duty and desire. I used the word *balance* as the solution to reconciling the paradox. I take language very seriously, and I think semantics are very important. How we define what success means to us can go a long way in helping us to create balance.

Martin Seligman's Well-Being Theory is not the only science behind a multi-component theory of well-being. The Gallup Poll group has weighed in with similar studies. Gallup's Tom Rath, in his book, *Well-Being, The Five Essential Elements* [60], writes, "much of what we think will improve our well being is either misguided or just plain wrong." Rath actually claims that intense focusing on any one aspect of our pursuit to wealth or happiness can be detrimental to our well-being. He says that our total well-being is a product of how all of the elements interact [61]. Gallup devised a study to find out what people thought the best possible future for them would look like. The two most common themes that showed up in their initial study were wealth and health. Once again, as in Seligman's studies, these answers were the ones that were measurable and tangible.

In a follow-up study, titled Wellbeing Finder, they used the best questions from their last 50 years of research to assess various life situations over time. What they found was five distinct statistical factors, similar, but not identical to Seligman's. The five elements were:

1) Career Wellbeing: what you do every day, or how you spend your time.
2) Social Wellbeing: having strong positive relationships.
3) Financial Wellbeing: managing your economic life.
4) Physical Wellbeing: having good health and enough energy to get things done on a daily basis.
5) Community Wellbeing: the engagement you have with the area in which you live and work.

According to the Gallup study, 66% of people are doing well in at least one of these areas, but just 7% are thriving in all five. Rath says, "If we are struggling in any one of these domains, as most of us are, it damages our well-being and wears on our daily life. When we strengthen our well-being in any of these areas, we will have better days, months and decades. But we're not getting the most out of our lives unless we live effectively in all five [62]."

Ever since I walked into that lecture hall at the Pankey Institute, I have obsessively tried to bring balance into my life. I have taken the long view, rather than focusing on short-term benefits. Total well-being is a long-term benefit that depends more on balancing the elements than about focusing on winning, wealth or fame. For me, success became about living a life worth living. But it all started with a change in perspective that led to a change in attitude.

Prior to my Pankey experience, I followed the timeless wisdom that the harder one worked, the more successful one would be, and that would lead to happiness. I grew up with a very potent work ethic. I believed hard work was the answer to all of life's problems. Although that led to some degree of success, it wasn't the answer I was eventually looking for. Once I began to focus on my own well-being, my life began to open up.

Once I prioritized my happiness over my striving to achieve more and more, a funny thing happened – I began to thrive. I felt better emotionally and physically. I took better care of myself. My work became less burdensome and more enjoyable. Then, the greatest irony of all, I became more pleasant to be around, my work-life flourished and, most importantly, my overall success improved. All because I put happiness first. Like they tell you on airplanes, if the oxygen mask drops, put yours on first, so you can help others.

As an offshoot of placing happiness first, I began to focus on different types of goals and challenges. I began to focus less on daily production goals. I still had them, because they play a role in the financial systems I placed in the management of the practice. However, they were no longer worshipped like the Golden Calf. What I came to realize was that the more we produced, the more I wanted to produce. Achieving one goal only led to setting the production goal even higher. The treadmill just kept going. By putting happiness first, I changed my perspective on goals. My goals shifted from external to internal goals. I created new challenges. I began to take more continuing education. I stretched myself by learning new techniques, communication skills, public speaking, photography, and most importantly, what it takes to be a leader. The reward was exactly what L.D. Pankey had promised at the center of his Cross of Dentistry – the spiritual reward of high achievement and life satisfaction.

For me, this level of personal success is quite gratifying. My early successes could only be counted by how much income I produced, or how many crowns or veneers I had placed in a month or a year. It's funny to listen to dentists at meetings, discussing how many new patients they get, or how much they get for a crown, or how many implants they placed. These are their measures of success; transactional sales statistics. I'm not judging, but I have learned that there are other ways to measure success. Don't get me wrong, though; material success or fortune can lead to happiness, as many studies have shown.

When I wrote my first book, I received another level of success. I was being asked to speak. I challenged myself to learn how to write and speak better. The dental industry acknowledged me at a different level. Once again, that level brought great satisfaction and, once again, it brought on the treadmill to write and speak more and more. People recognized me at most of the conventions. All of this felt good. I was happy with this social level of success, or the fame aspect of success. Once again, like fortune, fame can certainly work for some, as well.

There is a third type of success. I call it self success. Others cannot see it. It doesn't appear on your monthly statements or in the bookstores. It just means that you have achieved what you want to achieve. Remember, my simple definition of a leader is someone who achieves a worthy goal and inspires others along the way. A life of achieving worthy goals for their own sake is my personal definition of success. In the end, I am proud of my accomplishments, happy with my work and, most importantly, fulfilled and satisfied.

I began my leadership journey while in my early 40s. When I turned 60, a few years ago, I seemed to have developed a new perspective about life that was, at first, a bit confusing, because it felt unnatural and foreign. Most of my life, I was concerned with the material rewards, but now I was much less interested. I came to hear about a condition known as geri-transcendence. The term comes from the words "gero" (old age in Greek) and "transcendence" ('to climb over' in Latin). According to Swedish gerontologist Lars Tornstam

[63], the developer of the theory, "geri-transcendence is a developmental stage that occurs when an individual who is living into very old age shifts their perspective from a materialistic and rational view of the world to a more cosmic and transcendent one, normally accompanied by an increase in life satisfaction."

I felt relieved that someone had described what I was feeling. But I was hardly in old age. I was still young. I kept thinking about that, as I noticed colleagues of mine that were still searching for happiness by accumulating more and more. They are never satisfied as the treadmill keeps going and going. I began to wonder if we could only reach this transcendence through natural aging. I thought about how lucky I was to have reached this place earlier. I decided that there are many roads to Rome, and that a better way to achieve life satisfaction was to commit to the Hero's Journey that Joseph Campbell had described.

Campbell, in his *Power of Myth* interviews with Bill Moyer, told a story about his own retirement. While sitting around one day in Hawaii, he noticed that the conversations between the men and women consisted of the same old stuff they had always spoken about. There were considerably fewer men around the pool than women, he noticed. He realized that if someone had reached the age of 70 and still had not transcended the values of a younger life, "they may never get it."

For me, I think that defining success as self success made all the difference. There are times when sales success, social success and self success will conflict with one another. As we consciously evolve, if we evolve, then the wisdom of self success will develop. But I do believe it is a conscious evolution.

The last thing I want to do is impose my personal values on the reader. I believe and respect what L.D. Pankey said about success: that it is a personal matter.

Conclusion

"Before you are a leader, success is all about growing yourself. When you become a leader, success is all about growing others."

Jack Welch

"Everything can be taken from a man but one thing: the last of the human freedoms – to choose one's attitude in any given set of circumstances, to choose one's own way."

Viktor Frankl

I hope by, now you, that are beginning to appreciate how complex this idea of leadership can be. I also hope that you can appreciate why I spent so much time on the idea of happiness and well-being preceding success. Some readers may be overwhelmed by the leadership journey, although I believe that the whole idea is simple, but not easy. It mostly requires a conscious attempt to take control of our lives.

In this chapter, I wrote about the "why" and the "whats" of well-being, but the bigger questions for most of us seem to fall around the "hows of happiness." There is more than enough advice out there on how to develop happiness. Pankey, as mentioned, said "success is a personal matter." I don't think that information is readily usable. One of my mentors used to quote motivational speaker Zig Ziglar: "Your attitude determines your altitude." Once again, an empty platitude for me. Harold Wirth, one of the Pankey Institute's legendary teachers, would approach students with the daily greeting: "How's your PMA? (positive mental attitude). Although the emphasis on attitude is undoubtedly correct, it lacks an action verb. The one piece of advice that rings most true for me is the Viktor Frankl quote, above. It speaks to me because of one word: *choice.* And choice implies action and control. I also believe what a Texas preacher, Charles Swindoll, says: "Life is 10% what happens to you and 90% how you react to it."

The latest science proves this to be true. For those who are not endowed with Carolyn Dweck's growth mindset or an internal locus of control, it comes down to making choices that give us control of our destiny. In a 2005 study, University of California at Riverside, psychology professor Sonja Lyubomirsky [64] studied twins, to determine the capacity of people to change their levels of happiness beyond fixed factors like genetics or life circumstances. The study showed that on average, happiness is 50% genetics, 10% environment or circumstances, and 40%, as Pankey suggested, is up to the individual. The study determined that intentional activity – in other words the actions leaders take to be effective – offers "the best opportunities for sustainably increasing happiness [65]." So, as Viktor Frankl claimed many years ago, happiness is a choice.

One of the key traits of a leader is to stay focused. It is easy to get distracted in this day and age. Another trait that leaders exhibit is thinking long-term – focusing on what really matters in the long run. In this new, highly connected, world, it is difficult to stay focused on long-term values, rather than getting distracted by the next new thing. There is a famous study, known as the marshmallow test, conducted at Stanford University by Walter Mischel in the late 60s and early 70s. In the study, four-year-olds were given a marshmallow, but were told that if they waited seven or eight minutes before eating it, they could have two marshmallows rather than one. Fourteen years later, when these kids were tracked down, those kids who waited turned out to be better learners, more popular, and still able to delay gratification in pursuit of their goals.

That ability to delay gratification, according to Dan Goleman, hinges on a cognitive skill: concentrating on the good feelings that will come from achieving a goal and ignoring tempting distractions. That ability also lets us keep going toward that goal, despite frustrations, setbacks, and obstacles. And that is the tie-in to leadership. Observing this trait in four-year-olds was an early indicator of success. In our quest for success, the road will never be clear. This is the problem with the insecure path.

Leaders will have rocky times. There will always be failures. The ability to persist despite frustrations allows leaders to resist the temptation toward security and comfort.

The modern terminology for this trait is *grit*. According to Wikipedia, grit "is a positive, non-cognitive trait based on an individual's passion for a particular long-term goal or end state, coupled with a powerful motivation to achieve their respective objective. This perseverance of effort promotes the overcoming of obstacles or challenges that lie within a gritty individual's path to accomplishment, and serves as a driving force in achievement realization."

Whether it is the ability to delay gratification, willpower or grit, some level of self-control is needed to achieve long-term well-being and effective leadership.

In the next chapter, I will discuss the role of passion in achieving long-term success and the role our education system plays in our ultimate success.

References and Notes

1 "Elusive Butterfly" is a popular song written by Bob Lind, released as a single in December 1965. It was his description of happiness as a songwriter.

2 Martin Seligman (2004). *Authentic Happiness: Using the New Positive Psychology to Realize Your Potential for Lasting Fulfillment*, 1st edition. Atria Books.

3 Martin Seligman (2012), *Flourish: A Visionary New Understanding of Happiness and Well-being*. Atria Books; reprint edition.

4 Ibid.

5 Karl Pillemer (2012). *30 Lessons for Living: Tried and True Advice from the Wisest Americans*. Plume; Reprint edition.

6 Bronnie Ware (2012). *The Top Five Regrets of the Dying: A Life Transformed by the Dearly Departing*. Hay House; Reprint edition.

7 Maslach C and Jackson SE (1981). The measurement of experienced burnout. *Journal of Occupational Behaviour* **2**: 99–113.

8 Shiva Kapoor, Manjunath Puranik and SR Uma (2014). Burnout in Dentistry: An Overview. *International Journal of Advanced Health Sciences* **1**(8).

9 Forrest WR (1978). Stresses and self-destructive behaviors of dentists. *Dental Clinics of North America* **22**: 361–71.

10 Cooper CL, Watts J and Kelly M (1987). Job satisfaction, mental health, and job stressors among general dental practitioners in the UK. *British Dental Journal* **162**: 77–81.

11 Looking at the opposite of those words would be looking at a lost, lonely, disconnected state. That would be the negative, and hardly what we want to do with our lives.

12 Campos JA, Jordani PC, Zucoloto ML, Bonafé FS and Maroco J (2012). Burnout syndrome among dental students. *Revista Brasileira de Epidemiologia* **15**: 155–65.

13 D. M. McMahon (2006). *Happiness a History*. New York: Grove Press.

14 Christopher Peterson (2012). *Pursuing the Good Life, 100 Reflections on Positive Psychology*, 1st edition, pp. 4–5. Oxford University Press.

15 Martin Seligman (2004). *Authentic Happiness: Using the New Positive Psychology to Realize Your Potential for Lasting Fulfillment*, 1st edition. Atria Books.

16 Martin Seligman (2012), *Flourish: A Visionary New Understanding of Happiness and Well-being*, p. 16. Atria Books; reprint edition.

17 Barbara Fredrickson (2008). *Positivity: Groundbreaking Research Reveals How to Embrace the Hidden Strength of Positive Emotions, Overcome Negativity, and Thrive*, 1st edition. Crown Archetype.

18 Emma Seppälä (2016). *The Happiness Track: How to Apply the Science of Happiness to Accelerate Your Success*, pp. 40–41. HarperOne.

19 Roy F. Baumeister and Ellen Bratslavsky Catrin Finkenauer (2001). Bad Is Stronger Than Good. *Review of General Psychology* **5**(4): 323–370.

20 Lao Tzu (author), Stephen Mitchell (ed, 1994). *Tao Te Ching*. Harper Perennial; compact edition.

21 Clayton Christensen (2012). *How Will You Measure Your Life?* Harper Business.

22 Daniel Goleman (2005). *Emotional Intelligence: Why It Can Matter More Than IQ*. Bantam Books; 10th Anniversary edition.

23 Daniel Kahneman (2011). *Thinking, Fast and Slow*, 1st edition. Farrar, Straus and Giroux.

24 Breakthrough Ideas for Tomorrow's Business Agenda. *Harvard Business Review*, April 2003

25 Peter Drucker (2008). *Managing Oneself*, 1st edition. Harvard Business Press.

26 Carolyn Webb, *How to Have a Good Day: Harness the Power of Behavioral Science to Transform Your Working Life*, Crown Business (February, 2016), p. 20.

27 Matthew Lieberman (2007). Social Cognitive Neuroscience: A Review of Core Processes. *The Annual Review of Psychology* **58**: 259–89.

28 Ryan R.M. and Deci E.L. (2000). Self determination theory and the facilitation of intrinsic motivation, social development, and well-being. *American Psychologist* **55**(1): 68–78.

29 Blatt, S.J. Quinlan, Donald, M., Chevron, E.S., McDonald, C. and Zuroff, D. (1982). Dependency and Self Criticism: Psychological Dimensions of Depression. *Journal of Consulting and Clinical Psychology* **50**(1): 113–24.

30 John J. Ratey (2008). *Spark: The Revolutionary New Science of Exercise and the Brain*, 1st edition. Little, Brown and Company.

31 arnoldbakker.com (2016). *Work engagement.*

32 www.gallup.com, November 7, 2012.

33 Mihalyi Csiksentmihalyi (1997). *Finding Flow, The Psychology of Engagement With Everyday Life*, p. 38. New York: Basic Books.

34 Ibid., pp. 31–32

35 Jim Loehr and Tony Schwartz (2003). *The Power of Full Engagement, Managing Energy, Not Time, is the Key to High Performance and Personal Reward.* Free Press.

36 Ibid., pp. 18.

37 Mehl, M.R., Vasire, S., Holleran, S.E. and Clark, C.S. (2010). Eavesdropping on happiness: Well-being is related to having less small talk and more substantive conversations. *Psychological Science* **21**: 539–541.

38 Olivia Fox Cabane (2012). *The Charisma Myth: How Anyone Can Master the Art and Science of Personal Magnetism.* Portfolio.

39 Ibid.

40 Paul Bloom (2010). The Moral Life of Babies. *The New York Times*, May 9, 2010.

41 Ibid.

42 Franz de Waal (1996). *Good Natured: The Origins of Right and Wrong in Human and Other Animals*, 1st edition. Harvard University Press.

43 Richard Leider (2015). *The Power of Purpose: Find Meaning, Live Longer, Better*, 3rd edition, p. xxi. Berrett-Koehler Publishers.

44 Lee Eisenberg (2016). *The Point Is: Making Sense of Birth, Death, and Everything in Between*, pp. 98–99. Twelve.

45 This question is suggested by Carmine Gallo in his book *The Storyteller's Secret* (St. Martin's Press, 2015).

46 In my book *The Art of the Examination*, I recount the story of a conversation heard in the cafeteria of Tufts University while I was at my first interview for dental school.

47 There are many stories about L.D. Pankey as well, which inspired him to begin to understand the importance of communication skills in dentistry.

48 Paul Henney, Lynn Carlisle and Robert Frazer have devoted much of their careers to the ongoing mission of Bob Barkley.

49 William T. Brown (2010). Thoughts on Bob Barkley's article, "On Becoming a Humanistic Dentist." dental-intelligence.com/wp-content/…/Brown-Article-on-Barkley_v2.pdf

50 Simon Sinek, *Start with Why: How Great Leaders Inspire Everyone to Take Action*, Portfolio Hardcover; 44329th edition (November 13, 2009)

51 Nick Craig and Scott Snook (2014). From Purpose to Impact. *Harvard Business Review* (May): 106–111.

52 Joseph Campbell with Bill Moyers (1991). *The Power of Myth.* Anchor.

53 Alexandra Levit and Dr. Sanja Licina (2011). *How the Recession Shaped Millennial and Hiring Manager Attitudes About Millennials Future Careers.* Career Advisory Board, DeVry University.

54 Sone, T., Nakaya, N., Ohmori, K., Shimazu, T., Higashiguch, M., Kakizaki, M., Kikuchi, N., Kuriyama, S. and Tsuji, I. (2008). Sense of Life Worth Living (Ikigai) and Mortality in Japan: Oshaki Study. *American Psychosomatic Society* **70**: 709–715.

55 Schaefer, S.M., Morozink Boylan, J., van Reekum, C.M., Lapate, R.C., Norris, C.J., Ryff, C.D. and Davidson, R.J. (2013). Purpose in Life Predicts Emotional Recovery from Negative Stimuli. *PLoS One* **8**(11): 1–9.

56 Andrew Zolli (2013). *Resilience: Why Things Bounce Back.* Simon & Schuster, Reprint edition.

57 Barbara Fredrickson (2003). The Value of Positive Emotions. *American Scientist* **91**: 330–335.

58 Robert, O. Nara (1981). *Building the $100,000 Dental Practice.* Prentice Hall.

59 Martin Seligman (2011). *Flourish: A Visionary New Understanding of Happiness and Well-being*. Free Press, Reprint edition.

60 Tom Rath (2010). *Well Being, The Five Essential Elements*, 1st edition. Gallup Press.

61 Ibid., pp. 4–5

62 Ibid., p. 7.

63 Lars Tornstam (2005). *Gerotranscendence: A Developmental Theory of Positive Aging*, 1st edition. Springer Publishing Company.

64 Sonja Lyubomirsky, Kennon M. Sheldon, and David Schadke (2005). Pursuing Happiness: The Architecture of Sustainable Change. *Review of General Psychology* **9**(2): 111–31.

65 Ibid.

7

Passion is the By-product of Mastery – A New Curriculum

"Better to light a candle than to curse the darkness."

Chinese Proverb

"Better to light a candle than to curse the candle that others light."

Chris Peterson

Passion – The Fire of Desire

I have an admission to make. I can only make this admission through self-reflection by looking back on a 47-year career that began with my admission into dental school in 1969. I am not sure that I actually chose dentistry, or that dentistry chose me. Most of you reading this probably know what I mean – not all of you, because for some there were truly great reasons to go into dentistry besides parental and peer pressure. It's a decision we make before we have all of the facts. I knew a little about dentistry, but mostly I knew that I wanted to have a good life, make a good living, and that I liked the natural sciences. I had good grades in high school and college and there was this well-worn path of other students like myself that went before me. But, looking back I never truly had a passion for teeth.

So I chose dentistry for all of the wrong reasons, but good reasons nonetheless. Dentistry would provide me with the opportunity to make a good living. Dentistry was a helping profession, and I would feel that my work provided a valuable service for people; that was always important to me. Mostly, dentistry would provide me with autonomy, and the ability to control my own hours and schedule. I had grown up watching friends and family becoming slaves to their work, and that was the last thing I wanted. So I chose dentistry, and I don't regret my choice – but I had to do a lot of extra work to get the things I went into dentistry to get. Passion for teeth did not drive me and, when I graduated from dental school, I still didn't have a passion for teeth.

After dental school, I joined the US Army as a captain in the dental corps. It was easy duty. I learned a bit more about oral surgery and endodontics. At Fort Dix, New Jersey, we were lucky enough to have a training program for dentists. For a short time, our commanding officer was Dr. Jay Siebert, the future Dean of Penn's School of Dentistry. I had much of my own dentistry done while in the military, by a highly qualified prosthodontist whom I would still consider to be one of the best I ever knew. But there were other officers who taught me more valuable things about myself and leadership than the dental ingredient.

The Complete Dentist: Positive Leadership and Communication Skills for Success, First Edition. Barry Polansky.
© 2018 John Wiley & Sons, Inc. Published 2018 by John Wiley & Sons, Inc.

The oral surgeon in charge of Walson Army Hospital at that time was a great guy. Most of the dentists at Fort Dix considered him a friend, as well as a senior officer. He ran the hospital's oral surgery department and set the rules. But four months into my tour of duty, he got sick and was transferred. His replacement was the extreme antithesis of him – a pure disciplinarian who set up rules that everyone complained about. He was a tyrant who took pleasure in making sure everything went by the book. One new rule was that if a dentist was on call, he or she had to come in for the patient, no matter the reason, and no matter what time of night. The surgeon had at his disposal a sergeant who would act as a triage officer, but his nature was to never make a decision. The dentists hated this system. They would get calls at all hours of the night; they had no say in deciding who could wait until sick call at 7 am the next morning. The sergeant would call them for everything from mild gum inflammation to temperature sensitivity.

One night I was on call. In the middle of a deep sleep, at around 2 am, my phone rang. I was groggy and dazed. I asked the sergeant what the problem was. He said it was actually my patient whom I had done an amalgam filling on, earlier that day. His tooth was sensitive. Understand this; soldiers would always show up at the hospital whenever they wanted, claiming to be in pain. I knew this, and I knew the patient and the circumstances. I told the sergeant to give him some mild pain medication and go to sick call in the morning. The sergeant barked that there would be hell to pay if I didn't come in. I ignored him and went back to sleep.

But there *was* hell to pay. The colonel called me into his office the next day. He reported me to the base commanding officer as well as to my own commanding officer. He promised that I would be served with an Article 14, which is when a soldier commits a single act of "serious misconduct." Serious misconduct is an offense which could be punished by a punitive discharge. So I was that close to being discharged from the military and, even worse, from being court-martialed. But I was saved. The commanding officer in charge reversed the process, and began to take a look at the surgeon for letting the sergeant's insubordination get by. It seemed that the sergeant was making a routine of becoming a clone of the colonel. I became a hero instead of a victim.

Looking back, I realized how important being a master of my own destiny was to my future. I still did not have a passion for teeth, but I certainly displayed a passion for autonomy. I was displaying at the time how important was the freedom to make decisions on controlling my own destiny. You may be reading this and saying that I may have been guilty of insubordination. That may be true but, as far as leadership traits are concerned, sometimes leaders must express what is right for them. If I didn't have that trait, my career may have turned out a lot differently.

The most popular self-help book in publishing history is *Think and Grow Rich*, by Napoleon Hill. The book was written in 1937, and as been viewed as the bible of self-improvement by just about everyone in the motivation field. The popular book *The Secret* is an updated version of the same themes that Hill wrote about years before. *Think and Grow Rich* is composed of 17 laws of success, centering around the idea that thoughts are things, and that whatever we can conceive, we can achieve. One of Hill's first laws is about living with a definite purpose. Purpose, as discussed earlier, is one of the elements of well-being. It was described as "whatever makes your heart sing," or "gets you up in the morning." Hill writes about developing a burning desire as your purpose. I am not sure he realized the difficulty that dentists have today in keeping their desire burning. If this was worth writing about in 1937, so you can imagine how important it is for young dentists today.

Dr. L.D. Pankey understood clearly the difficulty dentists had in sustaining their desire or passion for dentistry throughout their career. For me, this has been the greatest struggle. To continue to ward off the powerful feelings of frustration, boredom, impatience, fear and confusion was a real and definite battle for me. Many times during my early career, before I relied on advice and counsel from mentors and coaches, I was saddened by all of the dentists who reported how much they loved their work and couldn't wait to get to the office every morning. I thought I had chosen the wrong profession – that something was wrong with me.

When I was exposed to Dr. Pankey's philosophy, I learned about what he called the Ladder of Competency. This was his way of categorizing the profession. Imagine a ladder, or some other ascending prop – maybe a mountain or a big hill. The top of the ladder represents the high point of a dentist's potential. It is the place where most dentists aspire to be when they enter dental school. When we leave dental school, we enter this hierarchy at the stage of the student, with years of focused learning ahead of us in our climb upward. Dr. Pankey estimated that only 2% of the dental population reaches the highest level, which he called *master*. Dr. Pankey and Napoleon Hill both would have agreed with the words of the German philosopher, Johann Wolfgang von Goethe:

> "Everyone holds his fortune in his own hands, like a sculptor the raw material he will fashion into a figure. But it's the same with that type of artistic activity as with all others: We are merely born with the capability to do it. The skill to mold the material into what we want must be learned and attentively cultivated."

Pankey believed that 2% achieved mastery, and 8% were on the road to mastery. He called them the *adept*. Thirty-six percent remained as lifelong students, but the remaining 54% he labeled indifferent, or even apathetic. His choice of words is very telling. A look in the dictionary tells us that indifference means uninterested, removed, and apathetic, among the many words that describe someone who is disengaged from their work. This bothered Dr. Pankey. It bothers me. Anyone who is deeply involved with their work and their profession is troubled by this displeasure in a profession that potentially holds the key to one's future and general well-being. I presume this is why Dr. Pankey spent his life trying to teach dentists how to create a better life.

Climbing this ladder toward mastery proves more difficult than it appears. It is not simply a matter of "just doing it," as the famous Nike TV ad claims. It is also not just a matter of reading inspirational stories of great dentists and their successes. Today, for many, climbing the ladder toward mastery is more like the mythological figure, Sisyphus, who was punished by being forced to roll an immense boulder up a hill, only to watch it roll back down, repeating this action for eternity. For many dentists and other professions, the punishment lasts only 40 years. Pankey's number of 54% indifference is probably higher today, considering the conditions. And this problem is not confined to dentistry.

In a Gallup World Poll of 47,000 employees in 120 countries [1], only 11% reported engagement in their work, down from 17% reported in a similar poll in 2005. Among the 2010 interviewees, 62% reported that they were not engaged – that is, they were emotionally detached and likely to be doing little more than is necessary to keep their jobs. And 27% were actively disengaged, indicating they viewed their workplaces negatively, and were liable to spread that negativity to others.

A very recent Gallup Well-Being Index was the subject of an online article by Elizabeth Mendes, "*America's Life Outlook Better Than in 2008, but Not Best* [2]," and indicated that life ratings for all age groups declined in October 2012, revealing that whatever issues were causing Americans to be less optimistic about their lives recently were affecting everyone, regardless of age. That's sad.

Where people live on this ladder is not an all-or-none phenomenon. The ladder is like a continuum. Very few people are totally disengaged or indifferent, and few people are totally engaged all of the time. It's like any other character strength or virtue; they all live on a sliding scale. Our job is to create the virtues that allow us to spend more time at the higher levels of the ladder, and it may start by enhancing motivation, rather than restraining it.

In my early years of practice, as I mentioned, I thought I was the only one who felt disengaged from dentistry. Today I am seeing this displeasure expressed more freely. Dentists are "coming out", so to speak. They are actively complaining about the difficulty of earning a good living and more importantly the difficulty of fighting off third party involvement and strong competing forces. I have seen numerous blog posts by dentists who have left dentistry because of these difficulties. Yet, regardless of the conditions, I believe it is a matter of leadership skills to overcome the obstacles along the road to mastery.

Passion is the Opposite of Apathy and the By-Product of Mastery

If apathy and disengagement are the problems, then passion is the answer. Yet, when I ask dental students and young dentists about their passion for dentistry, it seems universal – they all love it. So why the disconnect? Are the ones who say they love dentistry confabulating, or creating stories that justify their decision to choose dentistry as their life's work? In truth, studies have shown that we do not come out of school with a passion for dentistry. It must be earned over time, and it is a product of mastery. It is interesting to note that the word passion comes from a Latin verb, *patior*, meaning "to suffer and endure." Are images of Sisyphus coming to mind? These days, passion refers to pursuits we enjoy, as opposed to any sense of sacrifice and endurance.

In a recent book, *So Good They Can't Ignore You*, author Cal Newport cites a few studies that put an end to the "follow your passion" myth. The first study concluded that career passions are rare. Five hundred and thirty-nine Canadian students were asked if they had passions and, if so, what were they? The results showed that they indeed had passions, but 84% had passions unrelated to choosing a job. The top five passions were dance, hockey, skiing, reading and swimming. Only 4% had any relation to work or education [3].

The second study concluded that passion takes time. This study, published in the *Journal of Research Personality*, made the distinction between a job (a vehicle to pay bills), a career (a path toward increasingly better work), and a calling (work that is an important part of your life and vital to your identity). Recall the stonecutter. This study showed that when interviewed, people were split evenly in how they looked at their work. The defining trait of a calling? When asked, they said more years on the job and experience. Those who considered their job a calling were around long enough to become good at what they do, and to have consistent feelings of efficacy and the ability to create relationships. Hence, creating passion takes time and, as mentioned earlier, they take the time to create their own stories.

So what is mastery? The dictionary tells us that it is *full command* of a subject of study. Pankey knew this because, in his Cross of Dentistry, when he described the "work" of dentistry, he included both technical and behavioral components of the domain. In other words, the dentist could not reach the level of master, or even adept, without gaining *control* over the behavioral skills, including communication and presentation.

In support of the idea that mastery takes time, author Robert Greene, in his book *Mastery* [4], explains that our brains have a particular quality or grain and, when we take the time and focus on the depth of our subject of study, we are working with the grain and we will develop mastery. He claims, "We infallibly move to higher and higher levels of intelligence. We see more deeply and realistically. We practice, and make things with skill. We learn to think for ourselves. We become capable of handling complex situations without being overwhelmed. In following this path we become *Homo magister*, man or woman the Master, and to the extent that we believe we can skip steps, avoid the process and magically gain power through political connections or easy formulas, or depend on our natural talents, we move against this grain and reverse our natural powers [5]."

In other words, Greene is saying that the road to mastery follows a natural process, and our brains have developed to take us there. We need to feel in control of our lives. Yet, he says that most people abandon the process in favor of expediency, distractions, the opinions of others, and fears.

In further explanation, Greene tells us how the human brain is wired for mastery. He claims that humans evolved through two biological advantages. The first is having one of the most remarkable visual systems in nature. This allowed man to distinguish between friend and foe, and to have the ability to survive. Man's eyes developed in the front of his head, the most advantageous position for defending himself. The second biological advantage is that man is a social animal. Social intelligence helped man survive through group cohesion and cooperation. Both of these traits – vision and social intelligence – enabled humans to survive, create and master their domain. Hence, the mastery process is inherent in the human brain. Being in control of our lives is not just some nice thought; it is a biological requirement.

Engagement in our work, and having the ability to make decisions through freedom of choice is not only a biological imperative but, when it is blocked, neurologists believe, it leads to the base of the ladder of competency – apathy [6]. Making choices, and making decisions that gives us the feeling of control in our lives, is the essence of self-motivation. A series of studies during the 1990s in nursing homes showed that patients were able to make choices that rebelled against the rigid schedules, menus and strict rules the nursing homes tried to force on them [7]. Some of the patients were even called "subversive," as I may have been called in my army days. This book may even be called a small act of subversiveness.

But consider the alternative – *emotional detachment.* As I stated above, neurologists now believe that, when there is no sense of reward from taking control, emotion goes dormant, because we forget how good it feels to make a choice. Control and choice are the rewards of autonomy. If our choices are meaningful, then we are more in control of our lives. I will have more to say on this in the next chapter, on creating a new paradigm for dental education, self-motivation and protecting the provider's freedom of choice.

L.D. Pankey described three traits that a dentist needs to fulfill patients' needs. Those traits are care, skill and judgment. When we look at the three traits through the lens of mastery, we can say that skills would be more technical in nature. Alone, they wouldn't be enough to create success. The technical skills are easily taught and practiced. Often, after a period of time, many dentists say that the skills are so routine that, "we can train a monkey to do them." If it were just technical skills that created success, maybe monkeys could become dentists. But monkeys lack the other two components.

Care is not a biological trait common among primates other than man. You will rarely see two monkeys helping one another. Men and ants work cooperatively to build community. Caring for patients is what distinguishes dentists from one another, and it is a biological trait.

The last of Pankey's criteria is judgment. This is the time factor. It takes time – sometimes years – to develop the judgment necessary to practice the kind of dentistry that leads to mastery. If passion is born from mastery, and mastery takes time, how does a dentist nurture the mastery process to help fuel the passion that will drive his career? Before one can take on the job of mastering all three requirements, one must realize that it requires the internal locus of control that this book has stressed.

What is the Mastery Process? More Evidence of Control

In a study by bestselling author Dan Pink, *On the Surprising Science of Motivation* [3], he tells us that SDT (Self Determination Theory) claims we need three "*nutriments*" to feel intrinsically motivated for our work. Those three nutriments are autonomy, competence and relatedness. Let's take a look at these three, and see if they apply to dentistry. In a manner of speaking, the three nutriments are related to Pankey's care, skill and judgment.

Autonomy

By autonomy, Pink means the feeling that you have control over your day. Many years ago, I heard Dr. Peter Dawson explain that dentists would feel better about themselves and their work when they had control of the work, and were able to create predictable results. That was one of those moments that changed my career forever. It actually goes a lot further than just having control over your dentistry. Pink's criterion is to have control over your day – your time, your life. That could be a lot more difficult, because it means I would have to counter many of the forces that were working against my mission to provide complete care for patients. What forces? Insurance, staff, patients, the economy, business loans, to name just a few. I know few professions that spend the majority of days overcoming resistance. Like the nursing home residents, sometimes we feel like subversives, having to hurdle over the obstacles in order to complete our mission.

Really, having autonomy is the only way to do meaningful work. It's the meaning our work has that is engaging. How many times do we sit at the chair thinking, "Why am I doing this?" Recently, I went through some old patient photographs, and was reminded of how much good I did for patients through the years. That is what made me most happy. Occasionally, I still treat patients that do not exhibit the trust or appreciation and ownership that is required to reach fulfilling results.

How to get this kind of control? Through choice. By exercising our freedom of choice, we can control our destiny. Another way is systems and policies. Yes, systems and policies for everything in your practice. I will have more to say about how to put systems and policies together in a later chapter. I became so obsessed with creating systems that I actually wrote a book about my primary and most fundamental system, *The Art of the Examination*. I also have policies concerning insurance, patient identification, treatment planning, and just about any practice management thought you have ever had. Every policy and system I create is based upon discerning what I want, then making good choices in order to accomplish my most meaningful dentistry. Slowly applying these policies and systems leads to autonomy, and is the first step toward creating passion.

Time management systems are key to controlling how your day goes. Everyone in dentistry is concerned with time. How long will this procedure take? How fast can you get my crown back? Can I get my teeth before Christmas? All of these time issues convert to stress on everyone, from staff to the laboratory. Controlling every aspect of your work will lead to better time management. My practice has become what Dan Pink calls a Results Only Work Environment (ROWE). Everything we do focuses on results, without placing time constraints. In time we have become a performance-based culture, rather than one that just sings the platitudes of good service. Learning pain management skills and splint techniques, and making excellent provisionals, goes a long way when it comes to time management. This is where skill development merges with autonomy.

There is another way to achieve autonomy – that is, to learn the social skills necessary to deal with the forces that today's dentist must face. The social and political codes of his own office and the dental community do not work to give the typical dentist the autonomy he needs to practice and grow toward mastery. These skills take time to develop. Dentists who are not free to practice their own style of dentistry lose the ability to problem-solve and the ability to make simple day-to-day decisions. Eventually, this will lead to burnout, emotional detachment and apathy.

Pankey's judgment criteria never gets fully developed when there is no freedom or autonomy to practice. Creative solutions that require the best technical dentistry never get applied with any consistency. The time factor diminishes, and growth slows down. Autonomy is a necessary nutriment for the growth and development of a successful engaged dental practice, but autonomy can only be obtained through freedom of choice.

Competence

Competence is the feeling that you are good at what you do. It is a feeling of self-efficacy and once again, being in control of the work. It is a component of well-being, but it is not the same as self-esteem. Self-efficacy means you are capable of carrying out the tasks necessary for success. Self-esteem is an overall view of yourself.

Earlier, I mentioned that that are just two fears that people have: the fear of not having enough, and the fear of not being enough. That sounds like duty and desire again. Building self-esteem is very important when building your passion for dentistry. In dental school, we were taught the fundamental technical skills to enter the profession. These skills, known as hard skills, require a certain amount of practice. After a while, we tend to get better at the hard skills. Learning them requires a teacher and some feedback. Dental schools do this well (hopefully). The problem is that these aren't the skills that will get the dentist where he wants to go in practice and life. For that, we need soft skills. In the words of coach extraordinaire Marshall Goldsmith, "What got you here won't get you there [8]." It is the soft skills that will get you there.

Soft skills are those that usually involve communication, like leadership, listening, interviewing, trust-building and storytelling. They are also the skills of self-improvement and self-management. These are not taught in dental school. I guess the dental schools think we are going to make this up with continuing education or coaching. Soft skills actually take more practice than learning hard skills, because the failure rate is so high, and most people generally give up (unlike Sisyphus, who kept rolling the boulder up the hill, day after day), when they feel any level of anxiety when there is a "failure to communicate."

Dr. Tracy Orleans, a health psychologist at the Fox Chase Cancer Control Center in Philadelphia, found that two out of three physicians were pessimistic about their patients' ability to change. This would translate to poor compliance by patients. Orleans says, "This pessimism is the single biggest obstacle to getting physicians to help their patients with their health problems." Healthcare professionals are in the business of getting people to change by overcoming resistance. If these two-thirds of physicians don't believe their patients will change, they stop trying.

Coaching can help develop the soft skills, but mostly it is a matter of trial and error until, through "pattern recognition", we get it right. Pattern recognition is the ability to read, recognize and react – like a great quarterback (leader) who practices the fundamentals like passing and running (hard skills), but takes it to another level when he learns to read defenses, and communicates with his teammates (soft skills). Pattern recognition takes time to develop, and it takes making many mistakes and learning from those mistakes. That's where competence and resilience in the soft skills makes all the difference.

Make no mistake, fundamental hard skills are very important, and you can't reach success without them. In order to light your fire for dentistry, however, the soft skills are also necessary. Becoming competent in the hard and soft skills is necessary to develop mastery. Many dentists go into private practice, and have to learn these softer skills on their own. The very best usually take advantage of coaches and mentors. I have always been in favor of an apprenticeship for dentists. It is a good idea to work with a successful dentist to help coach you through those tough days when there is no one to turn to. Cynicism and depression can certainly knock you off the road.

Competence is Pankey's skills set. Of course, as mentioned, Pankey considered the behavioral social skills to be just as important as the hard skills.

Relatedness

The third nutriment, relatedness, is the feeling of connection to other people. Dentistry is about people. Pankey said, "I never saw a tooth walk into my office." Dental practice is all about people. A tenet of the Pankey Cross of Dentistry is to "know your patient." Whom we work with, and whom we work for, are paramount to maintaining passion for our work. Whether it's staff or the patient, we must be able to work in harmony with people. Jim Collins, author of the bestseller *Good to Great* [9], makes two comments about working with people.

The first is his idea of getting the "right people on the bus." This idea is to work with staff and patients who have high levels of appreciation for what you are trying to accomplish. This goes along with another idea that he wrote about: "First who, then what," referring to the fact that people you work for (or in the case of dentistry, we might say "work *on*") are more important than the work you are doing.

Taking the time, as part of your examination process, to get to know your patient, may be the most important thing a dentist can do in practice. There is a phrase I use that describes this nutriment well: "It's never about you; it's always about them." It is *them* that makes the dentistry worthwhile; in order to engage ourselves with our work, we must connect to others. The late positive psychologist and bestselling author Chris Peterson concluded, in much of his research, that "happiness is other people." In the end, that's all that matters. Peterson was known for the phrase, "Other People Matter."

Recently, I was going through years of dental photographs while cleaning out my desk drawers. I stopped at patient after patient, rethinking their stories. Some had left the practice, while many had stayed. Some had completed dentistry, while many did not. While going through the photos, I thought about what Clayton Christensen, author of *How Will You Measure Your Life* [10], said about finding fulfillment in your life. We will not please everyone and we will not succeed with everyone, but we can measure our success by the numbers of people we have helped in our lives. Going though those photos that day reminded of how much meaningful dentistry I did, and how many people I helped. Sometimes we focus on the wrong things – the difficulties and the struggles – but, in the end, other people matter.

There is a formula that I once read about called the critics math formula. It states: 1 insult + 1000 compliments = 1 insult. This is human nature. This is the human brain's natural tendency toward negative bias. We tend to focus on the few patients that we don't reach, the ones who didn't accept treatment, when the reality is that we have affected so many more in a positive way. Negative bias is self-inflicted resistance.

Relatedness is L.D. Pankey's "care" factor. My studies at the Pankey Institute helped me to develop my care, skill and judgment over time. As I grew, I also developed the autonomy to practice and develop my skill levels, and provide care for some of the best people in the world – my patients. I don't know if I could have survived all these years in dentistry without the freedom to do it my way.

When I wrote the *Art of the Examination*, I wanted to describe a process that led to patients accepting comprehensive dentistry. The one skill above all that was most responsible, and the most difficult to master, was face-to-face communication, or presentation. I truly believe it is an art and, once mastered, it will be the key to your success. Presentation takes time, and requires significant leadership and communication skills, but it will give you the autonomy to stay on the road to mastery and sustain your passion for dentistry.

I have a obsessive passion for understanding occupational satisfaction. It has led me to study ideas that relate to success, happiness, mastery and passion. I have developed an affinity for the study of positive psychology. It is the study of what makes life worth living. Positive psychology is not pop science; it is science, which requires checking theories against evidence. It is not self-help or any secular religion, and goes way beyond the ideas of Napoleon Hill.

One of my mentors, Dr. Irwin Becker, was always suspicious of speakers who would spout *pop psychology*. For many years, that was all that was available to help people improve themselves. Inspirational speakers, storytellers and bloggers can fill people with platitudes and false hope. Today, there is plenty of science that supports strong self-improvement and leadership development – knowledge that wasn't available in Pankey's day. It is ironic that positive psychologist Chris Peterson, in his book *Pursuing the Good Life* [11], lists 13 points that have been scientifically confirmed by positive psychology in its short history. One of those points is "That good days have common features: feeling autonomous, competent and connected to others." Just how Dan Pink described the three nutriments of passion.

In the next chapter, I will present my thoughts on why we need to reform dental education. We need to teach dentists how to develop the traits, skills and the self-motivation to sustain the long career they are being trained to do. We can no longer train dentists to become great technically and ignore the most important aspects of career development.

References and Notes

1 The State of the Global Workforce 2010, Copyright © 2010 Gallup, Inc.

2 Elizabeth Mendes (2012), *America's Life Outlook Better Than in 2008, but Not Best*. www.gallup.com, November 7, 2012.

3 Cal Newport (2012). *So Good They Can't Ignore You: Why Skills Trump Passion in the Quest for Work You Love*. Grand Central Publishing.

4 Robert Greene (2013). *Mastery*. Penguin Books; Reprint edition (October 29, 2013).

5 Ibid.

6 Charles Duhigg (2016). *Smarter Faster Better: The Secrets of Being Productive in Life and Business*, 1st edition, pp. 35–37. Random House.

7 Ibid.

8 Marshall Goldsmith (2007). *What Got You Here Won't Get You There: How Successful People Become Even More Successful*. Hachette Books; Revised edition.

9 Jim Collins (2001). *Good to Great: Why Some Companies Make the Leap ... And Others Don't*, 1st edition. Harper Business.

10 Clayton Christensen (2012). *How Will You Measure Your Life?* Harper Business.

11 Christopher Peterson (2012). *Pursuing the Good Life, 100 Reflections on Positive Psychology*, 1st edition, pp. 4–5. Oxford University Press.

8

A New Beginning – A New Curriculum

"The chief purpose of education is to teach young people to find pleasure in the right things."
Plato

"Management is doing things right; leadership is doing the right things."
Peter Drucker

"The function of education is to teach one to think intensively and to think critically. Intelligence plus character – that is the goal of true education."
Martin Luther King, Jr.

The mission of the Pankey Institute is to *"inspire dental professionals to narrow the gap between what is known and what is practiced."* I have always been impressed with that mission statement. It embraces the essence of my definition of leadership, as stated earlier, to set worthy goals and inspire others along the way. I am not sure about the individual missions of each dental school, but it would seem plausible to me that the goal should be to convert knowledge into practical application, or what Stanford University professors Jeffrey Pfeffer and Robert Sutton call closing the knowing-doing gap [1]. At the Institute, I have heard through the years that they just teach what we learn in dental school, but from the perspective of making it work. The expression they use is "getting it off the shelf."

Professional schools, from business schools to medical and dental schools, claim that they produce leaders, yet that is not evident in the various curricula for professional development. As discussed in the previous chapters, leadership is vital in all professions and organizations. The inadequacy of curricula for leadership development has left a void in the marketplace that has been filled with inexperienced and under-qualified people, teaching leadership that is out of context with each field. Leadership is broadly defined as the ability to move individuals toward a goal or a vision. But what goals? What people? What is specific to dentistry can only be taught by people with leadership experience in the field, which is why it must be under the auspices and support of a good dental education. The dental community has recognized the need for leadership development, yet there are very few schools that provide dentists with the training to practice in the ever-changing real world of dentistry.

Dentists generally seek leadership advice through their own personal reading and continuing education, under the heading of practice management. Generally, they seek successful dentists who function as mentors and role models. The one problem with that is they copy a certain style of leadership, which may not be appropriate for their own personality style. As mentioned earlier, just learning scripts and situations may get you close, but that is not real leadership.

The Complete Dentist: Positive Leadership and Communication Skills for Success, First Edition. Barry Polansky.
© 2018 John Wiley & Sons, Inc. Published 2018 by John Wiley & Sons, Inc.

There are many different leadership styles. When I first began my journey into practice management, I would try to copy every successful dentist I met. I would ask questions about how to handle every difficulty, from staff issues to case presentation. I could never get a handle on how to manage the day-to-day running of my practice. I would ask myself, "What would _____ do?" I would even say, "What would L.D. do? The problem was that I was me. I had to develop my own style.

Recently, I read that narcissists make good leaders. I had always been taught that modesty and humility were the traits that made a good leader. Then I thought about Steve Jobs and Donald Trump, both highly successful leaders, yet both have "likeability issues." Narcissistic leadership is a style of leadership that can be very effective, but it doesn't fit everyone's personality. Early in my career, I worked with a dentist who was a master at persuasion. At first, I listened to his scripts and watched his mannerisms, almost to perfection. In the end, I abandoned his style to develop my own. There are many different theories and styles of leadership, including servant leadership, authentic leadership, transparent leadership, heart-led leadership, and the one that I prefer – charismatic leadership.

I like charismatic leadership, because it is a blend of warmth and caring with presence. In Part III, I will explain why charismatic leadership fits my personality. Leadership literature is filled with descriptions of various types of leadership. The key is that any style that is developed should be principle-based. In Chapter 3, I described Covey's definition of principles as rules or laws that hold up over time. In other words, the principles of leadership and communication are timeless, and they transcend any style. Another way to look at this, for dentists, is that form follows function. Your style (form) will mimic the basic human principles that guide you. To me, this is the first rule of leadership development. I like to say, "Firm in principle, flexible in procedure."

When I think about leadership for dentists, I think about how they can be most effective and still achieve a high level of well-being. I don't like to overcomplicate things. Leadership is simply achieving worthy goals and inspiring others along the way. The three most important categories for dental leaders to work on are character, communication, and the actual work of dentistry. Yes, there are traits that are subcategories of each one, and those traits are the subject of the rest of this book. The main question now is, "is leadership important, valuable and necessary enough to be taught as part of a dental school curriculum?" We do know that dental educators think so, and so do dental students.

In a 2012 study conducted by Russell Taichman D.M.D., and Joseph Parkinson D.D.S., the authors surveyed all US Deans of Academic Affairs to determine where, in the various curricula, leadership is taught and emphasized [2]. What they found was that leadership is taught, but not directly. It is ill-defined, and obscured as being part of other disciplines, such as practice management, community outreach programs, and public health. Leadership, as a discipline of personal and self-management, is generally not considered as a topic for dental school education.

The study defined leadership as having the ability to move toward a goal, but many programs considered the leadership training to move communities toward greater oral and systemic health. In today's "real world" of dentistry, it would behoove most dentists to have the specific skills needed to move people forward, like "good communication skills, the ability to self-reflect, critical thinking, problem solving skills, ethical behavior and professionalism [3]."

In 2011, the authors of the study invited all of the Deans for Academic Affairs, at all of the US Dental schools, to participate in an eight-question survey about the leadership curriculum at their school. Approximately 54 surveys were sent out, but only 22 were returned, and one of them only answered the very first question: "Is the term 'leadership' part of the mission/vision statement of the institution?'" Recall that the Pankey Institute's mission statement is quite indicative of a need for leadership. I found it quite revealing that less than half of the deans responded to this very legitimate study. Figure 8.1 is a copy of the questionnaire sent to the

Question	Text of Question
1.	Is the term "leadership" part of your mission/vision statement at your institution? a. Yes b. No ***Response-62%-Yes***
2.	Is leadership training part of the current curriculum at your institution? a. Yes b. No (If no, can you please specify as to why?) ***Response-71% Yes but 4 said to faculty only. Some said only as an elective.***
3.	If leadership training is part of your curriculum, what is the primary focus? a. Our focus is on leading a dental team b. Our focus is on other aspects of leadership (If other aspects please specify). ***Responses: 12 of 19 respondents said leading a team. Others said for practice management or leading the profession or organized dentistry.***
4.	If leadership training is part of your curriculum, in what courses or academic settings is the training provided? A Text response is requested. ***Responses: 8 of 16 responses said it fell under "practice management" setting. Others said it was included in behavioral science, community dentistry, ethics and professionalism or in clinical settings.***
5.	What areas of dentistry does your leadership training program focus on? Please check all that apply:

Question 5 table:

	Emphasis			
	No	Some	Moderate	Strong
Academic dentistry				
Public Health				
Practice Management				
Healthcare Delivery				
Legal Aspects of the Profession				
Business				

Question 6: How many hours in your curriculum are specifically devoted to leadership training? Please check one box per academic year (D1, D2, D3, D4):

Hours	0–2	3–9	10–49	50 or more
D1				
D2				
D3				
D4				

Question	Text of Question
7.	How are leadership competencies evaluated to address CODA Standard 2–19: "Graduates must understand the basic principles and philosophies of practice management, and have the skills to function successfully as the leader of the oral health care team."? a. Not evaluated b. Examinations / Practicals c. Objective structured Clinical Examinations (OSCE) d. Per Feedback e. Other (Please specify) ***Responses-See below for discussion.***

Figure 8.1 Questionnaire with responses.

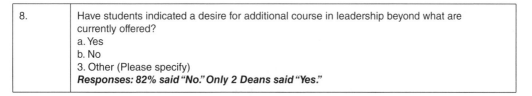

8.	Have students indicated a desire for additional course in leadership beyond what are currently offered? a. Yes b. No 3. Other (Please specify) ***Responses: 82% said "No." Only 2 Deans said "Yes."***

Figure 8.1 (Cont'd)

individual institutions. I added the responses to each question, and inserted the results to questions 5 and 6 below in Figures 8.2 and 8.3. Note that the questions were straightforward and only required a "yes" or "no" answer. Note the responses that came back.

From the standpoint of leadership development, it is worth noting that, in many cases, there is little or no leadership being taught as part of practice management or academic dentistry.

The sixth question is very telling as to the amount of time is spent on leadership development through four years of dental education. This was an obvious failing in how leadership development is viewed by dental educators. The real proof comes from how students are tested for any level of proficiency in leadership, communication, or even practice management, if you like that terminology. Generally, proficiency in all subjects is determined by testing but, in the case of this very vague curriculum, the responses included the following: "peer feedback, exams and rotation ratings, a practice plan as part of community-based training, development evaluation of a project, portfolio, examinations, feedback and faculty evaluations in clinical settings, exams and feedback. [4]"

In Part I of this book, I discussed the problems that exist in this changing "real world" of dentistry. This study tells me that the curricula, and the requirements needed to complete a dental education, are inadequate for young dentists to practice in today's environment.

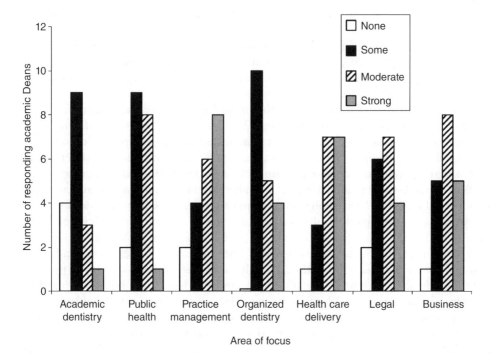

Figure 8.2 Response to Question 5.

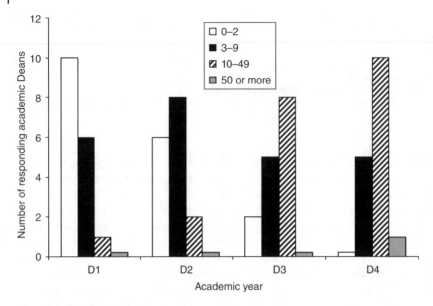

Figure 8.3 Response to Question 6.

The answer to question 8 is where the rubber meets the road. Eighty-two percent of the Deans said that students did not request additional leadership courses. The other Deans claimed that students did ask for more training in different formats, "*including workshops and that is why few students understand the value of leadership training at this particular stage of their education. Of those that do, they desire more. Those that do not, want less* [5]."

Think about that. The people in charge of education have literally abdicated taking responsibility for this very important content needed to prepare young dentists to practice in the real world.

According to the authors of the study, "only through dynamic leadership will oral health professionals be in a position to guide the current transformations in dentistry." While they agree that the competencies may not be easily taught, they are all in agreement about the necessity.

The most interesting part of the study was that most Deans agreed that the students saw no need for leadership training and development. The study cited a report that the majority of dental students surveyed claimed they were interested in leadership development [6]. When I think about my own dental education, I can understand why dental students may not understand or appreciate the immediate importance of leadership skills as part of a curriculum. When asked, these students reflect on their school days, and say that leadership skills are a crucial aspect of their professional responsibilities once they get into the workforce. We are certainly seeing the results of a lack of leadership training at the level of dental education.

In another study, conducted by dental students from the University of Michigan School of Dentistry [7], it was concluded that the leadership responsibilities necessary to practice effectively include skills in communication, independent learning, and vision casting. They referenced many recent publications that claim dental schools should consider implementing leadership development as part of their core curriculum. These programs, they say, should fulfill the requirements of the Commission on Dental Accreditation (CODA) [8]. Their conclusion is that leadership education is essential in the overall development of a dentist.

So why the disconnect between what the educators are doing and what they believe is necessary to develop better dentists? I believe, and it should be, that the role of dental education is, above all, to teach dentists to become competent technicians. This takes time, so fitting leadership development into a curriculum is difficult from a time standpoint. The second reason, I believe, is that the entire leadership community has failed to define leadership, and to provide tangible, measurable parameters that will fill CODA's requirements. I also believe that, from the start of organized dentistry, there has been a scarcity of dentists with comprehensive dental leadership skills. If there is a scarcity because of the overemphasis of technology, for good reason, then who is there to teach it? But that doesn't mean that the need goes away.

The leadership community, as discussed earlier, has made things even more complicated by not providing any standards. Leadership development, as stated, is mostly taught by unlicensed coaches and consultants. That is one of the reasons I looked toward the field of positive psychology and well-being, to help provide the measurable parameters to build positive institutions that can help create a curriculum that can be taught not only in dental schools, but in other professional schools as well.

The goal for leadership development is to help dentists to become more self-motivated, by helping them to obtain more control of their day-to-day decision making. Self-motivation is the reason why success breeds success. Preserving providers' freedom of choice is paramount to providers' sense of control of their destiny. Through the years, whether it has been the economy, or the third parties, or the newer corporate models, it seems that provider freedom of choice and decision-making ability is being adjusted to fit the pressing cultural demands. Dental education, I believe, whether it teaches technical dentistry or leadership, must take a greater role in helping dentists to protect their freedom of choice.

It is not that dental schools have totally denied the need for leadership development. Harold C. Slavkin, the ex-Dean of the University of Southern California's School of Dentistry, attempted to create a leadership development program at USC. He concluded that, from his perspective, "there is no infallible step-by-step formula for becoming an effective or transformational leader." He stated in an article that leadership signifies the act of "making a difference [9]." Although he states that there is no infallible method to develop leaders, he goes on to state that he believes leadership can be taught and learned.

In the final analysis, the authors of the 2012 study, Taichman and Parkinson, believe "that a failure to plan, foster and invest in the development of future dental leaders is a grave mistake and places our profession at risk." They go on to conclude that a failure to invest in leadership development could hasten an erosion of the stature of our profession while, at the same time, placing decisions and processes into the hands of others, who may not place as high a value on oral health: "We therefore feel that it is essential to find time within the rigorous curriculum regulated by the ADA accreditation standards that leadership training of future dental leaders be expanded [10]." Leadership training and development is the new frontier in dentistry. It may just be the critical ingredient for preserving the future of dentistry in this age of complacency.

This book is my attempt to define and describe a set of competencies, in a systematic fashion that can be developed into an effective curriculum for dental students and others who are in an oral health environment. Any endeavor to define leadership competencies must go beyond the accumulation of knowledge and the development of competencies. It must also teach methods of action that actually get results through effective leadership. It must fulfill the fourth arm of Pankey's Cross of Dentistry: the application of the knowledge.

In general terms, L.D. Pankey described many of the competencies and skills that fall under the field of leadership. Under the heading of "know yourself," Pankey may have placed the competencies of self-reflection, vision casting, articulation of mission and goals, optimism, value clarification, enthusiasm, ethics, professionalism and social responsibility. The "know your patient" arm of the cross might include skills in communication, motivation, persuasion, negotiation, writing, photography, case presentation and public speaking. Included under "know your work" may have been critical thinking and problem-solving (diagnosis and treatment planning), time management, systems thinking and brainstorming. As you can see, leadership encompasses many traits and competencies – and, yes, it takes time to learn them.

It is generally accepted that training professionals to become leaders is a difficult endeavor. Most professional schools make the promise in their brochures that they develop leaders, yet that is far from the reality. The truth is that many in the leadership industry wonder how effective leadership training really is. According to Kristin Hedges, the author of *The Power of Presence* [11], the leadership industry admits to a large gap in knowledge and actually performing like a leader. Mostly compelling concepts are presented during rousing meetings by dynamic speakers but, once the attendees go home, they forget 50% of what was presented, and most never get to implement.

The latest statistics reveal that the US spent over $70 billion on leadership and corporate training in 2014 [12], up from a 2012 study that claimed over $14 billion on leadership development training. There are thousands of books published each year, including this one, that address leadership development. Most of the books and programs say the same thing. The principles and fundamentals of leadership are fundamentally timeless – unchanged and unchanging. The problem is not with the knowledge, it is with the implementation. In order to close the gap between what dentist leaders know and what they do, it is necessary to take the focus away from programs, compelling concepts and entertaining speakers, and put the emphasis on processes that can lead to desired results. These processes lie in the day-to-day activities in dental practice.

One of the problems is that most leadership in dentistry is taught through a business model. The results most dentists concern themselves with from a leadership point of view center around the financials, such as daily production and collection. If the results centered around the end-user – the patient – then the whole approach would be different.

As I mentioned earlier, I own a dental laboratory. When a technician brings me a case for my advice, I generally find that the treating dentist didn't follow a process or a system, and now had boxed himself and the technician into undesirable circumstances. I find the same with dentists whom I coach. It is rarely a technical problem but is, rather, an issue with not following protocol. The number one issue is not doing a comprehensive examination. That process – the exam, treatment planning, diagnosis, and case presentation – goes a long way in teaching most leadership competencies.

In a business model of teaching leadership, the financial well-being of the practice takes center stage over the long-term well-being of the patient. Once again, form follows function. If dental schools would emphasize the "clinical systems" that are now being taught in a way that is disconnected from leadership issues, within a context of leadership development then, through the four-year curriculum, the young dentist would see the relevance of each and every competency – even the business skills. This is another example of the wholism that I mentioned earlier.

Leadership, at its core, is about maintaining behavioral change. Under current training, these new behaviors are not sustainable. There are all kinds of dashboards and software applications that remind dentists to achieve daily behaviors, and to create habits that will sustain good leadership.

Leadership development is not like technical dentistry. It takes place over time. Dentists need to be exposed to leadership in dental school, and to continue their education over time. It is an ongoing process. Continuing education programs can be developed or work in conjunction with dental schools for the lifelong process. I used to say, "you can't learn to ride a bike in a seminar." I think that sentence describes what we are facing today. In other words, leadership is an ill-defined topic, and if you Google the term "leadership", you will find 84 million hits. So where do you begin to teach leadership to dentists? That's what the rest of the book is about.

Before leaving this part of the book, I would like to make a distinction between leadership development and leader development [13]. Leader development enhances personal growth and is more directly related to the benefit of greater well-being, happiness and success, as discussed in Part I. Leader development, according to the researchers at the Center for Creative Leadership, has identified certain qualities and capabilities that continue to improve over time through leader development. Some of these capabilities, which will be explored later, include: self-awareness of one's strengths and weaknesses; balancing the demands of personal and professional life; the ability to grow and learn; a sense of ethics and integrity; developing personal initiative and responsibility; and an optimistic attitude. Other competencies include: the ability to create and maintain positive relationships; the ability to grow and develop others; and management skills like setting and achieving goals, planning, and the ability to initiate change and growth.

Leadership development promotes organizational growth, which helps groups develop as a whole, as well as creating and developing more organizational leaders. Leadership development is more about developing alignment and keeping the team on track. Although this is important, I believe everything starts with development of the individual dentist as a leader. In keeping with this distinction, I will focus mainly on the leader competencies necessary for success.

Some of the material in this book may appear to be of the self-help genre; however, I believe that it is more than just pop-psychology. As a matter of fact, I don't think viewing it as such can be much help. I listened to an expert on burnout once, and his solution was very close to psychotherapy. Although that may or may not help in some cases, I don't believe it addresses the universal problem of professional burnout that we are seeing today. Another attempt that we see is physicians and dentists limiting their practices to do only certain types of dentistry, or procedures on very specific patients. This is what has sometimes been called "concierge practice." Although this is how I began my attempt to control my life and practice, and it can be effective, I don't believe that it is the universal answer to what is becoming a public health issue.

In a recent interview with the US Surgeon General, Vivek Murthy, at the 2016 annual meeting of the Association of Heath Care Journalists, he said, "The suicide and burnout rate is very high, and this is concerning to me because we are at a point in our country where we need more physicians, not fewer; we need more people entering our profession, not fewer. If we have people burning out, it really goes against our needs. As I think about the emotional well-being for our country, I am particularly interested in how to cultivate emotional well-being for healthcare providers. If healthcare providers aren't well, it's hard for them to heal the people for whom they are caring [14]." This has been a long time coming. It may be the start of a movement to search for the answers other than self-help, isolation and psychotherapy.

Jerome Groopman M.D., the chief of experimental medicine at Beth Israel Deaconess Medical Center in Boston, and the author of the bestselling book, *How Doctors Think*, says that the vast majority of misdiagnoses, about 80%, are due to cognitive errors. He believes that the time pressures put on doctors these days can interfere with their cognitive abilities, and as you will see in the next chapter, one of the hallmark issues of bad leadership is cognitive errors [15]. What we are beginning to see is that more and more of the problems with healthcare are coming back to the issues of provider well-being. The problem is too big to ignore. My solution is to find methods that help healthcare workers to begin their well-being journey in the professional schools. I am a dentist, but I believe that every profession – medicine, law and education – should find ways to provide training for future professionals. It may take time, it may cost money, but I can see no other way to address this growing serious problem.

The key for any culture is to create conditions that best enable all humans to flourish and to prosper. In cultures that existed in the past, it was the job of philosophers, religious leaders and politicians to create the conditions that would enhance all human growth and flourishing. If you followed the 2016 road to the presidency, you are aware that most people are languishing. We see it in our practices everyday. What we see on Facebook is not the reality of today's dental profession. Dentists are distressed at every level. Compared to 50 years ago, as I noted with the changing roles of dentists, we are in a cultural mismatch, yet the profession continues to believe that the answers lie in more technology and more data. In other words, we want to continue to control our lives and culture through more force. It sounds logical and rational, but taking a softer step back, and applying the principles of human nature, may just be what the doctor ordered.

Our lives and practices show up on a daily basis. Day-by-day, drip-by-drip, we make decisions based on our emotions and intuition, while ignoring all rational thought. This is why the concept of emotional intelligence has become such a big part of a leader's armamentarium. Optimism and confidence is down within all of the professions. Someone once said that humans are not predominantly rational beings, nor are they solely emotional beings. Leaders must understand the nature of who they are, and create a balance between emotions and logic – care and competence, warmth and presence.

In one hundred years, will the beginning years of the 21st century be known as the Age of Happiness? Prosperity? Equality? Or Freedom? Hardly. If anything we are losing our freedom of choice. Michael Puett, author of the book *The Path*, says we may look back and call this the Age of Complacency: "A time when people were unhappy and unfulfilled; when they witnessed growing crisis but failed to respond, feeling there was no viable alternatives." Leaders must begin their quest by understanding that their day-to-day activities must begin by changing their behaviors from just a cliché of learned responses to more appropriate responses to daily life and practice. By reducing everything we do to what we have always been doing, because we just don't know any better, is just another excuse to maintain the *status quo*. And where has that gotten us? That is why leadership is necessary at every level.

This book is my plea for leader development to be taken more seriously by the dental community – a new curriculum, which merges the technical and rational work of dentistry with the softer emotional side of dentistry, to produce leaders who will take mastery to a more universal level. It is this *way toward mastery* that must be emphasized. If we recall Fredrickson's *Broaden and Build Theory* on positive emotions, and view it through the filter of a legendary quote by Confucius: "It is not the way that broadens; it is that humans broaden," we can see we must remove the barriers along the road to mastery.

References and Notes

1 Jeffrey Pfeffer and Robert Sutton (2000). *The Knowing-Doing Gap: How Smart Companies Turn Knowledge into Action*, 1st edition. Harvard Business School Press.

2 Russell S. Taichman, and Joseph W. Parkinson (2012). Where is Leadership Being Taught in U.S. Dental Schools? *Journal of Dental Education* **76**(6); 713–720.

3 Ibid.

4 Ibid.

5 Ibid.

6 Victoroff KZ, Schneider K, Perry C (2008). Leadership development for dental students: what do students think? *Journal of Dental Education* **72**: 982–988. [PubMed: 18768440]

7 Lior Aljadeff, BS, Rachel E. Krell, BA, Amy B. Lesch, BA, and Harold M. Pinsky (2013). The Importance of Leadership Development in Dental Education: Student Perspective. *Compendium* **34**(5).

8 Taichman RS, Parkinson JW, Nelson BA, *et al.* (2012). Leadership training for oral health professionals: a call to action. *Journal of Dental Education* **76**(2): 185–191.

9 Slavkin H (2010). *Leadership for health care in the 21st Century: A personal perspective. Journal of Healthcare Leadership* **2010**(2): 35–41.

10 Russell S. Taichman, and Joseph W. Parkinson (2012) Where is Leadership Being Taught in U.S. Dental Schools? *Journal of Dental Education* **76**(6): 713–720.

11 Kristin Hedges (2011). *The Power of Presence: Unlock Your Potential to Influence and Engage Others.* AMACOM (November 18).

12 John Bersin (2014). *Spending on Corporate Training Soars: Employee Capabilities Now A Priority.* Forbes.com, September, 2014.

13 Van Velsor, E and McCauley, CD (2010). Introduction: Our view of leadership development. *The Center for Creative Leadership Handbook of Leadership Development*, 3rd Edition, pp. 1–22, San Francisco: Jossey-Bass.

14 Joyce Frieden (2016), Editor for MedPage Today, April 12th.

15 Michael Z. Hackman and Craig E. Johnson (2013). *Leadership: A Communication Perspective*, 6th Edition, pp. 15–16. Waveland Press, Inc.

Part III

Leadership Ethos

"Your reputation is who people think you are, your character is who you really are."

John Wooden

"True leadership is moral authority, not formal authority. Leadership is a choice, not a position. The choice is to follow universal timeless principles, which will build trust and respect from the entire organization. Those with formal authority alone will lose this trust and respect."

Stephen Covey

"Example is leadership."

Albert Schweitzer

L.D. Pankey studied philosophy after returning from the European Dental Conference in 1932. He went to that conference because he needed a fresh outlook on the practice of dentistry, not unlike what many dentists are going through today. The economy was weak, he had just moved to Coral Gables, Florida, and he was tired of extracting teeth and just making dentures. He knew there was a better way to practice. Upon his return, he enrolled in Northwestern University. He took courses on the examination, diagnosis, treatment planning and occlusion. He also took general philosophy courses. That is where he became a student of Aristotle's philosophies.

Aristotle is one of three ancient philosophers (the others are Plato and Socrates) who are credited with developing the foundation of all Western thought. The general philosophy of all three, it can be said, is the basis for all of liberal arts education. Aristotle was born in 384 BC, on the northern coast of Greece. His father, Nichomachus, was a physician. Aristotle left his home to study in Athens at Plato's Academy, Greece's premier learning institution. He was an exemplary student but, after Plato died, Aristotle went on to create his own school, The Lyceum, where he taught subjects ranging from science and math to philosophy and politics. During this time, Aristotle broke away from his mentor and wrote his immortal *Nichomachean Ethics*. In that book, he prescribed a moral code of conduct for what he called "good living."

The Lyceum may be considered a rival school to Plato's Academy. Plato was what we would call, today, an existentialist or idealist. Plato just accepted what existed, while Aristotle challenged that viewpoint by questioning everything. He became a master at scientific observation, a systematic investigator who constantly sought the answers to the structure of reality. Aristotle's philosophies left a legacy of organized thought, which not only has become the basis

The Complete Dentist: Positive Leadership and Communication Skills for Success, First Edition. Barry Polansky.
© 2018 John Wiley & Sons, Inc. Published 2018 by John Wiley & Sons, Inc.

for the scientific method and liberal arts education, but also the basis of what has become a formula for living the good life, or what I have been calling the life worth living.

Underlying everything we learn in school is always the question of how to live; no matter what period of time throughout history, the question of human flourishing has taken center stage. Although every civilization leaves behind the artifacts of their specific cultures, in the form of artwork, architecture and technology, it is how the people lived that truly defined each culture. The philosophical questions that Socrates and Aristotle tried to answer were the same as Confucius, the Buddha, and even Jean-Paul Sartre in 20th Century Europe. The questions are timeless, and every one of us seeks the answers, even today. These questions are the same ones that today's positive psychologists are studying in the classrooms at Harvard and Stanford. The questions boil down to, *"How do I build a proper world where everyone has a chance to flourish?"* and *"How do I live my life? [1]"*

Those questions were the ones that I was asking when I began my journey at the Pankey Institute, and I believe they were the same questions that L.D. Pankey was asking when he opened his practice in Coral Gables.

I am sure that Pankey was fascinated by Aristotle's systematic thought process, which included not only the rational components of thought, but the emotional side as well. We owe a debt of gratitude to Pankey for taking Aristotle's deeply profound philosophy and attempting to make it useful for dentists. That was no easy task. But even when I first attended the Institute, the language of Pankey's philosophy was in the language of the ancient Greeks. I had a difficult time applying words like *virtues, eudaemonia, phronesis and ethos, pathos and logos* to my everyday world. Let's face it, reading the Nichomachean Ethics is not your everyday reading material.

I believe that the heart of Pankey's message was lost in translation, and continues to be confusing to many trying to navigate their lives and careers. Students I have met throughout the following years, including myself, would cite the various Crosses with a sense of understanding Dr. Pankey's complete philosophy. The philosophy needs a way to make it more accessible to today's students, because it is timeless, and based on human universal principles. It needs a language makeover; or else the main message of the Institute will be what it has been since its inception – occlusion. L.D. Pankey was much more than that.

Let's take a look at some of the old language. Aristotle's eudaemonia may be his version of happiness. Not the happiness that is described as pleasure, but the happiness associated with the good life. It is not a feeling, but a state – *and a state with a moral dimension*, synonymous with living well and acting well, as it arises from being part of and being active in a connected social world. Achieving the good life requires the development of certain virtues. Virtues are traits or competencies of moral excellence, righteousness and goodness. Some of these traits might include integrity, self-awareness, responsibility, compassion, forgiveness, honesty and character. L.D. Pankey considered it a moral obligation to do a complete examination on all patients, and that might be all-inclusive of many virtuous competencies. In contrast to Aristotle's moral virtues, he also had intellectual virtues, and one such virtue is *phronesis*.

The dictionary definition of phronesis is the wisdom of determining the ends, and the means of attaining them. Today, we might say that a person who exhibits phronesis has practical wisdom, or the ability to create a purposeful vision and have the means to achieve it. This person then would be an expert at deliberating for the purpose of living well, and would be able to ascertain the appropriate moral virtues in any given situation. This would be the person who understands the relationship between his or her work and the decisions necessary for promoting the good life. Aristotle might have said that it's "about having the right feelings at the right time on the right occasion towards the right people for the right purpose and in the right manner." Herein lies the connection between Aristotle, L.D. Pankey and leadership. After many years of study, I have concluded that the most appropriate word for what describes the Pankey Philosophy is leadership. It is a philosophy of leadership.

Let us now turn to the three words that are a big part of the Pankey Philosophy: *ethos, pathos* and *logos*. This is usually where I lose many of my audiences in describing the philosophy, yet these three words may just be the heart and soul of all leadership, and of everything that has been written in the field over the past 2500 years. As I have described leadership earlier as the ability to accomplish worthy goals and to inspire others along the way, I imply that the leaders must have certain competencies: to create worthy goals (vision), and to inspire or communicate that vision.

Many in the leadership field have defined leadership as "human symbolic communication that modifies the attitudes and behaviors of others in order to meet shared group and individual goals and needs [2]." In other words, leadership is about influence, and influence is about communication. The number one tools at a leader's disposal are language and visual symbols that project a message. Leadership at most levels is about our willingness to interact with others. In my experience, leadership can best be understood and taught from a communication standpoint. Leadership is at the core of human experience, and it is more than just an academic exercise – it requires phronesis, or practical wisdom. Ethos, pathos and logos are the practical components of Dr. Pankey's philosophy. Essentially it is how we apply our knowledge.

The remainder of this book will dissect ethos, pathos and logos. Stephen Covey, in *The 8th Habit: From Effectiveness to Greatness*, groups these three words as the Greek philosophy of influence [3]. Ethos refers to one's character, or Aristotle's moral virtues. It is about who you are. Ethos is about your ethical nature and personal credibility. Ethos answers the question that everyone wants to know: "Can I trust you?" It is about trustworthiness, honesty and integrity, as well as your competency that surrounds your knowledge and skills of dentistry.

The competency factor is important. It is the reason why knowing our work is such an integral part of the philosophy. Patients not only want to know that you care about them, but that you are competent to do the work, as well. Many dentists can talk the talk, but not all can walk the walk. Cowboys who just look the part are said to be "all hat and no cattle." Who you are is deeply connected to how well you do your work. There are numerous traits and competencies that make up one's ethos. That is the subject matter of Part III.

Under the heading of ethos, we should take a look at what would make a bad leader. Sometimes, we can get a good view of what it takes to be a leaders by looking at the flip side, or what are some of the traits of bad leadership. Anyone who has practiced dentistry for any amount of time will be able to identify bad leadership. Many researchers in the leadership field have begun to categorize traits that may contribute to toxic leadership, which include:

- *Selfishness*: these are leaders who use their position for their own gain. I have discussed narcissistic leaders in another chapter. At times they may be effective, but mostly they are self-absorbed. They may appear to be knowledgeable, but it may be a ruse to sound convincing. We all know narcissistic leaders who demand obedience, respect and admiration. Nothing is more important than accomplishing their own personal goals.

  There is another group of selfish leaders who are considered Machiavellian. These leaders are very skillful at manipulation, and use any means available to achieve their goals. Through my years in dentistry, I have met many manipulative Machs who teach dentists their brand of leadership. When young dentists are in survival mode, it is easy to be influenced by these types of leaders. Selfishness is behind many of the shameless behaviors we see members of our profession commit. Good leadership, as you will see, is about being other-focused and, as you will recall, being other-focused is one of Barbara Frederickson's qualities for maintaining positive emotions.

- *Cognitive errors* – from poor decision-making. Why do dentists make poor decisions? Sometimes they don't have all of the information to make good diagnoses or create effective treatment plans. Sometimes dentists takes their lead from less informed people. At times, the dentist relies on poor employees. The worst cognitive errors occur when dentists rely on information from suppliers and salesmen, rather than their own instincts.
- *Environmental factors* – unlike the above two factors, which are internal, the environment can be a source of poor leadership. Dentists who are under pressure to produce will frequently make poor decisions. When there is pressure from outside sources like insurance companies, dentists may feel they must do what they are being told under the restrictions of the insurance policy. Of course this is not an excuse. Good leaders would not allow themselves to be swayed by any standards other than their own. Some organizations actually encourage unethical behavior. I will have more to say about this when I discuss the leader's role in creating a culture.

Harvard University's professor Barbara Kellerman has made a career out of defining "bad leadership." She states that bad leadership falls into two categories – ineffective and unethical [4]. She defines these poorly skilled leaders as ineffectual because they lack strategic or tactical planning. I would like to point out at this juncture that poorly skilled does not necessarily mean "bad hands." Dentists who have graduated from dental school do so on their manual abilities. It is the strategic planning that gets tested in the real world. She goes on to define unethical leaders as those who cannot distinguish between right and wrong, often engaging in behaviors that maximize their rewards while harming others (see selfishness). Some of the qualities that Kellerman says are true of bad leaders include: incompetence, rigidity, intemperance, callousness or uncaring, corrupt, and just being plain evil.

In the final analysis, the matter of ethos tells people who you are. I am reminded of the famous quote by Ralph Waldo Emerson: "Who you are speaks so loudly I can't hear what you're saying." As I will explain, that is why ethos or character is the first requirement of good leadership. That's my segue into Aristotle's second requirement – pathos, the requirement that is about them. Pathos is about empathy.

Pathos means persuading by appealing to the listener's emotions. The magic of emotional appeal is often spoken about in sales seminars. Pathos implies to your audience that you can feel their pain – you have empathy. You understand their needs and have made them a priority. The very best way that someone conveys pathos is to become an extraordinary listener and a skilled storyteller. By uncovering what really matters to people, we can then express emotionally how we feel through the use of a story. Habit 5 of Stephen Covey's classic book, *The 7 Habits of Highly Effective People* [5], expresses this idea of pathos in one sentence: "Seek first to understand, then to be understood." If ethos is compared to self-concept, then we can compare pathos to the art of building strong relationships. If ethos is the trust and credibility side, then pathos is the emotional side and the heart of your influence.

An opinion that is expressed throughout practice management circles is the importance of the doctor-patient relationship. Another way to look at that is through the lens of the leader-follower relationship. Many emphasize the importance of the doctor/leader in most relationships, but the relationship is a collaborative effort toward shared objectives. We rarely see the patient as someone who brings contributions to the relationship outside of the fee. We depend on the patient's compliance and cooperation, in order to achieve our very best work. By shifting some of the spotlight from the dentist to the patient or the staff, our perspective changes, and so does the level of communication. In shared leadership situations, responsibility for achieving goals is distributed evenly throughout the group – doctor, patient and staff.

Finally, the last requirement, logos, means "word" in Greek, refers to the logical or rational component of your presentation. Dentists usually refer to the treatment plan as the logos part.

That portion of your examination in which you have invested so much time and energy, that you cling to like a treasured heirloom, the treatment plan that you will go to your death to defend – well, that's your logos. It's your claim to fame. It's your justification for even sitting down with your patient. It's the well-thought-out logic of every single step you will take to bring your patient to that perfect conclusion. It's technical dentistry and everything we know about the work of dentistry. It's what you spent all those hours in dental school for, and what you continue to spend all your money on when you take a continuing education course. It is the *raison d'être* for dental school. Logos was Aristotle's favorite technique of the three. Remember, he was a master of reasoning, a brilliant logician, and a great persuader in his own right. After all is said and done, doctor, you had better know your work, or else we become "all hat and no cattle."

Aristotle believed that salesmen were the most important citizens of ancient Athens. They were the true leaders of Athens, because salesmen, more than any other profession, understood rhetoric. Rhetoric is the study of effective use of language – the leader's toolkit. According to Aristotle, rhetoric is "the ability, in each particular case, to see the available means of persuasion." When you consider that 82% of dentists in America are entrepreneurs – that is, they own their own dental practices – then it might be a good idea for them not only to learn how to do fine dentistry, but to learn how to sell it as well.

Ethos, pathos and logos are the essential ingredients of good leadership. Notice the sequence. Recently I saw this whole concept played out in my office – a real-life embodiment of ethos, pathos, and logos. Ernie, a 20-year veteran patient/friend in my practice, came in for his hygiene appointment. Ernie had recently returned to the practice after suffering through an extremely painful incident in his life. His eldest son took his own life. Ernie followed his son home one night and watched as he drove his vehicle into a tree. Ernie, as you can well imagine, had a nervous breakdown. His life was put on hold. Teeth were no longer a priority.

In time, with the help of expert psychiatric care, he got his life back. On this particular morning, Ernie came in very distressed; you might even say agitated. Evidently, he hadn't taken his medication, and he was having some family issues that needed to be resolved. He had a dental appointment, but he wasn't really in my office for his teeth. Ernie needed help. He commandeered my office by asking my staff and me to assemble in my private office. He stood behind my desk and said that he loved every one of us. He told me that he trusted me like a brother. He then said that he needed to speak his mind and get things off his chest. Ernie then told us his rules. No one could speak until he gave us permission, until he had been heard. I envisioned a scene from the movie, "*Dances with Wolves*," when the Indian chief passed around a "talking stick." Finally, Ernie said, if we did this, he would do anything we recommended, including readmitting himself into a mental hospital.

The morning ended well. Ernie was admitted for psychiatric care, and he has totally recovered. He is doing fine and keeps his appointments – the old Ernie is back. A few days after the hygiene event, I realized that Ernie, even in his altered state, had demanded what Aristotle described: ethos (his trust in us), pathos (his need to be listened to), and logos (our final recommendation – the treatment plan). What I really found remarkable was the order of each component that Ernie described. Ethos and pathos were prerequisites for logos. In other words, the order of requirements was just as important as the requirement itself: ethos, then pathos, and then logos.

This is the natural order of things. First your credibility and trust, then establish empathy and finally you make your case logically. Most people get it backward. They go straight to logos, the left brain logic of their ideas. When they meet resistance they become frustrated and blame staff and patients, by continuing to convince other people of the validity of their logic without taking ethos and pathos into consideration.

I want to make this distinction because, in applying ethos, pathos, and logos, it needs to be in that sequence. In learning ethos, pathos, and logos, we need to learn the rational, logical dentistry first, or else we will become all hat and no cattle.

That is why our dental education focuses on the technical. The responsibility of our dental school education is to provide you with the tools to enable technical competence. That is the major requirement of being a dentist. Inevitably it won't get you to the pinnacle of success. In other words it is what got you "here," but it won't get you "there." Some have called this technical competence or technical intelligence. L.D. Pankey called it "know your work," and Aristotle called it logos.

Pathos, or "know your patient" in modern psychologic language, has been renamed "Emotional Intelligence" (EQ or EI) by author Daniel Goleman. It includes all of the competencies that help build relationships, including self-awareness, self-regulation, motivation, social skills and empathy [6]. The other intelligence of a good leader, moral intelligence (MI), is one that is the least popular and most difficult to apply because, unlike the other two, it is values-based. That point opens up many questions about a person's individual values and goals. It creates moral dilemmas, as you will see. Yet, as you will also see, moral intelligence is still based on human universal principles.

Authors Doug Lennik and Fred Kiel call technical intelligence the "threshold competencies," because they are the price of admission to the leadership ranks [7]. They call the other two – moral intelligence and emotional intelligence – the *differentiating competencies*. These two, the ethos and the pathos, knowing yourself and knowing your patient is what will differentiate you as a leaders and enable you to have a rewarding and sustainable career in dentistry. At times, you will realize that the specific skills and competencies will blend into one another, because developing traits like empathy, compassion and forgiveness must be realized at the "self" level before they can be applied to others.

Let's begin our description of the three dimensions of leadership with a discussion of the competencies of moral intelligence.

References and Notes

1 Michael Puett and Christine Gross-Loh (2016). *The Path: What Chinese Philosophers Can Teach Us About the Good Life*, p. 18. New York, NY: Simon and Schuster.
2 Michael Z. Hackman and Craig E. Johnson (2013). *Leadership: A Communication Perspective*, 6th edition. Waveland Press, Inc.
3 Stephen R. Covey (2005). *The 8th Habit, From Effectiveness to Greatness*, pp. 129–131. Free Press; Reprint edition.
4 Barbara Kellerman (2004). *Bad Leadership*. Boston: Harvard University Press.
5 Stephen R. Covey (1989). *The Seven Habits of Highly Effective People*. Fireside Book, Simon and Schuster.
6 Daniel Goleman (2011). *On Leadership. HBR's 10 Must Reads, What makes a Leader*, Harvard Business Review Press.
7 Doug Lennick and Fred Kiel (2005). *Moral Intelligence*, 1st edition, p. 5. Pearson Prentice Hall.

9

What Adam Smith Knew

"The only thing worth writing about is the human heart in conflict with itself."

William Faulkner

"True leadership is moral authority, not formal authority. Leadership is a choice, not a position. The choice is to follow universal timeless principles, which will build trust and respect from the entire organization. Those with formal authority alone will lose this trust and respect."

Stephen Covey

"Why was Lincoln so great that he over-shadows all other national heroes? He really was not a great general like Napoleon or Washington; he was not such a skillful statesman as Gladstone or Frederick the Great; but his supremacy expresses itself altogether in his peculiar moral power and in the greatness of his character."

Leo Tolstoy, quoted in *The World,* New York, February 7th, 1908

I am a blogger. At least once per week, I sit down and compose a blog post for the dental community on TAOofDentistry.com. My topics are random, but they usually are about the soft skills dentists need to practice successfully. Because it is a public domain, patients, at times, will read the posts. Occasionally, I receive letters from patients who feel that they need to vent after going to the dentist. Honestly, I usually find these letters filled with a lot of anguish, and the patient looking for guidance in seeking some kind of resolution to their being treated improperly. Many of the letters are like the following I received from Ellen (name changed):

Question:

My daughter had a bad toothache and she is no longer covered under my plan. Samantha is now 19 years old. She works and pays for her own way. I found a new dentist for her. The receptionist said the dentist is the best, and they will work with her budget there. I explained that she is paying out of her own pocket. The dentist started the root canal the day he examined her. I wanted to wait, but the dentist said she is in pain and needs the root canal started. When we went home that day I did some research on Dental Discount Plans. I took out a plan that this dentist accepts. The office would not accept the plan for the root canal $1,400, but they accepted the discount for the temporary and the permanent crown. She wound up paying $2,400 all together from start to finish. I helped her pay the balance, but it was a struggle for me to come up with the extra money she needed. It wasn't easy but we managed to scrape

---

The Complete Dentist: Positive Leadership and Communication Skills for Success, First Edition. Barry Polansky.
© 2018 John Wiley & Sons, Inc. Published 2018 by John Wiley & Sons, Inc.

the rest of the money together. When the root canal was completed she had a cleaning and a few x-rays taken. The dentist said Samantha had rotted roots in another tooth, and she needs another root canal. I thought not again, this poor kid doesn't have this kind of money, but she does have the Discounted Dental Plan to start with this time. She is receiving the discounted root canal, but now the office manager has tacked on an additional $250.00 for lab fees, which were not charged for the previous root canal they finished the week before. I do not feel this is fair to tack on additional fees for the office to try and make up for the discounted dental plan. If they do not want patients to use a discounted plan they should not say they accept the plan and then find a way to get extra money out of their patients. My daughter doesn't want me to say anything because she still needs her permanent crown and she said she will feel uncomfortable. I am holding my tongue but this is my daughter and I don't want her to be taken advantage of. Is there anything I can do about the $250.00 lab fee charge that all of a sudden they are charging her? I could really use some advice.

I showed the letter to some of my dental colleagues, and asked what they thought. Many could see both sides of the issue. It's hard to find fault with the dentist, who is trying to get a patient out of pain. Many of the dentists acknowledged the tough situation the mother was in, and that it was a mistake to seek help from an outside source like the Dental Discount Plans, which have skyrocketed in this new economy. Some dentists pointed their finger at the mother, claiming she should take more responsibility for her daughter's health. Many wondered what the extra $250 charge for a lab fee on a root canal consisted of. Yes, there may have been some holes in the story, which should tell us why communication is so important.

My thoughts were different. The letter sounded more truthful to me than just another story of another patient complaining. The story showed a lack of empathy on the part of the dental practice. In today's world of business we see this all the time. I saw a mother and her child needing a quick solution to a long-term problem, and yes, neglect was probably the cause, but that is no reason not to extend all of the help we are capable of providing. People fill hospital beds because of things they did to themselves like overeating and smoking. Is that any reason to treat them without empathy. The other issue that clouded my vision is that I truly see this behavior within our dental community all the time. I guess this is why "know yourself" and ethos is such a big part of leadership. This letter to me was a failure in leadership at the first level of ethos, and then carried through the practice as a failure in pathos. It wasn't, like so many, a failure at the dental level. Here is what I wrote to the mother:

Ellen

There were probably many other ways to handle your daughter's case. In this tough economy, dentists see this all the time. Dentistry is expensive. First, realize that the Discounted dental people are not your ally. They are strictly a fiduciary agency, who "bargain" with dentists to take lower fees. That being said, dentists are under pressure to accept these plans.

A dentist who truly has the best interests of his patients at heart will generally not align himself with third parties, and will create situations where the dentistry is accessible at fair fees.

The dentist could have – should have – started by getting your daughter out of pain by just doing a simple pulpotomy, without committing her to the root canal. That fee may have been about $300, which would have been applied to the final root canal.

THEN…

A complete examination should have been done which would have revealed all of her problems – and you both could have sat down with the dentist to discuss ALL options.

A successful pulpotomy could last for more than 6 months – so no one is under the gun to make quick decisions.

Now you have a situation where the treatment is out of order, and the bills are piling up.

My advice: forget the discount dental plan. Find an ethical dentist – principle-based – and calm down – start again.

As far as any recourse, sad to say, these are tough times in dentistry – you can complain to your State Board, but there is no malpractice. This falls under caveat emptor.

One of the reasons I write my blog is to help correct these things that our industry has become way too complacent about.

Good Luck

Earlier, I wrote about the paradox of duty and desire. In order to reconcile that paradox, we must make choices. Those choices are the essence of moral leadership and ethos. In the situation above, which sadly occurs all the time in dentistry, the dentist must make choices, and they are, generally, not easy. But that is what leaders do. Most dentists are in business, and are asked to make tough decisions every day. Every decision has a consequence. Our lives depend on the choices we make.

Most dentists seek business advice from practice management people and consultants. Their advice is generally the advice of "management issues," and only looks at economic consequences and considerations. Time management, money management – the management of things. People management is a tougher game, and that is the difference between management and leadership. That is what led leadership guru Warren Bennis to say, "Managers are people who do things right and leaders are people who do the right thing. Both roles are crucial, and they differ profoundly, I often observe people in top positions doing the wrong things well." That's what makes this whole game so difficult.

In Chapter 2, I implied that Adam Smith may have been the first behavioral economist. He began his career as a moral philosopher in 1759, with the publication of his first book, *The Theory of Moral Sentiments*, which eventually led to his later, more popular book, *Wealth of Nations*. The very choices that leaders are being asked to make is between the economics of daily practice and doing what is right for everyone. The daily practice of dentistry involves making tough choices. Our values will guide us, and that is why value clarification is so important. Keep in mind that not everyone shares the same values. One of the jobs of a leader is to clarify his or her own values, and make sure that team members and patients are in alignment – hence the term, "shared values". But the real question is whether we truly know the difference between right and wrong – between right values and wrong values.

Robert M. Pirsig, author of *Zen and the Art of Motorcycle Maintenance: An Inquiry into Values*, said, "Peace of mind produces right values, right values produce right thoughts. Right thoughts produce right actions and right actions produce work which will be a material reflection for others to see of the serenity at the center of it all." At the end of the day, it is not the knowing but the doing that makes all of the difference. Through their actions, leaders create a culture and an environment that is the reflection of their good work.

Adam Smith would argue that because we are endowed with an impartial spectator that at some level we know the difference between right and wrong. He would argue that the human brain is hard wired for morality. Adam Smith would have been an advocate for Moral Intelligence (MI).

We are endowed with a moral compass, and Dr. Peter Dawson's WIDIOM rule is a good example of this. Asking ourselves how we would treat ourselves or our loved ones should answer our most significant moral decisions (Would I Do It On Me?). That question alone acted as my GPS system for many years. Recall that selfishness is the telltale sign of bad leadership. Self-interest is not selfishness. WIDIOM implies that we will treat ourselves well because of self-interest, but that does not mean selfishness. Hillel, the first great BCE Jewish sage of the Talmud, asked, "If I am not for myself, who will be for me? If I am only for myself, who am I?"

I have already mentioned the work of anthropologist Donald Brown [1], who has studied human universal concepts all over the world. His research found that the moral codes of all cultures include recognition of reciprocity, responsibility, and the ability to empathize. All of the world's religions preach common values: commitment to something greater than self, responsibility, respect, and caring for others. In other words, at some level there is a universal moral compass. If we are born with the hardware of a moral compass, then why is it that we often disagree about what is right and what is wrong? It comes down to the moral software, or what we learn from our parents and our culture.

New York Times columnist David Brooks has weighed in on the values issue in his book, *The Road to Character*. He asks readers to describe the moment that America's values changed. For him it was the 1969 Super Bowl, when the New York Jets played the Baltimore Colts. The quarterbacks of both teams came from small steel towns in Western Pennsylvania, but were born ten years apart. Those ten years represented two different moral cultures. The older man, the Colts quarterback Johnny Unitas, came from a strict religious moral background – a Catholic school in the old tradition. He was a walk-on who earned everything he got. During the off-season he worked as an insurance salesman, earning $125 per week. To Johnny Unitas, football was just another unglamorous job, like being a plumber. David Brooks compared Unitas to Joe DiMaggio in baseball, "who came to embody a particular way of being a sports hero in the age of self-effacement [2]."

I grew up in the sixties. I remember the younger quarterback, Joe Namath very well. He came to be known as Broadway Joe when he became the Jets quarterback after a stellar career at the University of Alabama. Instead of black high-top sneakers, Namath became a fashion plate on the field, with white shoes and long flowing hair, in contrast to the Unitas crew-cut. To the understated, soft-spoken Unitas, Joe Namath was an outspoken center of attention, who filled the tabloids with headlines. Namath became his own brand, and represented a lifestyle that many young people of the day admired. His brashness led him to predict a victory in that Super Bowl over the heavily favored Colts. And his prediction came true – Broadway Joe became a superstar and a cultural icon. Essentially, both of these men represented prototypes of two different moral cultures.

To David Brooks, this Super Bowl marked the beginning of what he calls the "Big Me" era, which emphasizes external success. It was the beginning of changing how we describe ourselves – whether we use what he calls résumé virtues or eulogy virtues. The former are the ones you list on your résumé, the skills you bring to the job market and contribute to external success. The eulogy virtues are deeper. These are the virtues that make up your legacy – the ones that are at the core of our being, or who you really are. These are the virtues that Donald Brown called the universal moral compass – kindness, honesty, responsibility. Yet Brooks tells us that, in our modern culture, we are more concerned with the résumé virtues – in the economics, rather than the morality. He warns us that in order to live a more meaningful life worth living, like Aristotle, it pays to focus more on the eulogy virtues.

Aristotle, L.D. Pankey and David Brooks are not the only ones who have instructed us in ways to live a better life. The 21st century has become a revelation of changing values and beliefs. Every day we are being tested on how much we can stretch the nature of right and wrong. Yet, if we are hard wired for morality, why should we be so confused by this postmodern view of morality?

Each of us must determine what is right and wrong for ourselves. In order to do that, we must educate ourselves and reflect on the moral nature of things. We must use our empathic skills to serve others. We must live by a set of guiding principles based on well-thought-out values and beliefs, rather than doing what is expedient and just based on getting more fame and fortune. We must become morally discerning.

In Chapter 2, I mentioned the story that the late author David Foster Wallace told about two fish swimming, and they pass an older more wiser fish who asks, "how's the water?" After they pass the older fish, one of the two turns to the other and says, "What's water?" Foster told that story at a commencement speech at Kenyon College in 2005 [3]. Wallace had been trying to make the point that our values and beliefs are shaped by the culture in which we live. After a while, we take cultural values and beliefs as normal, everyday occurrences. We live in the age of business and success, and so many of our decisions are based on the values of business and success. Yet it is the principles, the unchanging principles of natural law, the human universals, that should guide our daily decisions. Wallace's speech was a plea for the young graduates to understand the purpose of their college education, to learn how to think, rather than be swept away by the popular beliefs and values of the time.

According to Doug Lennik and Fred Kiel, authors of the book, *Moral Intelligence: Enhancing Business Performance and Leadership Success* [4], the definition of Moral Intelligence is "our mental capacity to determine how universal human principles – like those embodied by the "golden rule" – should be applied to our personal values, goals, and actions." Returning to the letter above, I understand it may be confusing to many just where the leadership broke down. Was it an ethical matter? A communication issue? A lack of empathy for the mother and daughter's circumstances or objectives? Or was it a breakdown in the dentist's ability to break the work down into an organized sequence of events that made sense to everyone? Most of us, including myself, make a quick judgment about the dentist's ethics. Certainly, the public takes that position – but a leader sees the bigger picture.

The bigger picture is that leadership consists of all three components: the ethical, the empathic communication, and the complete understanding of the nature of one's work. It requires the awareness of understanding the simple first question that the public is asking every one of us, "Who are you and can I trust you?" There is no doubt that, through the years, the public has lost confidence in many of the professions. We live in a post-professional society, and the public expects more from us. As we go into the future, leadership at these three levels will do more to determine your success and well-being than any one determinant alone. And it starts with ethos. We may be able to fool ourselves at times, and we do, but we can never fool the public.

There is a fictional town in Minnesota called Lake Wobegon (woe be gone?). It is said to be the boyhood home of its creator, Garrison Keillor, the news reporter from the radio series *A Prairie Home Companion*, where he says, "all the children are above average." The Lake Wobegon Effect describes the human tendency for people to overestimate their achievements and capabilities in relation to others. In other words, most of us like to think of ourselves as above average. Generally, this occurs because we derive our sense of self-worth in contrast with other people. This phenomenon has been observed among drivers, CEOs, stock market analysts, college students, and state education officials, among others. Experiments and surveys have repeatedly shown that most people believe that they possess attributes that are better or more desirable than average.

Yes – even dentists. I know it's hard to believe, but it occurs when we think about our own competencies in moral, emotional and technical intelligence.

The Lake Wobegon Effect is a type of cognitive bias. A cognitive bias refers to a systematic pattern of deviation from norm or rationality in judgment, whereby inferences about other people and situations may be drawn in an illogical fashion. Princeton behavioral economist Daniel Kahneman and his colleague Amos Tversky first described cognitive bias in 1972. It grew out of their experience of people's inability to reason intuitively with greater orders of magnitude. The brain uses these cognitive biases to produce mental shortcuts called heuristics that are the results of these quick information-processing rules. Through the years, many cognitive biases have been investigated and described [5]. It just so happens that the Lake Wobegon Effect is known in the scientific community as the *illusory superiority effect*, whereby people overestimate their own qualities and abilities, relative to others.

This principle of human nature may be one reason why knowing ourselves is not as easy as Socrates, Aristotle and L.D. Pankey told us it would be. It may be one of our biggest barriers to becoming better leaders. I find myself getting into sticky conversations with dentists, when I suggest that they take a closer look at their abilities in moral and emotional areas. They are generally ready to accept technical deficiencies but, in the areas of moral competence, they seem to think they are doing very well. Even reading this right now may be making some readers uncomfortable, especially in light of the story that opened this chapter. If we can somehow learn the moral and emotional competencies, it will make our jobs that much easier because, as you will see when people sense that a leader really cares about them, the human brain secretes the hormone oxytocin, which increases trust levels exponentially [6].

I could simplify (reduce) this chapter to just saying, "do the right thing" or "be a mensch." But that would be just another example of reductionism.

Learning moral competencies is a lifelong process. It began in childhood. It continued through adolescence and even into our golden years. Because the cultural values have changed so much, we need constantly to be reminded to stick to principles. We learn the moral competencies everyday in our day-in-day-out decisions that usually involve high emotional circumstances. We learn to become more competent on a patient-by-patient, person-by-person, case-by-case, situation-by-situation basis. That is why I propose we learn and study moral and emotional competence in dental school and beyond. The rest of this part of the book will discuss some of the many everyday competencies it takes to become an effective dental leader. The first one is simply to become more aware.

References and Notes

1 Donald Brown (1991). *Human Universals*. Philadelphia: Temple University Press.
2 David Brooks (2015). *The Road to Character*, pp. 240–243. Random House.
3 David Foster Wallace (2009). *This Is Water: Some Thoughts, Delivered on a Significant Occasion, about Living a Compassionate Life*, 1st edition. Little, Brown and Company.
4 Doug Lennick and Fred Kiel (2005). *Moral Intelligence*, 1st edition, p. 7. Pearson Prentice Hall.
5 Daniel Kahneman (2011). *Thinking, Fast and Slow*, 1st edition. Farrar, Straus and Giroux.
6 Paul J. Zak (2012). *The Moral Molecule: The Source of Love and Prosperity*. Dutton, The Penguin Group.

10

The Foundation of Ethos – Self-Awareness and Ownership

"I think self-awareness is probably the most important thing towards being a champion."

Billie Jean King

"Being self-aware is not the absence of mistakes, but the ability to learn and correct them."

Daniel Chidiac

"The range of what we think and do is limited by what we fail to notice. And because we fail to notice that we fail to notice, there is little we can do to change; until we notice how failing to notice shapes our thoughts and deeds."

R.D. Laing

One of my favorite movies is *The Bronx Tale*. The film is a violent crime drama set in the Bronx during the very turbulent 1960s – my time. On the surface, the movie is about a young Italian-American teenager coming of age as his life path is guided by two father figures – his biological father, played by Robert De Niro, the director, and a local mafia boss, Sonny, played by the writer Chazz Palminteri. It became one of my all-time greats because I love DeNiro, I grew up in the Bronx, I love the doo-wop music, and mostly because I love stories about father-son relationships and leadership.

Palmintieri based the movie on *The Prince* by Machiavelli. The big question was, "is it better to be feared than loved?" The teenager, Cologero, struggles with this question throughout the entire movie. A perceptive viewer can easily tell that Cologero's journey was a series of awakenings. His lessons were taught by two people who were very close to him, with two very different ways of seeing the world. In one scene, Cologero is yelling at someone in the street to collect a $20 debt when Sonny sees him and calls him over. Sonny asks, "What's going on?"

Cologero answers, "This guy 'Louie Dumps' owes me 20 dollars. It's been two weeks now, and every time he sees me he keeps dodging me. He's becoming a real pain in the neck. I mean, should I crack him one or what?"

Sonny says: "What's the matter with you? What have I been telling you? Sometimes hurting somebody ain't the answer. Is he a good friend of yours?"

Cologero: "No, I don't even like him."

Sonny: "Well there's your answer right there. Look at it this way – it costs you 20 dollars to get rid of him. He's never gonna bother you again. He's never gonna ask you for money again. He's out of your life for 20 dollars. You got off cheap. Forget it."

The video can be viewed on YouTube. The look on Cologero's face after learning the lesson is priceless. Sometimes, we need a little bit of help to become self-aware.

The Complete Dentist: Positive Leadership and Communication Skills for Success, First Edition. Barry Polansky.
© 2018 John Wiley & Sons, Inc. Published 2018 by John Wiley & Sons, Inc.

That scene teaches a few lessons. One, the obvious one, is that we get to choose who we want to work with. Other people, as mentioned many times, contribute to the way we feel about ourselves and our work. In my practice, I got rid of the Louie Dumps many years ago.

Another lesson is that most people pursue happiness – actually chase it. After all, doesn't our Constitution guarantee our right to pursue happiness? What Sonny taught Cologero was that there is something more important than chasing or pursuing – that is, prioritizing happiness. If you make well-being and happiness the priority of your life, that changes everything. In order to make that a priority requires a high degree of self-awareness. By making the intrinsic eulogy virtues more important than the extrinsic virtues like money, fame and power, you will build your character.

If you have been in dentistry for any length of time, you should have noticed how competitive the field can be. It's not only dentistry: I guess all of the professions tend to have this culture of trying to be superior to our peers. This pursuit of superiority can also be detrimental to our well-being. If you recall, in the last chapter, I discussed the Lake Wobegon Effect, or our tendency to believe we are better than average, especially in the areas that cannot be measured, like the moral, eulogy virtues. Well, it just so happens that the illusory superiority effect can actually blind us to our own foibles and failings. Thus, those with a high need for superiority may end up sacrificing long-term learning and growth, for the sake of short-term boosts in hubristic pride. You will always be chasing the 20 dollars.

Early in my career, I repeatedly came across a poem that brought the self-awareness/self-deception lesson home. The poem, which is still popular today, was written by Peter Dale Wimbrow in 1934. It is worth reading:

> When you get what you want in your struggle for self
> And the world makes you king for a day
> Just go to the mirror and look at yourself
> And see what that man has to say.
>
> For it isn't your father, or mother, or wife
> Whose judgment upon you must pass
> The fellow whose verdict counts most in your life
> Is the one staring back from the glass.
>
> He's the fellow to please – never mind all the rest
> For he's with you, clear to the end
> And you've passed your most difficult, dangerous test
> If the man in the glass is your friend.
>
> You may fool the whole world down the pathway of years
> And get pats on the back as you pass
> But your final reward will be heartache and tears
> If you've cheated the man in the glass.

The look on Cologero's face was as if he had an awakening of sorts, like Sonny had knocked him out of a stupor and, for the first time, he became conscious of another way of looking at the world. What I am suggesting in this chapter is that self-awareness is one of two starting-points in helping leaders tell themselves the truth.

When I was first introduced to the Pankey philosophy, I was taught a concept known as being "above the line or below the line." It was explained as a way of identifying patients. I will explain that concept in a later chapter with regard to patients. In a nutshell, imagine a line that distinguishes people according to certain traits that a dentist may find desirable, like a high appreciation for good dentistry, or taking total responsibility for their health. Obviously, these traits would define or clarify patients who would be very compliant and good candidates for excellent dentistry. The concept of "the line" can be applied to dentists and leaders as well.

Let's take a look at what a "below the line" dentist would look like. First, they would react to every circumstance out of defensiveness and a commitment to being "right". They would be driven by their own egos and, because of this, they would become defensive. Their stress levels would soar and they would become very ineffective. They would, from a leadership standpoint, be unconscious incompetents. But once awakened, they can shift their mindset to a level of consciousness that will improve their effectiveness over time.

The awakened dentist-leader is aware. Slowly, over time, they shift their behavior toward better leadership decisions. This not only increases their effectiveness, but also shows up in their work and their lives.

This self-deception, or leadership blindness, is actually the normal state of most people. It certainly was for me. It takes some crisis, or some problem, to make us aware that the first place we need to look is toward ourselves. Strangely, and sadly, this is exactly the behavior that most of us look for in our patients and our staff. We all look for that wake-up call. The need to be right, and to protect our egos, can blind us to what we really need. I see this again and again when speaking to and working with dentists.

When a dentist realizes that he or she is "below the line", that's the starting point of self-awareness. When we realize the truth in the Joseph Campbell quote, that: "He who thinks he knows, doesn't know. He who knows that he doesn't know, knows," that is the start of a new mindset. To be humble enough to ask for feedback is another step forward in growing into a leadership role.

One of the first things a conscious leader realizes is that every conversation and every decision is not made in a vacuum. In other words, every conversation is composed of content and context. Unconscious leaders react to the content, while conscious leaders place their attention on context. All conversations have both content and context. When Pankey proclaimed that he never saw a tooth walk into his office, he was making the distinction between content and context.

Content is the "what" that is going on in the story. It answers the question, "What are we talking about?" Context asks a different question: "How are we talking about the content?" In other words, if we are just talking about the tooth, we miss the context, which is the patient, and their objectives and circumstances. The context is always about the patient's story – not the tooth. Leaders run everything through the context of the whole story.

We see this all the time in dentistry. A new patient comes into a practice with a tooth issue. The dentist looks only at the tooth. They attempt to fix the tooth without understanding the true needs of the patient. In time – sometimes a very short period of time – the fixed tooth comes out because it was not a strategic piece of a bigger treatment plan. Or, the patient used all of their resources on that one tooth and, by the time they returned, the tooth was hopeless. Many dentists consider this normal behavior, but a conscious leader will find the context, and will create a method of getting more successful outcomes. Everyone wins: the patient, because their overall health will improve, and they will be given an opportunity to "wake up" as well; the staff, because they will observe their boss doing the right, meaningful job; and, of course, the dentist will reap the reward of satisfaction of doing the right thing – over and over again.

Self-awareness is the first step in getting to know ourselves. It answers the question of who we really are. It requires us to reflect on our beliefs, values, principles and goals. Most dentists go to work and try to be "everyone's" dentist, without discerning what kind of dentistry they enjoy doing, what they consider important, and who they enjoy working on, without giving any consideration to their own personal values and guiding principles. Marcus Buckingham, the author of the book *The One Thing You Need to Know* [1], says that the one thing successful people do is that they stop doing what they don't like doing. That directive is easier said than done. It requires a total self-assessment, sometimes known as 360-degree feedback.

This feedback includes a self-evaluation, as well as direct feedback from employees, peers, and even patients. Of course this type of feedback requires the dentist to give up all sense of ego and importance. It requires a significant degree of self-honesty and trust, in knowing that the people you are working with have your interests at heart.

Early in my career, during my burnout, my ego controlled my every action. I couldn't be wrong. I was arrogant, not only to my staff but to patients as well. Early on, after I realized that I had a problem, one of my assistants approached me and told me that I looked like "a wreck." I will never forget her words and, looking back, I realize that the feedback she gave me was most valuable. I believe that was one of the early occurrences that enabled my shift toward becoming a better leader.

After that incident, I actually sought more and more feedback. I would ask my staff how I was doing. I videotaped my case presentations and asked for critiques. Slowly, over time, I began to understand myself, and began to be more discerning about who I worked on and what kinds of dentistry I enjoyed doing.

Of course, this doesn't occur overnight. It's a process and, as you will see, it requires the other two components of leadership: knowing your patient and knowing your work. The point is that knowing yourself and self-awareness, not self-deception, is the starting point. Once I knew my values, goals, strengths and weaknesses, I could align them with my vision and mission through developing systems that brought about the results that led to fulfillment.

There is another foundational virtue that falls under the heading of "know yourself." It is what I call ownership or total accountability and responsibility. In their book *Extreme Ownership* [2], former Navy Seals Jocko Willink and Leif Babin explain the importance of every Seal accepting responsibility for the accomplishment of the mission. Today, both men run a business leadership training company, using the skills they learned in the Ramadi battles in Iraq. The one point they make over and over is that the leader is always responsible (this is what they call "extreme ownership." Basically, leaders must always "own" the mistakes and shortcomings of their teams). They call it extreme ownership because the default is usually just the opposite – shifting accountability and blame.

I meet so many dentists who continually play the role of the victim. They constantly blame their lives on things that are beyond their control, from the weather, the economy, their staff, their lab, and their patients, who just don't understand the value of dental treatment. When things don't go their way, they point their finger in an outward direction. They have an external locus of control, instead of the leader's internal locus of control.

After self-awareness, taking responsibility for everything is the next step in becoming a leader. "Taking responsibility for everything" is a nice platitude, like something you might read in a self-help book – but this is a book about leadership, and leaders master the art of controlling their thoughts and feelings. It takes attention and work, but the payoff is that leaders take control over their own personal well-being and happiness by never blaming someone else, or the circumstances, for how they feel. It means figuring out ways to be happy despite other's actions, and despite external circumstances. This is the essence of understanding the gap between stimulus and response. Most people respond with blame.

Our personal lives and professional lives are filled with uncertainty. Humans don't like uncertainty; we strive for control and predictability, yet some things are beyond our control. Except our response.

It's amazing to me that we react with the same cliché of responses whenever the same situations occur repeatedly. In most dental practices, it's *déjà vu* all over again, every day. Once the dentist understands that he or she has seen the same situation before, it becomes easier to slow down and take internal control of their thoughts, which will change the feelings that are associated with every situation, whether it is a cancelled appointment, poor fitting work from the lab, or an employee who does not show up to work. Every situation results in feelings that will lead to anger, anxiety or frustration, and that can shorten a dental career in one way or another.

Eleanor Roosevelt once said, "No one can make you feel inferior without your consent." She was speaking about developing internal control of your happiness. It just takes practice, I know, because I was one who would fly off at the first sign of stress. And I still see it in my colleagues and coaching clients. With practice, leaders develop what I call a reverse paranoia, or a feeling that the universe is conspiring to bring you good luck. Remember that every feeling we experience is preceded by some thought. If we are feeling anxious, it is because we think we are losing control. If we are getting angry or frustrated, it's because we think someone is blocking our progress toward our goals. That is why we blame the patient for cancellations, instead of changing the way we build value during our case presentations, or improving our methods of collection. Blaming staff and patients only satisfies our ego for a little while – it never fixes the long-term issues.

Taking extreme ownership is more a matter of maintaining composure and calm while getting hijacked by fatiguing emotions. Maintaining one's composure and cool-headedness is a sign of good leadership. Of course, this isn't something we can will ourselves to have. It takes practice, like all of the leadership competencies. One thing a leader should never do is to expect emotional control under all circumstances; everyone loses it once in a while. The advantage leaders have, as mentioned above, is that the same scenarios tend to occur repeatedly, so we can train ourselves to recognize the situation and continue to practice our response. In time, through persistence and consistency, the strength builds, like building a muscle.

There are other specific methods to help us take internal control. One tactic which has already been mentioned is "emotional labeling," – or, rather, to tame it is to name it. Labeling the exact emotion enables you to become familiar with it and to learn how to respond better, rather than going into a reactive, blaming posture. The first thing you will notice is that it reduces and slows down the intensity of the emotion; the gap between stimulus and response opens.

Another way of dealing with an emotional hijack is through the use of cognitive behavioral techniques (CBT), like cognitive reappraisal. This is reinterpreting a negative situation so that we feel better about it. It is changing our automatic responses, the cliché of responses I spoke of earlier. By first naming the negative emotion, we can slow down and recognize our usual and customary response. We can then challenge our beliefs about what happened, and change the way we look at things from a different perspective. In time, our automatic response to negative emotions changes. Essentially, we are becoming self-regulating; we are changing our perspective by becoming more aware. That is why self-awareness and ownership are twin brothers in building the foundation of ethos.

The father of cognitive behavioral therapy, Albert Ellis, developed a model for helping to slow down the emotional hijack. He called it the ABC model. Let's take a look how it may be applied in dentistry:

- Adversity – a patient cancels a two-hour appointment without notice.
- Belief – "That so and so … they have no regard for my time … what a jerk."
- Consequence – you begin to lose trust in patients. You tighten up your view on all patients.

Some year later, Martin Seligman, a disciple of Ellis, added a few more steps and called it the ABCDE model [3]:

- Disputation – this is the point where a leader is in the gap and provides some counter-evidence, such as, "maybe there was an accident or another serious emergency at home."
- Energization – that moment when the leader can celebrate that they didn't flip out, do something they might regret and lose their composure for the rest of the day. This is that moment of truth where all leaders are judged. The response has much to do with the culture that develops – a topic I will discuss in a coming chapter.

It is in these moments that our energy either gets replenished or it gets sucked out of us. Eventually, the negative emotions that develop from our daily adversities affect our general health and well-being. It is in these moments that leaders make the tiny choices that help them to survive and sustain over time.

By developing self-awareness and becoming more conscious, we accept ownership of our personal and professional lives. Author and philosopher Sam Keen had this to say: "Burnout is nature's way of telling you, you've been going through the motions your soul has departed; you're a zombie, a member of the walking dead, a sleepwalker. False optimism is like administrating stimulants to an exhausted nervous system." Leaders do not kid themselves with false optimism based on a "just world theory." They don't fool themselves by telling themselves how the world "should" work."

All of this thinking and taking control of our emotions can get exhausting. Studies have shown that we have only so much energy to apply toward building willpower, self-control, and consistency. Florida State psychology professor and researcher Roy Baumeister says that self-control and willpower is more than just a self-help metaphor. Self-control relies on glucose, because it is a limited energy source. Because self-control, self-regulation, and the creation of habits that help to develop leadership skills require physical as well as emotional energy, this would be a good time to review some of the things that leaders do not take for granted – that is, leading a healthier lifestyle.

Leading a healthy lifestyle can do wonders for increasing resilience and creating optimism. For me, as mentioned earlier, one of the first things I did during my burnout was to run. Running was just the beginning of creating a lifestyle that included a better diet, yoga, and weightlifting. All of that led to better sleep patterns, more energy and much less emotional exhaustion. Put simply, a healthy lifestyle led to a clearer head.

When I became a diabetic, I automatically cut out the foods that were unhealthy. I have often said that becoming a diabetic was the best thing that ever happened to me: instant awareness. Yet, there are many diabetics who don't take the disease seriously. The average American consumes a half pound of sugar daily. In contrast, I eat nothing with more than four grams of sugar. Everything is sugar-free. It made a big difference in the way I felt. For me, the obstacle certainly became the way.

Today at age 69, I can still work a full day and leave the office without feeling tired. It may sound difficult, but everything is related to habits. Once I broke the sugar habit, I never craved it again. The same thing goes for pasta and other heavy starches. The best advice I ever heard about diet, for diabetics and non-diabetics, comes from author Michael Pollan in his book *In Defense of Food* [4]. His three simple rules are, "Eat food. Not too much. Mostly plants."

Eating right, for me, means staying away from all processed foods that come in cans or packages. I am especially aware of foods that come in clear packages, which hang around the staff room and are just tempting enough to take a handful, like pretzels. I am notorious for hiding my staff's stash if they leave clear packages around. I usually bring in trays of fresh vegetables to take their place. And let's not forget those saturated and trans fats. The result for me has been control of my blood sugar for over 25 years, weight control with a BMI of less than 25 and, most important, an increase in vitality, energy and creativity. Now *those* are benefits. This is possibly why Marty Seligman added vitality to his Well-Being Theory (V).

Another trait that I have found in many leaders is that they move. They consistently exercise. Dentistry is a sedentary job. Sit-down dentistry can be hazardous to your health. Studies show that sitting for more than six hours per day is one of the worst thing you can do to yourself. Some say that sitting is the new smoking. Some studies say that sitting too much causes more deaths, worldwide, than smoking. Exercising daily will add more life to your years and help provide the energy needed to run a dental practice – not only physically, but mentally and emotionally as well.

After diet and exercise, sleep is becoming a most significant member of the heath triad. From the dental community's perspective, sleep is becoming a new area of treatment for helping patients with snoring and sleep apnea issues, so many dentists are learning the importance of sleep and sleep interruption for their own well-being. Studies show that people need between seven and nine hours of sleep to feel well-rested, and to perform at their best. Several findings show that when we get less sleep, we tend to make worse decisions. Just getting 90 minutes less sleep per night can lower daytime alertness by more than one-third. It also affects mood, and you are more likely to feel anxious and lose ability for self-control. A lack of sleep can remove the gap between stimulus and response, which means poor choices, like grabbing that bag of pretzels, blowing off the gym, and blaming others for things that go wrong.

It doesn't take much more than a blink of an eye to change a life. Just a change of perspective, or a new way of thinking, can make us more self-aware and more responsible. It is a shame for me to see how many dentists live lives of quiet desperation because they fail to take internal control of their lives and well-being. There is no doubt that dentists have always been subjected to adversities, like most professionals. These days, school loans are weighing young dentists down even more so [5]. I don't have the answer to the school loan problem, but I do believe that if we become better leaders and take internal control, then we will find better answers and create better lives for ourselves. The answers lie in leadership.

This chapter began with my commentary about a scene from the movie *The Bronx Tale*. If you are so inclined, take a look at that scene. We can learn a lot about life from Hollywood [6]. Life's lessons can come from anywhere. In that scene, I noticed how, within a blink of an eye, young Cologero changed his entire outlook on life. Just perspective. I also noticed how reactive he was, and how in control Sonny, the mafia boss, was. Leadership is not restricted to a dental practice. Leadership is a life skill, and is a big component of mastering the art of living. Sonny always looked cool, calm and collected. He had charisma. One definition of being cool is being marked by calm self-control. Contrary to popular belief, being cool and charismatic can be learned, and taking internal control of our emotional lives is the subject of the next chapter, on emotional intelligence and leadership.

References and Notes

1 Marcus Buckingham (2005). *The One Thing You Need to Know … About Great Managing, Great Leading, and Sustained Individual Success*, 1st edition. Free Press.
2 Jocko Willink and Leif Babin (2015). *Extreme Ownership: How U.S. Navy SEALs Lead and Win*, 1st edition. St. Martin's Press.
3 Martin Seligman (1991). *Learned Optimism*, 1st edition. Alfred A. Knopf.
4 Michael Pollan (2008). *In Defense of Food: An Eater's Manifesto*, 1st edition. Penguin Press.
5 Jessica Mai (2016). Too many millennials are facing buyers' remorse over one of the most expensive purchases they'll ever make. *Business Insider*, May 3rd, 2016.
6 Ryan Niemiec and Danny Wedding (2013). *Positive Psychology at the Movies: Using Films to Build Virtues and Character Strengths*, 2nd Edition. Hogrefe Publishing.

11

The Virtues of Emotional Intelligence

"You can't stop the waves, but you can learn to surf."

Jon Kabot-Zinn

"If your emotional abilities aren't in hand, if you don't have self-awareness, if you are not able to manage your distressing emotions, if you can't have empathy and have effective relationships, then no matter how smart you are, you are not going to get very far."

Dan Goleman

"For leaders, the first task in management has nothing to do with leading others; step one poses the challenge of knowing and leading oneself."

Dan Goleman

Dan Goleman is the undisputed father of emotional intelligence – but he did not invent the term. It was first used in 1990 by two psychology professors, John D. Mayer of the University of New Hampshire, and Peter Salovey of Yale. They first described emotional intelligence (EQ) in a 2004 Harvard Business Review article [1] as: "the ability to accurately perceive your own and other's emotions; to understand the signals that emotions send about our relationships; and to manage our own and other's emotions. It does not necessarily include the qualities (like optimism, initiative, and self-confidence) that some popular definitions ascribe to it."

It wasn't until 1995 when Goleman, a science journalist, published his mega-bestselling book, *Emotional Intelligence* [2] which, to date, has sold more than 5,000,000 copies worldwide, and was listed by *Time* magazine as one of the 25 "Most Influential Business Management Books" of all time. A summary of much of his work on leadership and emotional intelligence, *What Makes a Leader* [3], was published by the Harvard Business Review as one of only ten "must read" articles from its years of leadership publishing. Goleman's entire career, from the time he published and defined EQ for the business community, has propelled him to being the undisputed dean of emotional intelligence.

In the article, *What Makes a Leader*, he states: *"Most effective leaders are all alike in one crucial way: they all have a high degree of what has come to be known as emotional intelligence. It's not that IQ and technical skills are irrelevant. They do matter, but … they are entry-level requirements for executive positions. My research, along with other recent studies, clearly shows that emotional intelligence is the sine qua non of leadership. Without it, a person can have the best training in the world, an incisive, analytical mind, and an endless supply of smart ideas, but he still won't make a great leader."*

The Complete Dentist: Positive Leadership and Communication Skills for Success, First Edition. Barry Polansky.
© 2018 John Wiley & Sons, Inc. Published 2018 by John Wiley & Sons, Inc.

Many of us have seen dentistry change through the years. I have spent too much time discussing these changes and their causes throughout this book. One thing is for sure, technology is probably changing dentistry more than any other factor. It may be a worthwhile exercise for all young dentists to sit down and reflect what this profession will look like in ten or 20 years. We are beginning to see many of our tasks getting easier and more automated; that is what technology does, and it is a good thing. However, through the years, we see that our jobs and our roles change. This has happened before in our history, with the advent of any new technology. We are already beginning to see the greater roles our laboratory technicians are playing in our practices. I am lucky enough to work with an in-house lab that helps me tremendously in my day-to-day operations. But I also see what technology cannot and will not be able to do in the future.

Dental schools have done a wonderful job in preparing young people in the technical competencies, and many of us have a greater amount of technical intelligence, as Goleman states above. Technical intelligence is just a threshold competency – "an entry-level requirement" – especially as we meet our new future. In our new future, all jobs will change. I know, because of the intimacy of dentistry, that it is difficult for many of us to imagine that we can be replaced, yet it will happen. From dental assistants, hygienists and lab technicians, to the dentists and dental specialties, our jobs will change. The one thing that will never change, however, is human behavior. Every cultural change brings about new ways of performing work; culture and work are the variables, while humans are the constant. We have come to undervalue what only we can do.

The story of John Henry, the steel-driving man, is exemplary of how work changes. Henry was born a slave in the 1840s, and was freed after the Civil War. He worked for the Chesapeake & Ohio Railroad, and was known as the most powerful man working the rails. When it came to drilling holes by hitting thick steel spikes into rocks, he was beyond comparison. No one could match him, and many tried. But technology was changing things, and the new railroad would have to get beyond barriers that they had not seen before. The enemy in this case was Big Bend Mountain, and the bosses would have to drill right through it. Many men lost their lives drilling through the mountain, but John Henry worked tirelessly, pushing 10–12 feet every work day. No one could match him.

Then, one day, a salesman came along to the camp. He had a steam-powered drill, and he claimed it could out-drill any man. Well, they set up a contest then and there between John Henry and the drill. The foreman ran the newfangled steam-drill. John Henry, he just pulled out two 20-pound hammers, one in each hand. They drilled and drilled, dust rising everywhere. The men were howling and cheering. At the end of 35 minutes, John Henry had drilled two seven-foot holes – a total of fourteen feet – while the steam drill had only drilled one nine-foot hole.

John Henry held up his hammers in triumph! The men shouted and cheered. The noise was so loud that it took a moment for the men to realize that John Henry was faltering. Exhausted, the mighty man crashed to the ground, the hammers rolling from his grasp. The crowd went silent as the foreman rushed to his side. But it was too late. A blood vessel had burst in his brain. The greatest driller in the C&O Railroad was dead.

Some folks say that John Henry's likeness is carved right into the rock inside the Big Bend Tunnel. And that if you walk to the edge of the blackness of the tunnel, sometimes you can hear the sound of two 20-pound hammers drilling their way to victory over the machine.

The story is folklore, but its moral is that all of our jobs will change due to the changing nature of technology. In our own lifetimes, we have seen many jobs go by the wayside as industries have changed. From the obvious industries, like farming and journalism, to the airline, travel and automobile industries, work is changing – for the good and the bad.

Healthcare is a personal and intimate activity. It requires professionals to go beyond the physical and technical. It has a most important emotional component. This is what Dan

Goleman means when he says that it is the emotional intelligence that makes the leader. Those who focus only on the technical will go the way of John Henry as the future unfolds.

Before I move on to describe the elements of EQ, I want to mention the importance of cognitive intelligence. This is the subject of logos, the ability to organize our work through sequences, processes and systems. How we organize work is possibly more important than the technical component. Hopefully, I am making it clear that dentistry is more than prepping teeth, scaling teeth and taking impressions.

At the start of Chapter 9, I wrote about a letter I received from a patient about her daughter. I concluded that the dentist may have done a better job of understanding Aristotle's ethos, pathos and logos. At this point, we may be able to see better that it can be in any of the three areas – technical, cognitive or emotional – that the dentist might have done a better job. This is why I believe that dental schools must teach dentists leadership, and the components beyond the technical, to produce complete dentists who will survive in the future regardless of any technical advances.

Let us now take a look at some of the individual virtues of emotional intelligence. I also want to make clear that these virtues are just as practical as the technology. What good would this book be, if I only described the tools of emotional intelligence as spiritual attributes, rather than practical disciplines that we can take to the practice and to the chair, like so many of our science-based techniques? Many of the disciplines can be "deliberately practiced" and developed over time, just like any other dental technique, like tooth preparation and impression taking.

One note about leadership styles. When it comes to learning emotional intelligence, many of us look toward mentors for clues. Leaders come in various styles, from the subdued, quiet analytical introvert, to the authoritarian, outgoing socializer. This can become confusing. Many tend to fall back on our "fixed mindset," and tell ourselves that we just don't possess that kind of talent. The growth mindset must overcome that tendency, and realize that anything can be learned with a little effort. I will have more to say about this particular leadership trait in the next chapter.

I was not at the top of my class in dental school, but I was in the upper half. I witnessed an excessive amount of politics back then. I saw some of the very best students get rejected from graduate programs, while students who did not do as well got into some fairly elite programs. I thought it was unfair. In the last week of school, before graduation, I spent some time doing lab work with a student who was ranked in the top ten of my class. He had still not heard from a perio program that he applied to, and it looked as if he was going to go into the Army, like me. I thought it was unfair, and I told him so. I wondered who you had to know to succeed.

When I graduated and entered private practice, I observed the same thing. Success didn't naturally go to the very best clinicians. Of course, I naively felt this was unfair. I guess, looking back, I had the mistaken belief in the "just world theory" of life – that is, if you work hard and strive to be the best, you will be successful. I still believe that to be true but, as I have come to learn, there is more to the story than that. The work of Dan Goleman filled in many of the gaps.

As stated above, Goleman's definition of emotional intelligence defines three categories of competencies that make the very best leaders successful. Those with pure technical skills, like my friend in the lab, or others who have created careers only to derail, have an abundance of what L.D. Pankey called "skills." Recall that Dr. Pankey considered the complete dentist as one who possessed *care, skill, and judgment*. We all know these superstars. We meet them on the first day of dental school. They get into our heads and we begin to say things to ourselves like, "I'll never be as good as them, I don't have gifted hands." I know it was that kind of mental chatter that held me back while I was in school. It was classic fixed mindset language and yet, as I came to find out, being a successful dentist requires much more than "good hands."

Luckily, for me there was hope. Fighting the "hands" game would always be a losing battle. Don't get me wrong; I continued to take courses and get better at technical dentistry, but there was always someone better. My hope came in what Goleman calls the cognitive competencies, or those skills that centered around critical thinking, goal-setting, long-term vision and planning. Those life skills came easier to me and they, too, improved in time. Pankey would have called the cognitive competencies "judgment". This was one of my strengths, and it probably led me to write about the examination as a key practice system. But Goleman describes the third, and most important, competency as emotional intelligence, or what Pankey might have called "care." EQ is the ability to work with others and effect change.

In Pankey's time, that word was the best he had to describe what science now describes as emotional intelligence. Goleman's research has shown that emotional intelligence is actually twice as important as the other two in creating success and helping leaders to reach their goals. If cognitive intelligence helps us to define worthy long-term goals for ourselves and others, it is emotional intelligence that provides the way to get there. Emotional intelligence, as defined by Goleman's research, is comprised of five components – three inner components and two outer components. Since this section of the book is about ethos, or knowing oneself, I will describe the inner components – self-awareness, self-regulation and self-motivation. In the next section, pathos, or know your patient, I will discuss the outer components of empathy and social skills.

Self-awareness

Self-awareness is the first component of emotional intelligence, and is the starting point. It is so important that I devoted the whole last chapter to it and ownership. As a form of review, it is what Socrates meant by "know yourself." Too many leaders, as discussed, deceive themselves into thinking they are better than they truly are (the Lake Wobegon effect). According to Goleman, self-awareness "means having a deep understanding of one's emotions, strengths, weaknesses, needs and drives [4]."

A self-aware dentist understands his or her own strengths and weaknesses when it comes to taking on complex cases, or persuading patients to accept high-value complex cases. The self-aware dentist takes the time, and spends the money, to continually learn and improve to grow in his or her strong areas, and to help improve weaknesses, rather than deceive themselves about what is possible. A self-aware dentist will take the time to understand his or her long-term goals and values, in accordance with what is possible, and then create the systems and habits to succeed, rather than doing the short-term expedient thing.

Self-awareness requires a high level of honesty and integrity with oneself. It also requires a great amount of humility, to be open enough to realize that, in every area, there is room for improvement. To be open to feedback is a strength of the self-aware dentist. Asking for help from staff, as well as colleagues, is another trait of the self-aware dentist.

Self-regulation

It was just another quiet morning in Dental Clinic #3 at Fort Dix New Jersey. I was a captain in the Army Dental Corps, serving my two years after dental school. The morning started out like any other. Some patients had scheduled appointments, like any group practice, and others lined the hallway for sick call. I was on the second floor when a violent crash broke the stillness of the morning calm. The clamor and commotion was coming from the first floor. The entire clinic staff rushed to see what had happened. Once there, we all watched in shock as the periodontist melted down right before our eyes.

The periodontist was working with a new dental assistant. They were doing a routine surgical procedure, and the assistant kept handing him the wrong instruments. After a while, he became so frustrated that he placed his hand under the steel Mayo tray and flung it against the wall, causing the loud crash. The doctor continued to rant and rave about the ineptitude of the dental assistant, while the patient looked on with shock and surprise. He had lost it. There was no contrition. He continued to rant and rave about the unfairness of the clinic's policies. He never saw the distraught dental assistant crying in the corner, or the patient with a look of terror on his face. He was what some would call mind-blind.

Mind-blindness can be described as a cognitive disorder, where an individual is unable to attribute mental states to the self and other. As a result of this disorder, the individual may be unaware of others' mental states, or incapable of attributing beliefs and desires to others [5]. Popular author Malcolm Gladwell in his bestselling book *Blink* [6], asks the question to his readers: "have you ever experienced a 'mind-blind' moment?" I know I have, as I described in an earlier chapter when I broke up a dogfight. Gladwell goes on to describe the moment as where conditions become so stressful or confusing that your actions seem to bring on temporary autism. It's those moments when we seem to lose all control. That was the first and only time I witnessed mind-blindness in a professional setting, but I can say that there were many times when it got close.

Dentistry is difficult. Technically and emotionally. I am reminded of the classic book by M. Scott Peck, *The Road Less Travelled*. The latter is not a business or leadership book; I read it many years ago, to help me solve some of the emotionally difficult moments I faced on a daily basis at home and in my practice. The first words of that book taught me a lesson that has stayed with me throughout my career. It opens with these lines:

> "Life is difficult. This is a great truth, one of the greatest truths. It is a great truth because once we truly see this truth, we transcend it. Once we truly know that life is difficult- once we truly understand and accept it-then life is no longer difficult. Because once it is accepted, the fact that life is difficult no longer matters."

Every day, things have the potential to go awry. All of us have been in the situation that the periodontist went through that morning. Every day, we get to face the difficult patient, the difficult tooth or the crying child. Every day, we wake up and hope, or even pray, that the day will go without complications. We count the cars in our parking lot to make sure that the waiting room isn't too crowded, or that our whole staff is present and ready for action. We do everything to make sure things go well, yet we have a difficult time shutting off the mental chatter – waiting for the next shoe to drop. We are prisoners of our feelings.

Leaders who have mastered this second component of emotional intelligence, self-regulation, understand the need to manage their emotions, because they will always be there, as Scott Peck tells us. Self-regulation, or managing emotions, is important for leaders, because more than anything it helps to build a culture of trust and fairness. As I will discuss in a later chapter, a culture of trust helps to build a calm, friendly environment, where production and happiness prevail. Emotional calm is a top-down affair in a dental practice.

The past few years have presented many private practices with different ways to practice that threatened their core values and basic philosophical principles. Staff members approached me many times to do things that might compromise my sense of values. I have to admit that there was pressure to change because of what I like to call "marketing adversity." The mental chatter was non-stop, but I held, and provided a foundation for stability that we would weather the storm and prevail. We adjusted, and still work with, our relationship-based philosophy. I attribute that to keeping emotions in check through self-regulation. We rolled through the changes and, as Jon-Kabot Zinn says, "You can't stop the waves, but you can learn to surf."

Dan Goleman actually makes the point that self-regulation leads to a higher degree of integrity [7]. He claims that many of the bad things that happen in an organization occur because of impulsivity, or doing the expedient, rather than the most long-term valuable procedure. Those with low-impulse control tend to look at short-term needs rather than doing what is best, and that leads to problems within the organization and, especially, at the leadership level.

Dentists who manage their emotions well do not come across as the best leaders. It is the brash, emotional types – the fiery ones – who get all of the attention, but it is a sign of intellect and maturity when a dentist develops self-regulation. Through the years, I have learned continually to do a better job to slow down my thought processes. I use techniques that have turned into daily habits, like journaling and recording my feelings. I also use meditation and physical exercise to slow down the mind. It works – and I can't recall a time when I was close to becoming mind-blind. Self-regulation is another of those traits that continue to get better in time with practice.

Self-motivation

What drove me to write this book was the preservation of the dentist's well-being and happiness. In that, I believe, I share the same motivation that inspired L.D. Pankey to create his philosophy. One of the key ingredients that can stand in the way of dentists reaching success is a fall-off in motivation through the years of practice. Sustainable self-motivation is another of the components of a leader's emotional intelligence that will help sustain the dentist through years of practice.

During my years of practice, I went through periods when I just wasn't motivated to get better. In the early years, I would take continuing education courses to help with technical skills or practice management skills. Some were helpful, while others were a waste of time and money. Along the way, I met many dentists on a similar journey, but many had different motivations. When I went to the Pankey Institute, I took great pleasure in not only what they were teaching there, but also in the quality of the students who attended the continuums. They seemed driven by a different spark, almost as if driven by a calling, more than what dentistry was providing for them.

What I found interesting was that these same people would show up at the same meetings and courses. Pankey students would also take Dawson courses and Frank Spear's courses. They were not only continuing education zealots, they were driven by a need to learn, and their drive was about achievement and accomplishment. Through the years, I have seen many of these dentists become leaders in dentistry. Many have become dentistry's finest teachers, writers and speakers. It is no accident, because it was self-motivation that got them there.

The problem is that, although those dentists are very visible in our community, they are in the minority. Most dentists cannot sustain the drive and, soon after dental school, lose their motivation. Most dentists only take the required amount of continuing education. Most dentists only take technical courses that they believe will make them into better dentists, without ever questioning the other factors that lead to happiness and success. Most dentists have bought into our culture's current definitions of success and, because they are good students and good rote learners, they follow the path laid out for them. The real leaders I have met along my journey were not only good students, but they challenged the status quo and took risks in every way – not wild and irresponsible risks, but risks that challenged the current way of doing things, in order to create better lives for themselves, their families and their patients.

Self-motivation is one component of emotional intelligence that can be worked on and improved, if we recognize some of the forces that are working against today's dentists.

In Chapter 6, I discussed Seligman's Well-Being Theory, which consisted of five factors: positivity, engagement, positive relationships, meaning and achievement. Many dentists focus on the last factor – achievement – and what that means as a criteria for success. Yet, without the necessary long-term motivation, achievement of worthy goals is difficult. For many, the achievements center around money and material possessions, but they find out that it never lasts. We are all human and, certainly, making money is a worthy goal, but I have found that the dentists whom I consider to be leaders create goals that involve learning and doing for the sake of doing themselves. They love to learn and they love to grow – and, of course, the money comes as a product of their growth.

There has been study after study showing that the key to self-motivation is to enhance and augment our opportunities and abilities to make decisions. Earlier I cited a study that showed that making decisions gives us a sense of control that fuels self-motivation. If you recall, it was a study conducted during the 1990s, and it showed that, when nursing home patients were able to make choices that rebelled against the rigid schedules, menus and rules that the institution set or tried to force on them, they were able to establish a greater sense of control in their lives. They were motivated to do more, and to become more creative.

Author Charles Duhigg in his bestselling book, *Smarter Better Faster* [8] says, "*Self-help books and leadership manuals often portray self-motivation as a static feature in our personality or the outcome of a neurological calculus in which we subconsciously compare efforts toward rewards. But scientists say motivation is more complicated than that. Motivation is more like a skill, akin to reading and writing, that can be learned and honed. Scientists have found that people can get better at self-motivation if they practice in the right way. The trick, researchers say, is realizing that a prerequisite to motivation is believing we have authority over our actions and surroundings. To motivate ourselves, we must feel like we are in control.*"

People who believe they have dominion over their lives live longer, more fulfilling lives yet, through the years in dentistry, we have witnessed a relinquishing of that control to outside forces. Duhigg quotes a group of Columbia psychologists in the magazine *Trends in Cognitive Sciences:* "The need for control is a biological imperative." We gain control by autonomy in decision-making. In other words, we should reward the rebel within each of us.

Earlier, I mentioned that the thing that propelled my journey was that I was doing meaningless dentistry. There was another factor that I remember, and I would express it to myself as being "the master of my own destiny". To make that happen would require me to make decisions. Some of the decisions were wrong. None were fatal. Mostly, I continued to make things happen by just exercising my freedom of choice and making decisions. The lesson was that I was in control, regardless of what happened. Some readers may be thinking that is because I am a risk-taker, and they are risk-averse. Risk-aversion is a human trait. Most people crave certainty; I know I do. Still, just the idea of making choices gives us the feeling of control over our lives and careers, and that's the payoff.

There is no such thing as an overnight success. No one course or book will bring instant fulfillment or achievement. Success is a journey. It takes times. After 20 or 30 years of experience, we might expect to be accomplished and fulfilled but, of course, life gets in the way. It was John Lennon who said, "Life is what happens to you while you're busy making other plans." I meet so many dentists who never get the 30 years of experience. What they get is their first year experienced 30 times. It's decision making, freedom of choice and self-motivation – the third component of emotional intelligence – that makes leaders into creative artists of their own lives.

Of course, life does get in the way. The road to success is filled with potholes and obstacles. Yet, most leaders know that the obstacle is truly the way to success. It is what provides for our best learning. Leaders are endowed with three traits that will get them through during the toughest times – when life happens. The next chapter will provide leadership tools that are necessary for the trip.

References and Notes

1 John Mayer and Peter Salovey (2004). Leading by Feel. *Harvard Business Review*, January 2004.
2 Daniel Goleman (2006), *Emotional Intelligence:10th Anniversary Edition; Why It Can Matter More Than IQ*. Bantam.
3 Daniel Goleman (2011). *What Makes a Leader*, pp. 1–21. HBR's 10 Must Reads. Boston, Massachusetts: Harvard Business Review Press.
4 Ibid. p. 7.
5 https://en.wikipedia.org/wiki/mind-blindness.
6 Malcolm Gladwell (2005), *Blink: The Power of Thinking Without Thinking*, 1st edition. Little, Brown and Company.
7 Daniel Goleman (2011). *What Makes a Leader*, p. 13. HBR's 10 Must Reads. Boston, Massachusetts: Harvard Business Review Press.
8 Charles Duhigg (2016). *Smarter Better Faster: The Secrets of Being Productive in Life and Business*, 1st edition, p. 19. Random House.

12

Grit, Optimism and Resilience

"Grit is living life like it's a marathon, not a sprint."

Angela Duckworth

"Over time, grit is what separates fruitful lives from aimlessness."

John Ortberg

"Success is how high you bounce when you hit bottom."

George S. Patton

"There is an interesting scientific dispute about realism and optimism. Some find that very optimistic people have benign illusions about themselves. These people may think they have more control, or more skill, than they actually do. Others have found that optimistic people have a good handle on reality. The jury is still out."

Martin Seligman

We sat down for dinner each night at six o'clock. Josh, my youngest son, was consistently late. It wasn't the lateness that bothered us, it was more that he had ripped another pair of jeans and had bloodied his knees. He carefully placed his skateboard in the corner and sat down at the table for dinner. His clothes were greasy and grimy, as if he had been working in a garage all day. His body was battered and bruised, but he showed no signs of pain or soreness. Incongruously, he would drip spaghetti sauce on his greasy tee shirt, and rush to take it off and get it into the wash. "Does sauce stain?" he would ask, and we all laughed.

Josh has grown up to be a fine young man, someone who has made me very proud. He owns his own dental laboratory, and is a key opinion leader in the dental laboratory technician field. He is a highly sought-after speaker, and has spoken throughout the world. He taught himself dental photography and public speaking – skills, as you will see, that are both very necessary for leadership in dentistry. Most of his expertise, including his implant knowledge, was acquired without the advantage of formal professional training. He wasn't an A student while growing up, and often got himself into trouble at school. These are not the traits you would expect to see in a book on leadership and success, yet he had skills that went beyond conventional academics.

One day, while we were on vacation on the tropical island of St Maarten, Josh asked me to buy him a boogie board, which is sort of a child's version of a surfboard, or an aquatic version of a skateboard. As luck would have it, a tropical storm rolled in on our first day of vacation. The tide had come up to the base of our hotel. When I awoke and looked out at the ocean, all

The Complete Dentist: Positive Leadership and Communication Skills for Success, First Edition. Barry Polansky.
© 2018 John Wiley & Sons, Inc. Published 2018 by John Wiley & Sons, Inc.

I could see were clouds and water – and Josh flying around on his boogie board. He never stopped. All day long, he was thrown around by the shallow waves. He tossed and turned as the waves came up and flipped him over, again and again. He just laughed it off and got right back on. He was eight years old. I always knew that some day he would succeed, because of that trait. I just didn't know what to call it. Today, the positive psychologists have given it a name: grit.

Josh was exhibiting the idea of deliberate practice. He has applied the same deliberate practice to the art of dental ceramics, and to cosmetics, photography, presentation, and public speaking. It was grit, rather than the accumulation of degrees, courses, and knowledge that accounted for his success. It was grit that kept Josh in the game. It was grit, more than talent. Through his own admission, he will tell you that he has met many technicians along the way who exhibited greater talent than he had, but who ended up getting out of the field or burned out, because they didn't put the same effort into every aspect of the field. We see the same thing in all fields, including dentistry. As mentioned throughout this book, we are seeing more and more dentists having their careers derailed for various reasons. In the end, the survivors will be the ones who get tough when the going gets tough. No job, career, or calling goes smoothly. Life is a series of peaks and valleys. The tools we need to survive the valleys are grit, optimism, and resilience.

Are grit, resilience, and optimism fixed traits that people have inherited, or can they be learned? I believe, and some science backs me up, that these traits can be developed and learned, like skills. They are more than just a disposition or a personality type. All people go through hard times, but only some rebound and actually thrive. There has been much written about younger people these days, and their sense of entitlement. I don't know if there is enough evidence to support such a bold and sweeping claim. I have seen young dentists with plenty of grit to take on big challenges, but I do believe that these skills are forged through surviving tough issues.

Most of the issues for leadership are beyond the technical skills of dentistry. They lie in the skills of leadership, management, and communication. I find the greatest frustrations that the young dentist experiences are the people issues. The people issues are what test the younger dentists. They know where to go to find out the answers to their dental problems. In my career, it was learning from adversity that helped me develop the skills to get back up and learn how to do things the right way.

Of course, this takes effort.

Of course, the first question we must ask ourselves is, "if I am going to put in all this effort, will it be worth it in the end?" To answer that question, we need the energy that is supplied by optimism. Optimism is the fuel behind resilience and grit. There is some evidence that where we stand on the optimism scale is genetically determined; however, we can all change the way we look at the world. Through the use of mindfulness and the cognitive behavioral techniques of explaining things better to ourselves, we can always reassess the lens through which we see the world. Our expectations prime our behavior. The late psychologist-author Wayne Dyer is famous for saying, "If you change the way you look at things, the things you look at change." I often use that quote while coaching young people.

One morning, while leaving my yoga studio, I asked one of the teachers what she was going to do after she graduated from college. I had heard rumors that Aly was going to go to medical school. She surprised me when she told me how tough the MCATs were going to be. I was taken aback. Bikram Yoga teachers have to go through 14 weeks of intensive training to become licensed. They have to perform under the most intense circumstances. I knew she was one of the best students in her class, and has become one of our best teachers. I asked her why she was changing her mind about medical school. She replied that she didn't know if it was going to be worth it to spend all of the energy and effort to study for the MCATs, only to fail.

Well, that became a coaching moment. But the driver of her attitude was her outlook. She needed an optimistic view of the outcome. What was the difference between learning yoga and becoming a doctor? Was it that she was able to see herself doing the postures during practice, that she knew she had what it would take if she just applied herself, and that becoming a doctor was too vague and the competition too great that she didn't know whether she had what it would take. Was she good enough?

Conversations like these are more prevalent these days than when I grew up. Maybe it's the culture or the times. It doesn't matter. It's optimism that will provide the fuel. It takes energy to get off the couch and out of one's comfort zone. It seems that we are living in the age of complacency these days. We settle. In her enlightening new book, *Grit* [1], positive psychologist Angela Duckworth tells us that we are distracted by talent.

Throughout our careers, we are taught that the most talented are the ones who become successful. Before I entered dental school, the only talent I exhibited for dentistry was my ability to carve a block of wax. I assumed that everyone who made it in had the same ability, more or less – and, of course, we all did well in college and on the dental boards. The journey up until that point was all about talent and staying within the rules. However, things changed once we entered dental school. It wasn't difficult to see who the "best hands" people were and, from the beginning, the talent issue was raised again.

But that is not what creates success in the real world, according to Duckworth. It's effort. It's work ethic. It's passion and perseverance. These are the components of what she has labeled *grit*. It takes grit to be successful in the real world of dentistry, which goes beyond learning how to do excellent dentistry, but also how to master all of the components of dentistry that I call dental leadership. Dental school certainly tests our self-esteem. We think it's talent, personality and style that will determine our career outcomes, when those things play a small role in how far we will actually go. So who becomes the most successful dentists? The ones with the best hands and the best grades? Are the schools preparing us to be our very best? Are book smarts more important than street smarts? How do we get the social, emotional and practical skills that I call leadership skills to function best in the real world?

Most dental and medical students learn to follow the rules of education from an early age. That is what is responsible for their success – but only so far. William Deresiewicz, author of the book *Excellent Sheep* [2], mostly talking about the elite Ivy League schools, writes how education should be a time for self-discovery, when people can establish their own values and measures of success, in order to forge their own path. He believes that our education should provide a time and place to mold character, in addition to careers. In other words, it is a time that students learn to build eulogy virtues in addition to résumé virtues. The question we need to ask ourselves is, "why do we go to school?" The way the system is set up now is to make a choice between learning and success. Education's purpose should be to teach students how to articulate its values. A genuine leader defines his or her path through their education.

Dental school is like getting processed through a system. "*The system produces students who are smart, talented, and driven but also anxious, timid and lost with little intellectual curiosity and a stunted sense of purpose,*" according to Deresiewicz. They are producing excellent sheep who achieve success, but who generally find themselves climbing through the wrong jungle without a sense of purpose. When they graduate, they seem lost, and in the continuation of what he calls credentialism, or the accumulation of as many gold stars as they can acquire. Most dentists, upon graduation, apply what they learned in dental schools in the most conventional manner. They never question the status quo. The times have so significantly changed, as far as the conditions for success go, that most dentists will reach their limit quickly.

The profession has done nothing to change this situation, because of a lack of leadership. Most dentists accept their jobs without questioning the defaults. The fee-for-service private practice model which was, at one time, the standard, is now the exception, because most dentists have accepted the conventional path to success. According to Adam Grant, author of the book *The Originals*, many of these *good students*, "become doctors who heal their patients without fighting to fix the broken systems that prevent many patients from affording health care in the first place [3]." In other words, it takes the other traits we have been talking about, in addition to taking the road less travelled. We must step a little out of bounds – not quite the "go along to get along" mentality that we are being taught in school. Leaders do not accept the default. They try to change the status quo. That takes grit.

I have always questioned why dentists so readily accept the system that has evolved into the status quo as acceptable. Grant explains, in his book, that justifying the default system serves a calming function. He calls it an emotional painkiller: "if the world is supposed to be this way, we don't need to be dissatisfied with it." That sounds like another version of the "just world theory" to me. Grant goes on to comment that acquiescing robs us of the moral outrage to stand against the injustice and to create a career and a life that could work. I should remind you that insurance and corporate dentistry are just another set of rules that have become the norm. They are man-made systems. We are constantly reminded that we don't have to accept those rules unless we choose to, yet they are slowly becoming the default, and readily accepted by many dentists – but not those who have chosen to become leaders.

If this sounds like too much pain and suffering, take heart. You don't have to be a daredevil skateboarder to become a leader. Many of us believe that we can't be leaders or entrepreneurs because it requires too much risk-taking, and most dentists, including myself, are risk-averse. Even the word *entrepreneur* literally means "bearer of risk." Sure, learning skills will require many of us to take emotional risks, but it just takes perseverance, discipline and consistency. No one gets hurt, but it takes some courage. It takes courage to learn how to deal with the day-to-day conditions dentists work under. Those who never take the time to learn leadership skills, and depend solely on their technical expertise and personality, eventually hit their limit. Taking the time to learn and apply all of the skills necessary for success requires patience, passion and perseverance – grit, optimism, and resilience. As the Japanese proverb tells us: "Fall down seven times, get up eight."

Dentistry is, on a daily basis, difficult work. Sometimes, the easiest part of the day is prepping teeth and taking impressions. Those technical tasks require focus and, for a few moments, we get to experience "flow" and total engagement. It's the day-in-and-day-out emotional conflicts that seem to wear us out. My biggest failures early on were about motivating patients and getting case acceptance. Over time, I was faced with a choice to give up and not present comprehensive cases, or to learn how to present better. I don't know if I could have had the career I had in dentistry without learning how to present effectively. Success breeds success. When my case acceptance improved, my desire to do better dentistry grew as well. My response to failure was to learn as much as I could about presentation. That led to studying communication, human behavior, cognitive psychology, photography, treatment planning, diagnosis, and so many other skills that seemed to have application in day-to-day dentistry.

According to the Merriam-Webster dictionary, grit in the context of behavior is defined as "firmness of character; indomitable spirit." Angela Duckworth, based on her studies, tweaked this definition to be "perseverance and passion for long-term goals." The terminology may be new, but the concept is as old as Aristotle. If grit is a character trait, then it is what Aristotle would have called a virtue. In the *Nicomachean Ethics* [4], Aristotle wrote, "*Ethical virtues are acquired by habituation; they do not arise in us from birth, but we by nature have the capacity to receive and perfect them. A good government attempts to legislate such that it helps to habituate its citizens to act virtuously. The way to become habituated in virtue is to perform virtuous actions beginning from one's early youth.*" So we are left with the question of how to develop grit as a character trait and virtue. Aristotle would say to make it a habit. To make something a habit requires effort.

Angela Duckworth's research tells us that grit, as explained above, is less about talent and more about effort. As the composer and lyricist Irving Berlin once said, "talent is only the starting point." In developing grit, Duckworth acknowledges that talent is important, but effort counts twice as much. As stated above, we want to believe that some dentists are more talented than others. I hear it all the time: "You're just an excellent communicator, or how do you know how to ask the right questions at the right time?"

Even in my son's lab, they look on in awe at his magnificent ceramics and photography. Most observers give all the credit to natural born talent, rather than the hard work that went into the excellent results. I am reminded of the famous story about Michelangelo. When someone called him a genius, his response was, "If you knew how much work went into it, you wouldn't call it genius." In anther famous reference to the famous artist, he said, "The greater danger for most of us lies not in setting our aim too high and falling short; but in setting our aim too low, and achieving our mark."

Learning the skills necessary to master dentistry requires effort through deliberate practice and habit formation. Angela Duckworth's Grit theory relies on two equations [5], both of which have *skills* as the main variable. The equations are as follows:

a) talent × effort = skill;
b) skill × effort = achievement.

She claims that her theory is incomplete, because it doesn't take into account the role of coaches and mentors, which I will discuss in a later chapter. The point of her theory, incomplete as it may be, is that effort is the predominant factor in creating success. In writing this book, and other books I have written, I keep a sticky attached to my computer that reads, "all writing is rewriting." Just keeping that in front of me reminds me of how much effort I will have to put in to finish a writing project. I have taken the same approach to every skill I have tried to master in dentistry. All learning is a struggle. Learning new skills requires patience, and very few skills can be mastered overnight without the struggle. Grit is what is necessary for the fight.

The sad truth is that most people give up way too early. They don't exhibit the persistence necessary for grit. One look at dieting and exercising tells us enough about people. Mastering dental skills – the soft as well as the hard skills – requires persistence. When I was diagnosed with diabetes, many years ago, I became committed to my personal health. I changed my lifestyle and made diet and exercise a priority. I still go to my local gym three days per week and lift the same amount of weight I started with 28 years ago. When people observe me bench pressing more than my weight, they ask how I can still do it. My answer is always the same: persistence and consistency. Effort, habit, practice.

Duckworth has concluded in her studies that people who are gritty have four psychological traits that can be developed over a period of time. The first trait is interest or passion. This is the reason I have written so much about clearing the path for dentists to maintain and sustain their interest in dentistry, even going to the point of passion and beyond. The way healthcare is set up these days, it is difficult to sustain the passion for many dentists.

The second trait is what she calls the capacity to practice. She tells us that those with a capacity to practice constantly remind themselves that, "whatever it takes, I want to improve." Most dentists truly do not understand the concept of deliberate practice. Anders Ericsson the father of the *Rule of 10,000 Hours*, which says that it takes 10,000 hours of practice to master any field, has recently clarified this as a myth. He claims that it takes the equivalent of 10,000 hours of *deliberate practice* – in other words, just putting in the time doesn't count.

In his recent book, *Peak* [6], he claims that a doctor with 20 years of experience who believes that they have reached a level of acceptable performance is no better, and possibly worse, than a doctor with only five years of experience. Those that believe that their skills are good enough, and choose to go on autopilot, are actually worse. In other words, as Angela Duckworth confirms, deliberate practice requires the person to push themselves out of their comfort zone to achieve any level of mastery.

The third trait is one we have already mentioned as one of the parameters of well-being – that is, purpose. People with grit don't quit, because underneath everything is a firm belief that their work matters. Duckworth says, and I agree, "interest without purpose is impossible to sustain over a lifetime." Your dentistry must be connected to the well-being of others to provide sustainable meaning and purpose. You must believe that your work makes a difference in the lives of your patients.

The last trait she calls hope. I call it optimism. Who could possibly survive in any career with a "what's the use attitude?" Hope or optimism is what is necessary when things don't go our way and, if you have been in dentistry for any length of time, you know that dentistry is about peaks and valleys. Things just don't go right every day. It is an expectation and belief that the effort we put forth will create better and better results. The results do not come immediately, hence the struggle. Recall Aly, my yoga teacher. Might she have needed a bit of hope?

Recently, I met a young dental technician who had just taken her certification test. I asked her how she had done, and she told me she had done poorly. I asked her when the next test was, and she said she wasn't going to take it again. I asked why, and she said it wasn't that important, and she could get a job without it. I wondered if she listened to herself. It's not about the job. It's about getting better, a sustainable career, or even a calling. Without the hope of improving those, this would be unavailable to her. This is why hope and optimism are the drivers of grit.

It is truly a shame that most people give up too soon. I once heard a motivational speaker say that most people suffer from GUTS – they Give Up Too Soon. I see it so often in all fields, but a leaders must not only have grit and be positive – they must also set the example for their patients and staff. Gritty people live by the thought, "winners never quit and quitters never win."

Martin Seligman, the architect of the Well-Being Theory discussed in Chapter 6, originally made his bones in 1964 by developing his "learned optimism" theory and writing about it in his first book by the same name, *Learned Optimism* [7]. The book was based on the original experiments that involved shocking dogs, and might be considered cruel and unusual by today's standards. Nevertheless, Seligman and his collaborator Steve Maier developed a very valuable theory [8]. Essentially, they showed that it wasn't suffering that created depression and helplessness and hopelessness, but rather it is suffering that you think you can't control. When we feel we have no control over our work or other people's behavior, we begin to feel hopeless, and lose any sense of control and optimism. Remember, 40% of our happiness is dependent on our ability to choose.

Seligman's experiment was the first of many since then that have shown how "suffering without control can produce symptoms of clinical depression, including loss of appetite and physical activity, sleep problems, and poor concentration [9]." Hopefully, I have explained how important it is, not only for dentists, but for all health care professionals, to maintain their control through total protection of their freedom of choice. Just saying it doesn't make it so. Protecting our freedom of choice, and enhancing our ability to use it in our everyday lives, is a mark of great leadership, and it needs to be taught and developed at the level of professional education.

When freedom of choice is exercised, or even believing that their are options, it leads to the feeling of control, and that there is not a sense of permanence in one's situation. With control, there is hope that whatever happens is just a temporary circumstance. Seligman believed, through his experiments with dogs, that humans too can learn to be helpless – or, better yet, they can learn optimism. Seligman's initial studies led him to his classic studies on optimism during the 1980s.

Seligman's initial studies on optimism in the mid-80s included one conducted for the Metropolitan Life Insurance Company. They commissioned him to better understand what traits certain salespeople had that enabled them to out-perform others. They wanted to identify people who:

• were better at handling frustration;
• took each refusal as a challenge, rather than a setback;
• were resilient, courageous, and would not give up;
• found solutions, followed through, and succeeded.

Seligman administered a test for optimistic mindsets. He found that those who scored in the top half for optimism sold 37% more insurance than those in the pessimistic half. Those in the top 10% of that optimistic group sold 88% more than those in the most pessimistic group. In 1995, Seligman repeated the studies across several industries. The results across all studies indicated that optimists outsold pessimists by 20–40%. Like Carolyn Dweck, who wrote about the growth and fixed mindset, Martin Seligman claimed that optimism can be learned. Seligman's research shows the power of self-fulfilling prophecies. The way a person explains events in his life, Seligman says, can predict and determine his future. Those who believe they are masters of their fate are more likely to succeed than those who attribute events to forces beyond their control.

It is interesting to note that Seligman says that the way we explain events to ourselves helps create our perspective and helps to predict our future. It makes me wonder if using language is a way to cultivate a leadership mindset that leads to success. Possibly a language that emphasizes effort over talent. I genuinely believe that dentists who succeed in the future will have to learn language beyond dental technical language. This may be true in all fields from law to medicine to computer science. The liberal arts education must be continued through one's professional education for professionals to survive and thrive. By combining the work of Carolyn Dweck and Martin Seligman, Angela Duckworth has created her own equation for grit:

growth mindset → optimistic self talk → perseverance over adversity [10]

Dentistry is difficult, and no one's career goes smoothly, no matter how it looks when you evaluate other's practices. That is why these traits are so important. Everyone stumbles; everyone struggles, especially with people issues. We all fall down and must get back on the horse. Resilience is the trait that enables us to get back up on the horse. Futurist and author Andrew Zolli, in his book *Resilience* [11], defines resilience as "the ability of people, communities, and systems to maintain their core purpose and integrity among unforeseen shocks and surprises." Zolli describes grit as a level of hardiness that is composed of a combination of optimism, creativity, and confidence, which empower people to solve problems and create success. In other words, optimism and resilience are key components of grit. Gritty people believe, in a nutshell, that everything will be all right in the end and, if it's not all right, it's not the end.

Before leaving this chapter, I want to make the distinction between perfection and excellence. Dentists are notorious for calling themselves "perfectionists", as if that is some kind of virtuous trait. Gritty people do not necessarily strive for perfection. Taking on difficult cases will cure most dentists of the need for perfection. Take the single central incisor as an example. The perfect single central in nearly impossible. Coach John Wooden used to say, "Perfection is impossible, but striving for perfection is not. Do the best you can. That is what counts." Doing the best you can leads to excellence. Perfection may be an ideal, or a standard to shoot for, but it is mostly impossible to reach. Perfection is chasing someone else's perception of an ideal or standard. Perfectionism has been linked to many psychological disorders like anxiety, low self-esteem, obsessive-compulsive disorder, substance abuse, and clinical depression. All of these are limiting factors to success and leadership.

Perfection is a result which is probably unachievable. Excellence is a process. I will have much more to say about process in the section on Logos. Leaders are process oriented, excellence then, like grit, resilience, and optimism is an attitude. The Greek word for excellence is arete, which is associated with the idea of fulfilling a purpose or function. Hence, excellence is another virtue in Aristotelian terms. As a matter of fact, the old Greek had something to say about excellence as a virtue, which seems to sum up this whole chapter: "Excellence is never an accident. It is always the result of high intention, sincere effort, and intelligent execution; it represents the wise choice of many alternatives – choice, not chance, determines your destiny."

Excellence allows us to fail and start again. It allows us the freedom of humility and vulnerability, both additional virtues of strong leaders. It allows for mistakes and failures that are required for learning, growth and self-improvement.

Recently, I had a patient return to my practice because she was dissatisfied. Three years prior to her return, we made her a crown over an implant and abutment for a single right central incisor. It was directly next to a natural left central incisor. The implant was placed by a competent periodontist who did an excellent job of preparing the site for an immediate placement. Matching the shade, shape, pitch, and gingival contours truly tested our abilities. After two try-ins, everyone was satisfied, but we could sense that the patient was not totally in agreement. We let her wear it for a short period. She came back and approved it for cementation. Three years passed. She never returned for any other treatment. My son and I used the case in our presentations to other dental professionals. All of the feedback was positive. Then she returned.

The patient was dissatisfied. She told a story about how she went for surgery and an anesthesiologist commented to her about how beautiful her smile was – except for the crown in the front. That was all the impetus she needed to complain. My immediate response was to remake the crown, because my aim is to always please. She was abusive both to me and to my son. We decided that we could never get it perfect. Recall the definition of perfect as someone else's standards. Three years had passed, and it was well beyond the statute of limitations.

I recalled the story I told earlier from *The Bronx Tale* – that for $20, I never had to see her again. We pursued excellence and got a great result. She wasn't happy, and that bothered us. The case tested our resilience, because we only want to make people happy. It tested our vulnerability and humility, because no one is perfect. It bothered me for a day or two, then we sent her a check and got right back on the horse. Stories like that are more common in dental practice than we would like to believe; I am sure you have some of your own.

As I am finishing this chapter, the news of the day included the passing of Muhammad Ali, arguably boxing's greatest heavyweight champion of all time. Over 100,000 people are expected to attend his funeral in his birthplace home of Louisville, Kentucky. Sure, Ali will be remembered for his legendary fights and fighting styles, but he will also be remembered for the same traits that we have been discussing in this chapter: leadership, grit, optimism, resilience, and excellence. All of those virtues led to the life of a champion. In an interview, he once said, "I know myself – I know where I stand, even when I am booed, I know other's opinions of me – I know my strengths. My greatest opponent is in the mirror." That is the essence of ethos.

References and Notes

1 Angela Duckworth (2016). *Grit: The Power of Passion and Perseverance*, 1st edition, pp. 15–34. Scribner.

2 William Deresiewicz (2014). *Excellent Sheep: The Miseducation of the American Elite and the Way to a Meaningful Life*. Free Press.

3 Adam Grant (2016). *The Originals: How Non-Conformists Move the World*, p.10. Viking.

4 Aristotle (2013). *Nicomachean Ethics*. CreateSpace Independent Publishing Platform.

5 Angela Duckworth (2016). *Grit: The Power of Passion and Perseverance*, 1st edition, pp. 42–45. Scribner.

6 Anders Ericsson and Robert Pool (2016). *Peak: Secrets from the New Science of Expertise*. Eamon Dolan/Houghton Mifflin Harcourt.

7 Martin Seligman (1991). *Learned Optimism: How to Change Your Mind and Your Life*, 1st edition. Alfred A. Knopf.

8 Angela Duckworth (2016). *Grit: The Power of Passion and Perseverance*, 1st edition, pp. 171–173. Scribner.

9 Ibid., p.173.

10 Ibid., p. 192.

11 Andrew Zolli (2012). *Resilience: Why Things Bounce Back*, 1st edition. Free Press.

13

The TAO of Dentistry and a Culture of Trust

"The final requirement of effective leadership is to earn trust. Otherwise there won't be any followers, and the only definition of a leader is someone who has followers."

Peter Drucker

"How can we create a cultural legacy of happiness? Let other people matter."

Christopher Peterson

"Our number one priority is company culture. Our whole belief is that if you get the culture right, most of the other stuff like delivering great customer service or building a long-term enduring brand will just happen naturally on its own."

Tony Hsieh, CEO, Zappos

Sometimes, I see dentists from a different perspective. I am the owner of a dental laboratory with my son. I am a hands-off owner, mostly acting as a sounding-board when he needs some guidance or wisdom. Generally, the most difficult problems he confronts are the people issues, rather than the technical issues. Through my own experiences of practicing dentistry for over 40 years, I have a unique perspective on many of the problems. After doing this for a few years, I came to see certain patterns that repeated themselves. I began to see how many of the problems appeared to be specific and incidental in nature but, in the end, revealed themselves as leadership issues that spread into cultural issues. Those cultural issues also repeated themselves, and resulted in workplaces that were troubled by high turnover, high stress and poor overall performance [1].

Up to this point in the book we, have been talking about the ethos of leadership. Getting to know yourself goes a long way in the development of a leader. The biggest payoff in knowing ourselves goes beyond the self-awareness, self-motivation and self-control that I have written about. The biggest payoff is the creation of a high-performing organization through the creation of culture. Ninety percent of business leaders agree that culture is critical to success. Most dentists believe that talent is the key to success. In the last chapter, we refuted the talent myth by giving credit to effort over talent. In this chapter, I will go one step further, and say that leaders who create high-performing, successful dental practices do it through building cultures of trust, excellence, and shared purpose.

You can recognize good culture instinctively. That is why I am able to recognize a dentist's real problems when they call our lab, as a matter of culture. When the dentist doesn't return telephone calls on important matters that concern the potential outcome of a big case, when the dentist shifts accountability to a staff member, when the dentist blames the technician for

The Complete Dentist: Positive Leadership and Communication Skills for Success, First Edition. Barry Polansky.
© 2018 John Wiley & Sons, Inc. Published 2018 by John Wiley & Sons, Inc.

everything that occurs, other than taking credit for a job well done – these are all leadership issues that get trickled down to cultural issues that infest the entire practice.

Some of those negative traits mentioned are traits we see in our patients, and we don't like them when we are on the receiving end of poor behavior. I find it interesting that the very same lack of virtues that many patients exhibit are the same traits that so many dentists exhibit. It is no accident that the very successful dentists are those who have developed the better virtues of leadership and who transfer those to their organization and to their patients.

In observing dental practices for many years, I have discovered that organizational culture may be the most important component of success. I have seen practices, and interacted with staff, where I walk away thinking that the monkeys are running the monkey house. By monkeys, I mean anyone other than the dentist. I have seen strong-armed staff members, demanding patients, spouses, and the codes and systems set forth by insurance companies, act as the dominating culture of a practice.

It is amazing to me that a dentist would spend his entire life and career living in a culture that he or she did not create. Creating a culture is the major responsibility of a leader. Some would argue that culture plays no role in the success or failure of a dentist; some would argue that the dentist has any control over creating culture. I would argue that a leader creates culture.

The first thing we must do is to define what organizational culture is. In a 2013, Harvard Business Review article [2], author Michael Watkins surveyed over 300 respondents on LinkedIn, in an attempt to define organizational culture. Before I reveal my definition of culture, let's take a look at some of his responses:

- *Culture is how organizations do things.* Two things come to mind for me with this definition. Firstly, many years ago, I read the excellent book *The E-Myth* by Michael Gerber. In that book, and in watching Gerber's videos, he explained, very simply, that an organization needs to explain clearly, to all concerned, the answer to the question, "How do you do things around here?" Very simply, he was defining culture. As you will see, my definition is similar, but it contains a slight distinction. The second thing that comes to mind is Aristotle's famous quote, which I mentioned in the last chapter: "Excellence is never an accident. It is always the result of high intention, sincere effort, and intelligent execution; it represents the wise choice of many alternatives – choice, not chance, determines your destiny."
- *In large part, culture is a product of compensation.* On this, I would agree as well. But I would also say that this is a core problem of many cultures. As previously mentioned, most dentists learn the business model of "production comes first." Most staff members see their work as a job. As you will see, when the dentist actively creates a new culture, they can change the prevailing paradigm so that it is not the ruling model, yet still maintain financial as well as psychological success.
- *Organizational culture defines a jointly shared description of an organization from within.* This definition is more closely aligned with one of the parameters of my personal definition. It includes the concept of shared values and shared purpose. This definition moves beyond the concept of job, into the possibility of a career, or even a calling.
- *Organizational culture is the sum of values and rituals which serve as glue to integrate the members of the organization.* This definition is even closer, because it attempts to answer the question of "why" the organization even exists. It also attempts to describe the organization's story. As you will see in a coming chapter, the role of "story" is to emotionally enlist all involved into the culture. The story carries the meaning of the organization.
- *Organizational culture can act as "civilization in the workplace".* Imagine for a moment that all cultures, in all businesses, placed the customer first. Imagine that the behaviors, values, and rituals involved were always other-focused. What kind of world would that be? How would our profession be viewed if the dental culture always placed patients first? What would that do for trust? Yes, great cultures build trust.

- *Organizational culture acts as an immune system.* Culture can protect a practice from some of the other problems that come up, such as high turnover, cash flow problems, excessive cancellations, or an oppressed staff (or doctor).
- *An organization is a living culture.* There is no doubt that the practice of dentistry has changed. The culture should be flexible enough to grow through the changes. The culture, which includes the behaviors, values, and beliefs of the practice, needs to be the guiding principles over time.

All of these viewpoints about organizational culture are true, to one degree or another. Hopefully, the definitions have revealed why leadership is so important. The one thing that I have discovered about culture is that the answer always lies within the leader. The leader is the answer to one question: "why?" By being the living, breathing concretization of why we come to work everyday, he or she becomes the motivation for keeping the culture alive and well. The total well-being of the organization is preserved through shared meaning, shared values, and shared purpose. The well-being of the doctor in a virtuous cycle helps create a thriving, prosperous, and flourishing culture. The key, then, is not money or production – neither the carrot nor the stick. The key to culture and motivation is the silent question all employees are asking: "Why?"

As you will see, once this question is satisfactorily answered it, leads to a second question that all employees and patients ask: "Can I trust you?"

There is no limit to the rewards one can reap if the foundation is strong. In his book *Who Says Elephants Can't Dance* [3], Louis V. Gerstner, Jr., the retired CEO of IBM, writes about the importance of establishing a culture that is the result of one person's vision. "*I came to see in my time at IBM, that culture isn't just one aspect of the game – it is the game. In the end, an organization is nothing more than the collective capacity of its people to create value. Vision, strategy, marketing, financial management – any management system, in fact – can set you on the right path and carry you for a while. But no enterprise – whether in business, government, education, health care, or any area of human endeavor – will succeed over the long haul if those elements aren't part of its DNA. A company's initial culture is usually determined by its founder's mindset – that person's values, beliefs, preferences and also idiosyncrasies. It's been said that every institution is nothing but the extended shadow of one person,*" he wrote. In dentistry, that one person is the dentist-leader.

If the message the dentist sends answers the question, "why do we work?" that will show up in the results. We cannot visualize the DNA of a culture outside of the results that are produced. Culture is like the background conversation that goes on within the daily practice. It is invisible, hidden in plain sight. Metaphorically, it is like the wind or a breeze – you can't see it, but you can tell its effects by the way it moves the branches of trees and scatters the leaves across the lawn. The culture drives motivation.

According to authors Neel Doshi and Lindsay McGregor, cultures that provide total motivation are more productive and more profitable [4]. Their research describes six sources of motivation that are derived from leadership that they call the motive spectrum. These six motives are divided into two categories: direct and indirect motives. The direct motives are directly connected to the work itself, and result in the highest levels of performance. The three direct motives – play, purpose and potential – give employees the highest levels of commitment to the work.

The motive of play is something that has already been discussed, under the concept of engagement. It is when we are driven to accomplish something just for sake of doing it as its own intrinsic reward. The dentist who does dentistry the way some people do things as a hobby exhibits the play motive. It is what Confucius meant when he said, "Choose a job you love, and you will never have to work a day in your life." Doshi and McGregor say that "play is the most direct and most powerful driver of high performance [5]." If the dentist/leader is truly engaged in his/her work as play, the culture will benefit.

The second direct motive is purpose. When the purpose is clear, it directly answers the "why" question, because everyone is on the same page in producing a clear outcome or mission, versus the activity itself. The work is driven by the good it does for people. This occurs when the values and beliefs about dentistry align with the work. Because purpose is one step removed from the work, the authors consider it the second strongest driver of culture. Purpose is the driver that most practice management people tell us is the one and only pure driver but, as you can see, there are multiple direct motives for a work culture.

The third direct driver is potential. This is an ongoing series of steps that get individuals and practices to higher places. Potential is about constant professional growth. For some, it may mean getting accredited by an organization, or changing roles from a dental assistant to a dental hygienist, or the dentist learning new techniques. It is constant growth and education. Many cultures place a high priority on potential and, for many, it is the driving force. Some dental practices can be cultures for learning leadership. Many dentists in their careers have hired staff that have come from such cultures, and they make all the difference in the world. These three motives form the heart of highly performing productive dental cultures, but there are three prominent drivers that are indirect, and are more the current norm in dentistry – emotional pressure, economic pressure, and inertia.

Production-driven practices generally use these three motives. They are recognizable from the complaints, the turnover, and the general discontent of staff and patients. The background conversation in these cultures differs significantly from the directly driven, intrinsically motivated cultures.

Emotional pressure, the first indirect motive, occurs when the values and beliefs of the dentist are misaligned from the work. It occurs when the dentist would rather be somewhere else, and is not working for the pleasure of the work. The dentist may have been driven to dentistry for the wrong reasons, or reasons that were not his or her own. We see emotional pressure in many workplaces. When your response to a worker is that you don't want to be there, their works suffers and we are the beneficiaries of poor service. Yet, it is difficult to see in ourselves. That is why the ethos of knowing ourselves is so fundamental to our success. We can kid ourselves, and hide the emotional pressure, but the second indirect motive – economic pressure – is more prevalent in our profession, and has the potential to destroy a culture.

Economic pressure occurs when the dentist's self-interests predominate over the work and the patients. It is when the dentist solely goes to work for the material reward. It occurs when every decision is guided by how much we will earn. Practice management people stress this, and I have always found it to be poor advice. It produces fear, and fear is the poorest of advisors. It is the hallmark of an autocratic boss and, as you will see, it is not the best recipe for long-standing, high-performing cultures. It occurs when the practice solely operates on numbers, budgets, data, and metrics. When the numbers don't appear, fear sets in. This is pure management without leadership, as you will see soon enough.

I may not earn brownie points with staff in this section, but the point I want to make is that money is not the prime motivator. It is the personal preference of the dentist whether or not to have bonuses drive the production. I have found this to be a temporary motivator. Real change and lasting performance comes from the intrinsic drivers, like the direct motives.

The third indirect driver is inertia. This is what L.D. Pankey called indifference. Essentially, it is what this book is trying to avoid, and why our well-being is so important. When the dentist's drive is dead, so is the culture. There is no management, no leadership, and the practice is doomed. It is the main threat to our well-being, and so prevalent in today's world, as already discussed in the Gallup Poll's conclusions on engagement in the workplace.

Author and motivational expert Dan Pink expresses it best in his book, *Drive* [6]: "In business we tend to obsess over the 'how' – as in 'Here's how to do it.' Yet we rarely discuss the 'why' – as in 'Here's why we're doing it.' But it's often difficult to do something exceptionally well if we don't know the reasons we're doing it in the first place."

Production is a major preoccupation for dentists. We set production goals on a daily, monthly, and yearly basis. It may seem counter-intuitive that organizations that nurture a culture of commitment and culture of trust are more productive than organizations that do not value the direct motives that lead to high trust and commitment.

Author Charles Duhigg studies productivity. In his book *Smarter Faster Better: The Secrets of Being Productive in Life and Business* [7], he explores the science of productivity, and why managing how you think is more important than what you think. Early on in the book, Duhigg defines productivity as the name we give to our attempts to figure out the very best uses of our energy, intellect, and time, as we try to obtain the most meaningful rewards for the least wasted effort. It's a process of learning how to succeed with less stress and struggle. It's about getting things done without sacrificing everything we care about along the way. His book is a worthwhile read for all dentists who are interested in leadership and productivity. Among the topics he writes about are goal-setting, decision-making and team-building, but the chapter of managing people through building cultures of commitment will do more for your productivity than most consultants would demonstrate.

Duhigg cites the work of two Stanford business professors, James Baron and Michael Hannan who, in 1994, had been studying how one would actually build a culture of trust in their organizations. Baron and Hannan had become missionaries for the idea that culture mattered as much, or more, to a company's success as building a strategy. They claimed that the way businesses treated employees was more important than the service or product produced. In other words, they believed that things would eventually fall apart unless there was a culture of trust. Duhigg noted that the two professors were sociologists, and had no proof to support their feelings, so they embarked on a study to see if their thesis held up.

Their project, which started in 1994 [8], ended up taking 15 years to complete. They examined over 200 firms, using every variable that might influence a company's culture. After collecting the data, they placed companies into five separate categories. The five categories, which have correlations to dental practice are:

1) The star culture. This model hired only the very best – the stars, if you will. They were hired with the idea that they would have total autonomy in their decision-making. In dentistry, we can look at this as the star dentist, or even the hiring of a star office manager or dental assistant.

2) The engineering culture. This was defined as being very similar to most dental practices, where the dentist has total control, based on his technical expertise. This group consisted of engineers who were given total control over all decisions, even though their major focus was on solving technical issues.

3) The third and fourth cultures were what the authors called a bureaucratic culture and an autocratic culture. These two cultures were very dependent on strong management and were very data-driven. Everything gets spelled out in these two cultures. The only difference between them is who is giving the orders. In the bureaucratic culture, it is rule by committee and, in the autocratic culture, it is by one person. Baron and Hannan describe these two cultures as "You work. You do what I say. You get paid."

4) The final or fifth category is what they called the culture of commitment. This is the culture that I grew up with. At one time, it may have been called a "mom and pop" culture. I know that times have changed, but sometimes the old customs contain wisdom that can still guide us today. The old ways were concerned with the values I have been writing about in this book.

As you will see, Baron and Hannan's study confirms that a culture of commitment and trust lead to long-term production and stability. They found that some of the other cultures produced successful business models but, over the long term, the only cultures that exhibited consistent winners were those built on commitment and trust. They claimed that "hands down, a commitment culture outperformed every type of management style in almost every meaningful way." The study went on to reveal that commitment culture employees wasted less time on internal rivalries, because everyone was committed to the business. In dentistry, that means committed to the patients rather than to their own agendas. Cultures of trust and commitment tend to know their customers better than the other management styles do.

Baron and Hannan concluded that the success of commitment cultures occurred because of the high level of trust among the employees and the customers. This confirms to me that the "know yourself" component of Dr. Pankey's philosophy can directly lead to a "know your patient" element. In other words, ethos will lead to pathos. The advantages of a commitment culture not only are more productive practices, but less time lost due to changing employees, layoffs and sick days. The number of broken appointments is lower, as a collateral element of the background noise of a commitment culture. Loyalty at every level reigns in the commitment culture. Baron hits the nail on the head when he says that, "Good employees are always the hardest asset to find. When everyone wants to stick around, you've got a pretty strong advantage."

Leadership is about being effective. There has always been a debate about the difference between leadership and management. As mentioned earlier, management deals with the harder issues – metrics, budgets, and data. Management is about discipline and rules, and always asks "what and how," while leadership is about people, creativity, flexibility, and asking the question "why?" Management is about an office manual and a rule book, while leadership is about protecting the culture and caring for all those concerned. Leadership is about explaining and communicating complex ideas to all concerned, so that there is universal buy-in at every level. Leadership is about long-term vision and goals, love and care, and big-picture thinking. A commitment culture is open-minded, and accepts leaders at every level. It's also about becoming a learning organization through inclusion and communication.

In developing a culture of commitment and trust, we need both leadership and management. Just using practice management as the guide will lead to stodgy, stale practices that breed negativity, a lack of growth and a culture of blame, as negative bias seeps in over time. Practices that grow do so through their cultures. I have always wondered why certain practices, through good times and bad, stay consistent in their numbers without trying. The answer is the culture. If you have a $100,000 per month culture, like magic, you will reach those numbers every month. If you can't break above $50,000 per month, I suggest you check the culture.

We need a balance of good leadership and good management to succeed. Learning leadership skills, like communicating better through listening, questioning and storytelling, giving short clear explanations, vision building, motivating, establishing direction, understanding people's needs better, and learning how to be creative in sequencing and planning go a long way toward building a trusting culture. The harder skills of practice management, like diagnosis, examination, problem solving, monitoring, budgeting, and time management are also necessary for success. Balance is the key.

John Kotter, the professor emeritus at Harvard Business School, is often called the world's foremost authority on leadership and change. In his most recent book, *That's Not How We Do it Here* [9], he discusses the difference between leadership and management in the form of a chart. The chart depicts four quadrants. On the lower right side, where management is very strong and positive, we notice that, if leadership is weaker, the culture will be well-run but very bureaucratic, or autocratic. This culture has a tendency to become stale and stodgy. We see many practices like this, with high turnover and poor patient retention. On the upper left, where leadership is strong but lacks good management, the practice is quite innovative and energetic, but with poor management, doesn't get very good consistent results, and appears chaotic. Once again, we see many practices that spend more time having a good time but never seem to get the job done and, mostly, never grow professionally.

The lower left quadrant is the least desirable. It lacks any form of leadership or management. Kotter calls these organizations "doomed". There are far too many dental practices that are doomed, and that has led to an influx of external forces that have taken over the profession. The cultures of trust and commitment that used to prevail in dentistry have now been influenced by insurance and corporate models that bring in their own management systems and leadership styles.

It's the upper right quadrant that is the most desirable, with a balanced blend of leadership and management that will be the most successful and rewarding. This culture of trust and commitment, based on both good leadership and management, will be the most innovative, adaptive, and energetic in the future.

Early in my career, I believed that strong management was the answer to my problems. Command and control seemed logical, but autocracy never worked for me. I took courses from some of the best practice management people around. We measured everything, and I still believe that what gets measured gets done. I also believe what Einstein said, "Not everything that counts can be counted." One day, while listening to a lecture on how to identify patients, I saw three words written on the blackboard. The words described the type of patient we want to attract to our practices – those with a high level of trust, appreciation, and ownership. Recognizing that "who" we serve is more important than "what" we do, I keyed in on looking for those values or traits. I later started a blog that I titled TAOofDentistry.com, because those words, trust, appreciation, and ownership (TAO), signified the type of people I wanted in my practice. It became my "way" of practice and, like the Chinese philosopher Lao Tzu, it represented my path to building a culture that has served me very well.

I believe that my culture of TAO, trust, appreciation of people, and the work we do, as well as a high level of thankfulness expressed daily and the ownership and responsibility levels expressed by staff, patients and suppliers, has led to a rewarding, and fulfilling career in dentistry. But my career is coming to an end.

I have been courting potential buyers for my practice over the last year. The one thing I notice, and want to avoid, is a drastic change in cultures. I have witnessed all of the cultures that Baron and Hannan described in their study. The corporates have come in and looked. A star has looked. Mostly, engineers have looked, but the biggest trend I see is still the over-reliance on strong practice management, mostly autocratic. My staff and my patients, who have grown up in the TAO culture, are not used to being treated in ways that offer them no freedom of choice. All of my policies and systems have been created with their autonomy in mind, yet we mostly reach our daily, monthly and yearly goals. I believe it's because of culture. When I tell the potential buyers that some of my staff have been with me for over thirty years, they step back in awe. When they see the number of sick days, and case acceptance rates, they are stupefied. It's the culture, I tell them. Culture trumps everything – culture is king.

A commitment culture of trust, appreciation and ownership can also be viewed as a model of leadership. The O component can be seen as the leadership ethos. Self-awareness, self-motivation, and complete ownership are the hallmarks of good leadership. The A component is another way to explain our appreciation for the work we do, and the gratitude we have for the people we work with and work for. Becoming a member of the dental profession embodies an enormous amount of responsibility in regard to the work we do. The A component then, can be seen as the logos of leadership. Finally, a culture of commitment is based on trust – the T component.

Trust is the pathos of leadership. In the next part, Pathos, I will demystify the pieces of the trust puzzle. You will come to see that what appears to be self-evident is a fairly complex set of skills that is the key to culture building, communication and solid leadership.

At the beginning of this part of the book, on leadership ethos, I claimed leadership was essentially about communication and influence. I hope you are beginning to see the various usages of language to describe what a leader's role can be. Aristotle's definition of ethos, pathos, and logos had to do with influence and persuasion. In closing this chapter, I want to describe those three words as they apply to persuasion and influence in dentistry.

Logos is persuasion through logic. Dentists love to explain difficult concepts, and call it "educating the patient." We believe that the logical explanation of our work trumps everything. However, it's just not true. It may just be the weakest form of persuasion. Using logos as the primary method of persuasion falls under what psychologists call the "Curse of Knowledge," another of those cognitive biases I referred to in Chapter 9. According to Wikipedia [10], "the curse of knowledge is a cognitive bias that occurs when, in predicting others' forecasts or behaviors, individuals are unable to ignore the knowledge they have that others do not have, or when they are unable to disregard information already processed." In other words, we use our entire knowledge base when explaining things to people who have no references.

Pathos is persuasion through emotion. There is an old expression, "people buy on emotion and justify on logic." In other words, logos must follow pathos. I know this sounds counterintuitive, especially to rigorously trained technical dentists, but science backs it up. Behavioral psychologist and author Jonathan Haidt [11] created what has come to be known as the "rider and the elephant" metaphor. He argues that humans have two sides – an emotional, automatic, and irrational side (the elephant), and an analytical, controlled, and rational side (the rider). The problem, according to Haidt, is that the elephant always overpowers the tiny rider. The key is to get the rider and elephant on the same directional path, by speaking to both the emotional and the rational sides of the human brain. The key to persuasion, then, is to speak to the elephant first, by appealing to the emotional side, then to speak to the rational rider, by explaining the direction and path through logic. The rider then acts as the person's lawyer, and describes the long-term logic. So appeal to the emotions first, then explain logically. People buy on emotion and then justify on logic.

In the end, though, what patients are buying is you. People buy you before they buy your dentistry. That is why Aristotle placed ethos first and foremost in his communication formula. Ethos is persuasion through identity. It is your beliefs, philosophy, history, and character that make you trustworthy. It is our story. Aristotle himself said it best in his work *Rhetoric*:

> "Of the modes of persuasion furnished by the spoken word there are three kinds. The first kind depends on the personal character of the speaker; the second on putting the audience into a certain frame of mind; the third on the proof, provided by the words of the speech itself. Persuasion is achieved by the speaker's personal character when the speech is so spoken as to make us think him credible ... his character may almost be called the most effective means of persuasion he possesses."

As we leave this part and head over to pathos, hopefully it is clear why Dr. Pankey advised us to know ourselves first. Lao Tzu, the famous Chinese philosopher, also advised, "Knowing others is intelligence; knowing yourself is true wisdom. Mastering others is strength; mastering yourself is true power."

References and Notes

1 Deloitte (2012). *Core Beliefs and Culture, Chairman's Survey Findings.* http://ow.ly/Gf8rQ.

2 Michael D. Watkins (2013). What Is Organizational Culture? And Why Should We Care? *Harvard Business Review*, May 15, 2013.

3 Louis V. Gerstner (2002). *Who Says Elephants Can't Dance? Inside IBM's Historic Turnaround,* 1st edition. Harper Business.

4 Neel Doshi and Lindsay McGregor (2015). *Primed to Perform: How to Build the Highest Performing Cultures Through the Science of Total Motivation*, p. 9. New York, NY: Harper Collins.

5 Ibid., p.7.

6 Dan Pink (2009). *Drive : The Surprising Truth About What Motivates Us*, 1st edition. Riverhead Books.

7 Charles Duhigg (2016). *Smarter Faster Better: The Secrets of Being Productive in Life and Business*, 1st edition, pp. 145–150. Random House.

8 James N. Baron and Michael T. Hannan (2002). *The Economic Sociology of Organizational Entrepreneurship: Lessons from the Stanford Project on Emerging Companies, The Economic Sociology of Capitalism*, pp. 168–203. New York: Russell Sage.

9 John Kotter and Holger Rathgeber (2016). *That's Not How We Do It Here! A Story about How Organizations Rise and Fall – and Can Rise Again*, p.147. Portfolio.

10 en.wikipedia.org, curse of knowledge.

11 Jonathan Haidt (2005). *The Happiness Hypothesis: Finding Modern Truth in Ancient Wisdom*, 1st edition. Basic Books.

Part IV

Pathos – Other People Matter

"All happy families are alike; each unhappy family is unhappy in its own way."

Leo Tolstoy

"The best way to find out if you can trust somebody is to trust them."

Ernest Hemingway

Dentistry is a people business, and people, above all, are emotional creatures. It is interesting to note the effect that other people have on us. Psychologist Chris Peterson once said, "Happiness is other people," and the philosopher Jean Paul Sartre said, "Hell is other people." Either way, how we feel about other people can affect our lives and practices. That is why it is so important to work with, and for, people we genuinely like to be around. Have you ever looked at your schedule in advance, only to see a patient on the schedule that you genuinely didn't want to work on, or a procedure that you didn't like doing? This leads to what the psychologists call *toxic inauthenticity*, and it can lead to serious health issues, such as high blood pressure and issues with longevity.

When I think about my career in dentistry, I think about the highs and lows, but mostly I think about the people who have created my best moments and my worst moments. One of those patients is Tom B. Many years ago, Tom came in for what was scheduled as a routine new patient examination – if there is such a thing. My dental assistant called me aside and said that there was a man who refused to sit down until he could speak directly with the doctor. I entered the room and introduced myself. This interaction occurred long before I had made the examination process my career focus. I acted as I hoped most dentists would act – with extreme care and concern about his obvious dental anxieties. I listened patiently as he reviewed his dental history and his desire to restore his mouth, which was in a sudden and rapidly advancing state of collapse.

He was in danger of losing his lower four incisors to periodontal disease. It wasn't imminent, but we both could see the handwriting on the wall. I immediately liked Tom, and what he needed was someone he could trust. I will never forget that first meeting, and I am sure that every dentist or dental professional reading this has had similar stories. Tom went on to become one of my very best patients, if not my very best patient. It is now many years later, and Tom is totally restored, with a combination of conventional crown and bridgework and implant dentistry. He has been the recipient of removable partial dentures and periodontal surgery. We have all seen these transformations. I have seen his son grow up and become a very successful young man. Tom retired and moved to North Carolina, but still continues to make his four month re-care visits by combining family visits with his dental appointments.

The Complete Dentist: Positive Leadership and Communication Skills for Success, First Edition. Barry Polansky.
© 2018 John Wiley & Sons, Inc. Published 2018 by John Wiley & Sons, Inc.

It's patients like Tom that make dentistry such a wonderful career. From the moment he entered my practice we both went through a process that can be described as leadership pathos, or what marketing experts refer to as the "know – like – trust" principle. The ultimate goal is a low fear – high trust relationship, that provides the milieu that determines all interactions that lead to a successful life. I know it's a bold statement to make, but the whole of life is all about relationships. The key to helping people and, in essence, helping ourselves to change and live better, lies in trusting relationships that are distinguished by high levels of communication.

Pathos, Aristotle's second component, is about appealing to the other's emotions. The magic of emotional appeal is often spoken about in sales seminars. Pathos implies to your audience that you can feel their pain – you have empathy and compassion. You understand their needs, their objectives, and their challenges, and have made them a priority. It implies that you care. The very best way someone conveys pathos is to become an extraordinary listener and a skilled storyteller. By uncovering what really matters to people, we can then express emotionally how we feel through the use of a story. Habit 5 of Stephen Covey's classic book, *The 7 Habits of Highly Effective People* [1], expresses this idea of pathos in one sentence: "*Seek first to understand, then to be understood.*" If ethos is compared to self-concept, then we can compare pathos to the art of building strong relationships.

Of course when we look at our own practices, as I mentioned earlier, we tend to focus on the "bad patients." When I use that term, I would like to make it clear that I am not talking about bad people. This is not about making judgments; it is strictly about the relationship. Some chemicals or drugs don't react kindly to one another. We must come to understand that we cannot be everyone's dentist. I am reminded of a patient, Barbara, who read a negative review about me online some years ago. When she came in for a checkup she told me she read it, and said, "I don't believe that. It couldn't be '*my* Barry Polansky.'" I laughed, because we always hear the term "my dentist" used by patients, who certainly have a dentist, but not a relationship such as the ones I like to create with my patients, like Tom or Barbara.

Jim Collins, author of the book *Good to Great*, uses an illustrious metaphor when he compares a business to a bus, and leaders to the bus driver. One of his leadership traits is called *getting the right people on the bus*. He claims, "Great vision without great people is irrelevant [2]" In a dental practice, those great people include staff members, patients, specialists and laboratory technicians. In order to put the right people on the bus Collins describes a concept he calls, "*first who, then what.*" It is a process for developing these most important relationships. In the section on ethos we discussed vision, mission and culture. It is the people that we work with and for that will determine our success. The first step, using the bus metaphor, is to get the right people on the bus. In order to do that, we need a process that will help us to identify those people, so that we can match their aspirations, desires, and skills to the mission and vision of the practice.

Collins describes the second step as getting the right people in the right seats. This is the heart of good management. The third step, and the one where many dentists make mistakes, is to get the wrong people off the bus. Just as patients refer to dentists as "my dentist," we also have the tendency to refer to all patients as "my patient." Remember, it is the strength of the relationship that creates the long-term value. Patients, staff members, and specialists who do not fit with the dentists shared values are not bad, as mentioned above – they are just the wrong people. The wrong people can certainly ruin the bus ride and, as Tolstoy says in the quote that leads this chapter, they can ruin the ride in so many different ways. The wrong staff member, the wrong patient, or the wrong colleague can make the journey tough.

That is why Collins advises us to shift the decision from "what we do" into a "who" decision. He believes that developing a solid process in order to discern our traveling partners can be one of the most significant things we do for our careers. Once our lives are filled with the right people, in the right culture, with shared values and complete understanding of their vision, it becomes less of a question of where your career is going and, instead, of how far you can go.

The majority portion of the next section will be about leadership behaviors, and skills that will help to develop great relationships and the emotional component of communication. The context of our lives and careers is other people and our relationships. Whether it is the culture we develop, or the white noise background of our environment, it's our day-to-day relationships that not only create our success but, more importantly, our personal happiness. There is no model of well-being that does not include positive relationships. Once again, I will refer to the David Foster Wallace parable about the two fish swimming and asking, "what's water?" The water is our own personal universe. Leaders create their own universe. They do it by building great positive relationships. Every conversation contributes to the white noise of that universe. Very few people agree on every matter. The leader's job is to understand the standards of his own life and practice, and to make sure that others buy in as well. He does this through compassionate communication.

The Urban Dictionary [3] defines the term "worlds colliding" as when two separate aspects or relationships in a person's life collide. I first heard that term on a popular Seinfeld episode. I remember thinking that my role as a leader was to make sure that my world didn't collide with my colleagues. I spent many years taking courses and reading books on how to communicate better in order to help create a better world for myself. Maybe that was my biggest mistake? Somewhere in my reading about leadership, I came across a fundamental question that every human being is asking as part of the universal white noise. That question is, "Can I trust you?" A few follow-up questions may be "Can I trust you to do your job properly?" and "Can I trust you to put me first over yourself?"

These questions are universal, primary and very emotional. Yes, they will require behaviors and skills to make sure we communicate our messages properly. Skills like empathic listening, motivational interviewing, appreciative inquiry, and visual storytelling all belong in the leader's toolbox. These tools, however, will not work, and will appear to be manipulative if they are not preceded by a new mindset. That mindset is to be other-focused, rather than self-focused. I feel it is so important that it deserves its own chapter before I get into the skills of leadership communication. It falls somewhere between ethos and pathos, because being other-focused is more of a leader's fundamental character virtue, rather than a specific skill. With it, all communication efforts will help to remove the barriers on the road of knowing, liking and trusting.

References and Notes

1 Stephen R. Covey, *The Seven Habits of Highly Effective People*, (Fireside Book, Simon and Schuster)
2 Jim Collins, Good to Great: *Why Some Companies Make the Leap...And Others Don't*, HarperBusiness; 1st edition (October 16, 2001), Chapter 3, p. 42.
3 Urbandictionary.com

14

Your Focus – Your Success

"The most important decision we make is whether we believe we live in a friendly or hostile universe."

Albert Einstein

"If you change the way you look at things, the things you look at change."

Wayne Dyer

"There is no self-interest completely unrelated to others' interests. Due to the fundamental interconnectedness which lies at the heart of reality, your interest is also my interest. From this it becomes clear that 'my' interest and 'your' interest are intimately connected. In a deep sense, they converge."

Dalai Lama

It takes a lot to admit that you are wrong. If you have ever met me, you probably have judged my personality as somewhere between bold, pushy, or self-assured. I am not sure if these personality characteristics are the ones that I want to project. I would much rather project the "real me." Abraham Lincoln said, "Reputation is the shadow. Character is the tree." Our character is much more than just our reputation – what we try to display for others to see. It is who we are, even when no one is watching. When we focus on people in general, then we can define personality in terms of individual differences – that is, the range of different styles of thinking, feeling and acting. I would much prefer being judged on my character, rather than on my personality – as long as I was certain about my character. Most people believe they are of sound moral character until they put themselves through the lens of "knowing ourselves." That is where we come to find self-deception. I know I did.

The very best leaders, through the traits mentioned earlier – self-awareness, self-regulation, and self-motivation and introspection – make an effort to ward off self-deception. Why all of the confusion about self-interest? Why are we so susceptible to this self-deception? One reason may have to do with the Lake Wobegon effect of illusory superiority as discussed earlier. Another reason may be the difference between the résumé and eulogy virtues that David Brooks described. Another may be the one given by Stephen Covey in his book, *The 7 Habits of Highly Effective People* [1].

Covey reviewed all of the success literature since this country's inception, and found that the first 150 years focused on a character ethic as the foundation of success. Virtues like humility, fairness, justice and the Golden Rule were taught in schools and at home. Those same virtues were first described by Aristotle [2] and later set down by Ben Franklin [3]. After World War I, there was a major shift in teaching success, from a focus on character to a focus on personality, which included techniques and tactics of communication for persuasion and sales.

And so began the self-interest culture that we are living in today – what has been called the norm of self-interest.

The character ethic challenges each of us to become the very best versions of ourselves, while the personality ethic depends on methods or techniques to bring about our success. However, that success, as we will see, is short-lived and not sustainable. Our self-interest culture is inundated with phrases such as, "only the strong survive," "fake it till you make it," and "sink or swim." It is popularized by books like *Looking Out for # 1* [4], by Robert Ringer, Rhonda Byrne's, *The Secret*, and *The Power of Positive Thinking* by Norman Vincent Peale – all bestsellers. The focus today is that, to be successful, then first and foremost we have to focus on ourselves. Although these traits of the personality ethic may lead to short-term success, counter-intuitively, science and research show that character traits of humility, compassion and empathy lead to long-term happiness and success.

The character ethic, character strengths, character virtues, and eulogy virtues, no matter what we call them, are what matters when it comes to building long-term success and well-being. As mentioned earlier, people buy you long before they buy your dentistry. Ralph Waldo Emerson said it best: "What you are shouts so loudly in my ears I cannot hear what you say." This is the reason why ethos always precedes pathos when it comes to leadership. Covey referred to this when he named those with strength of character virtues to have what he called *primary greatness.* Leadership requires that we have all three components of ethos, pathos and logos. Pathos, however, is secondary to ethos, and those who possess just pathos and great communication skills alone, Covey said, have *secondary greatness.*

The elements of the personality ethic – communication skill training, and education in the field of influence strategies and positive thinking alone, are still essential for success, but they are secondary to character virtues. There are many successful dentists who are highly skilled in their sales techniques, but who lack primary greatness or genuine goodness of character. Sooner or later, this generally effects most of their long-term relationships. Yet practice management coaches and consultants consistently teach dentists the language of sales, rather than discussing where the real rewards lie. It is character, above all, that communicates most eloquently.

Fred Kiel, who I mentioned in Chapter 9, defined moral intelligence as "our mental capacity to determine how universal human principles – like those embodied the in "Golden Rule" – should be applied to our personal values, goals, and actions." In one of the most important initiatives in the 20th century, according to renowned Harvard professor Howard Gardner, the research of Peterson and Seligman [5] to categorize the personal strengths and virtues of people into six categories includes 24 distinct character strengths. A discussion of each virtue is beyond the scope of this book, but the universal nature of these virtues goes a long way in applying the Golden Rule.

Some of the virtues include persistence – or what we described earlier as grit – integrity, or honesty and authenticity, and extreme ownership, vitality and zest, kindness, compassion, empathy, social and emotional intelligence, fairness and justice, humility, and modesty. They even include the virtue of leadership. In reading through the list of virtues, one thing stood out for me, and that was that these strengths always required the leader to be other-focused. The leader who practiced using a strong set of virtues always did so in the context of others. They are servant leaders.

In 2015, Fred Kiel wrote a follow-up book titled *Return on Character* [6]. Kiel wanted to offer solid evidence that demonstrates the connection between character virtues, leadership excellence, and organizational results. His landmark study confirmed what Aristotle, Ben Franklin, Stephen Covey, and L.D. Pankey had been saying for years, that strong character matters. Kiel studied more than 100 CEOs, and 8000 of their employees' observations. His findings showed that leaders of strong character achieved up to five times the return on assets (ROA), or how profitable an organization is, than do leaders of weak character. Although this "secret" seems intuitive, so many business leaders still believe that a winning strategy and a sound business model are what really matter. In other words, character development and education in building leadership ethos has been left out of the equation.

Kiel's study had to quantify the very subjective nature of character and leadership. He started by sifting through the very same *human universals* that anthropologist Donald Brown categorized in his inventory of all human societies throughout time. Seligman and Peterson had created a list of 24 character strengths. Kiel *et al.* whittled their list to four moral virtues – integrity, responsibility, forgiveness and compassion as their four human universal character strengths. They did this by sending anonymous surveys to employees at 84 US companies and non-profit organizations, asking how consistently CEOs and managers embodied the four moral principles. They also interviewed each of the leaders, in order to measure discrepancies in perception (measuring self-deception?). They then compared their findings to the financials of each organization, to see if there was a correlation between character and financial results. Their results were interesting for our purposes.

They categorized two ends of a spectrum that they called the ROC (return on character) Character Curve [7]. At one end, they found CEOs whom they called "virtuoso CEOs". The employees of this group gave their CEOs high grades in all four moral virtues. Their strong character review included standing up for what was right, expressing concern for the good of all concerned, and showing compassion and empathy.

The other end of the curve included the lowest scores. Kiel has called them "self-focused CEOs." Their traits included warping the truth for personal gain, and caring mostly about themselves and their own financial security, no matter what the cost to others. Employees reported that this group only told the truth about one half of the time, they could not be trusted to do the right thing and, more often than not, they shifted accountability away from themselves by blaming others. They frequently punished well-intentioned people for making mistakes, and were especially bad at showing care and concern for other people. Both of these types of leaders built corresponding cultures. In Kiel's study, the results showed up in the bottom line.

The study also revealed what I have been saying throughout this book – that self-deception is common when it comes to leadership, especially in the area of character strengths. In the study, Kiel asked the CEOs to rate themselves on the four character strengths. The self-focused CEOs gave themselves much higher grades than the employees did. This study, in other words, gave an accurate 360-degree feedback concerning character, leadership, and results. The CEOs who received the highest ratings from employees actually gave themselves lower scores, which the researchers interpreted as a sign of their humility and further evidence of their strong moral character. This is the value of 360-degree feedback and self-awareness. It is the reason why primary greatness is difficult to achieve, and why L.D. Pankey and all others who believed in the character ethic tell us this is the starting point.

Pankey used to say the best dentists had three attributes: care, skill and judgment. Judgment comes from years of experience while on the road to mastery. The skills are learned every day by conscientious dentists. Care was Pankey's word for being other-focused. In the end, care + skills + judgment = results. The virtuoso leader maintains a people-first, character-based culture. Many dentists put an overemphasis on learning effective communication skills and, though I will admit that those skills are important, a leader's true effectiveness comes from character development. The question, then, may be the same question as, "are leaders born or can leadership be learned?"

I believe it can be learned. I also believe that there is a worldwide trend occurring that emphasizes the teaching of character-building through positive education. In a recent lecture at IPEN, the International Positive Education Network, Dr. Martin Seligman, the founding father of positive psychology, acknowledged what he believed would become a sea-change in the future of education. He believes that the old models of psychology were based on a disease model, and made psychologists into victimologists. The new model of positive education places an emphasis on building the best version of people, and part of that building process is about building strong character. Seligman says, "Positive emotion alienated from the exercise of character leads to emptiness, to inauthenticity, to depression and, as we age, to the gnawing realization that we are fidgeting until we die." I believe that ethos and character-building is the start of leadership, and will lead to better and more fulfilling lives and careers in dentistry.

Can an old dog learn new tricks? I know I did. For the first 15 years of my practice, I was self-focused. When I learned, through self-awareness and a lot of pain, to put others first, I began to practice more meaningfully. Of everything I did, I believe this led to the biggest changes. I began to take more responsibility, I began to help people to improve their lives and the lives of their families, by seeing my role as more than just a fixer of teeth, and my practice began to take on a much more positive element. Yes, through building strong character, leaders can be developed.

Let's take a quick look at the field of emotional intelligence. I am a big believer in emotional intelligence, and try to practice all of the skills that are included, some of which will be discussed as part of pathos. But emotional intelligence is not a good indicator of character. Emotional intelligence is not the starting-point for leadership. Becoming other-focused is the starting-point.

So, with all of the emphasis on a self-interest culture, what is the downside? Why does self-interest fail to come through, in the long run, as a blueprint for success? In my 43 years of practice, I have seen my own self-focus backfire. I have also seen many colleagues whose lives and careers have not been as admirable as they may have been. Most casual observers may conclude that the self-focused leaders have successful careers and, if money is the only measuring stick, that may be true. But money is not the only gauge when we look at an entire career. Let's take a look at a few of the disadvantages of self-focus.

The first one is arrogance. No one likes a bully or a narcissist. Self-focus is the telltale sign of narcissism. Earlier, I discussed the question of narcissistic leaders and whether they could succeed. I admitted that they could succeed, but here I want to discuss the long-term effect of narcissism. Narcissists, in general, like to take on the leadership role but, because of their arrogance and self-focus, they have multiple blind spots. They take on too many risks, because they don't have a clear view of their own abilities. In the long run, many of their cases fail, because they bite off more than they can chew. Many of them believe that, because of their position of authority, they can just tell people what to do without getting to know them. Their case presentations are more lecture than discussion.

In the book *The Narcissism Epidemic* [8], author Jean Twenge tells us that self-focus can lead to an inflated feeling of superiority and entitlement. She says it brings on "a multifaceted trait that brings together vanity, materialism, lack of empathy, relationship problems, egotism." She believes that at the core of these problems is an inflated sense of self. Narcissism is on the rise. Narcissism scores of "college students have climbed steeply since 1987, with 65% of modern-day students scoring higher in narcissism than previous generations [9]." There are a few reasons for this in dentistry: the competition to succeed is higher than ever; courses in complex dentistry are given, and dentists are told to try new methods after a weekend course, never considering their true limitations; technology leads dentists to believe that human relationships are secondary; and we still believe in the outdated autocratic style of leadership.

Self-focus does not lead to long-term success. I have seen it over and over again. Arrogant dentists have ruined their reputation in the dental community, with patients as well as with colleagues. They have a difficult time maintaining relationships. People like people who are humble, agreeable, and compassionate – three traits of effective leadership.

Another disadvantage is the affect on relationships, as just noted. As noted earlier, in the section on culture building, some leaders build a culture with a bias toward blame. Once again, self-focus is the cause for blaming others. When something goes right, the self-focused leader will always take credit. When something goes wrong, he or she will never hesitate to throw others under the bus. This is another example of arrogance; dentists are notorious for throwing lab technicians under the bus. This leadership principle reverts back to the character virtue of extreme ownership and total responsibility, but you can see that the core issue is self-focus. All of these things lead to poor long-term relationships.

I always wonder about dentists who have high turnover, or who switch labs and specialists like they are changing shirts. I see the lab situation all the time now that I own a lab. I know a specialist – a very good practitioner – who consistently throws his referring dentists under the bus. His arrogance has led him to make some technical errors on some of my patients through the years. Some time ago, we had a screw loosen on an implant crown that we worked on together. When I sent the patient to him to take a look, he told the patient that I had not tightened the screw down enough. In truth, the implant was placed at too severe of an angle in order to avoid the sinus. I protected him, but his ego took over and he blamed me instead of just correcting the situation. This may sound obvious, but it happens more often than we think. In the end, I lost that patient. The specialist lost me as a referrer. His reputation has suffered through the years in our dental community. Self-focus hurts long-term relationships because it doesn't build trust – the ultimate requirement for lasting relationships.

In addition to poor relationships, self-centered leaders create a stressful workplace. When self-centered leaders have their self-esteem and ego threatened, they respond with bullying and anger. Because of their tendency toward anger, they are more prone to unethical activities [10]. Because of fragile egos, their anger and bullying lead to poor relationships. Self-centered leaders continually put pressure on their teams, which leads to a high stress, and an unproductive workplace. That workplace stress eventually leads to high turnover and instability.

Another downside of self-focus is that it undermines the very important character trait of resilience. Every dentist suffers failures, whether at the technical or the behavioral level. Self-centered leaders are very susceptible to illusory superiority, or the Lake Wobegon effect mentioned earlier. They always believe that they are way above average. When they do fail, as all dentists and leaders eventually do, their egos get crushed. Their self-worth is dependent on their success at work – hence, the bias to blame others, get angry and destroy relationships. When a self-centered dentist suffers a setback, it can crush them. Thus, even high self-esteem is not the cure for self-centeredness.

Finally, and probably the most important downside of self-focus, is the effect it has on the leader's health and well-being. This book has covered the negative health issues that have been documented by numerous studies, from burnout and depression, to high blood pressure, coronary artery disease, and increased morbidity and mortality. The point is that self-focus can create social isolation, loneliness, and poor relationships, which can effect one's health in the same ways. I hope I have made the point, at the start of this section, that self-focus versus other-focus is the filter through which pathos works. Every technique involved in the emotional component of leadership rises and falls on this point of view.

The hallmark traits of being other-focused are compassion and empathy. There is a distinction between the two traits. Empathy is understanding how someone else feels, and trying to imagine how that might feel for you – it's an approach to relating. For example, when the economy dipped after 2008, I began to see young patients in their 20s and 30s who had stayed away from the dentist, because they had just entered the job market and were financially strapped. Many had good habits from their youth. Many came in because of an emergency.

I began practicing 40 years ago, when dental fees were not as overwhelming as they are today. I have empathy for these young people. I feel for them, and I want them to get the same benefits of my comprehensive care that all of my patients receive. Empathy is the trait that drives compassion.

Compassion is the true pathos, or emotion. It is the experience of empathy. Compassion is what drives us to find solutions for people because we care about them. Recall that empathy is one of the human universals. We are biologically wired to love and be loved, and to want to be worthy of being trusted. Essentially, empathy and compassion are the deepest connection between people. It is through compassion that we find the purpose and meaning in our work – one of the components of the PERMA model of well-being. So, if science tells us that it is beneficial to be compassionate, and that compassion and empathy lead to success, then why do so many people believe in the norm of self-interest? Maybe not everything should be looked at through the eyes of a businessman.

You could look at the benefits of compassion as the opposite of self-focus. Kim Cameron, from the University of Michigan, wrote an article in the *Journal of Applied Behavioral Science* that concluded that organizations that have compassionate cultures "achieve significantly higher levels of organizational effectiveness – including financial performance, customer satisfaction, and productivity [11]." In other words, happier employees make for a committed compassionate culture and happier workplaces, not only improving the well-being of employees, but improving the health of client outcomes as well. Compassion, created by an other-focus mindset, benefits everyone.

Compassion, then, is good for productivity, your personal health, employee loyalty, and engagement but, of all the benefits of compassion, mostly it increases the status of the leader through building trustworthiness.

So is it true what they say, that "nice guys finish last?" Adam Grant, the youngest tenured and highest rated professor at the Wharton School of Business at the University of Pennsylvania has researched this question for his bestselling book, *Give and Take* [12]. He concluded that generosity and an other-focused mindset is more effective than selfishness and is critical for personal fulfillment, just as Fred Kiel's research resolved. He argues that kindness and compassion gives us a far greater long-term advantage than does self-focus. Grant calls leaders who put other's well-being first *"givers"*, or what Kiel calls the virtuosos. He calls the selfish ones *"takers"*. His research shows that givers are both overrepresented at the bottom and the top of the success ladder. He explains this by admitting that the takers will surpass many of the givers, unless the givers learn the skills that prevent others from taking advantage of them.

These leadership traits make it easy for others to work with them, because they build trust. Trust is crucial in order for people to feel safe. As I will explain in the next chapter, trust is ubiquitous. Whenever there are two points of view, and a decision must be made, there is some risk. After all, everyone has a point of view and a possible agenda. Leaders better understand the risk through empathy and compassion, and do their best to reverse the risk. Everyone is asking the question, "Can I trust you?" or, another way of saying it comes from the classic spy-dental movie, *Marathon Man*: "Is it safe?"

Recall the marketing concept of *know, like and trust*. This applies to leaders, as well. People feel much safer around others who they have come to know, like, and trust, through their kindness and compassion, both derivatives of having an other-focused mindset. Fear is the poorest of motivators. A culture driven by stress and fear can stifle drive and production. Think back to Chapter 10, and the question Machiavelli asked in *The Prince*, "is it better to be feared than loved" when it comes to leadership? Through the filter of compassion and empathy, my answer would be "both". However, *fear* may be too strong a word – the word I would use is *presence*. Fear may produce a bit of unwanted stress, but presence will prevent others from taking advantage, and it will project the answer to another question people are always asking: "Are you competent enough to get the job done?" Leaders project the confidence of knowing what they are doing through their presence, while still maintaining a safe and friendly environment.

Now that we have established the importance of taking a perspective of being other-focused, let's move on to a description of a leadership style I call charismatic leadership which combines two traits that will help produce trust: warmth and presence.

References and Notes

1 Stephen R. Covey (1989). *The Seven Habits of Highly Effective People*. Fireside Book, Simon and Schuster.
2 Aristotle (1999). *Nicomachean Ethics*, 2nd Edition. Hackett Publishing Company, Inc.
3 Benjamin Franklin (1996). *The Autobiography of Benjamin Franklin*, new edition. Dover Publications.
4 Robert J. Ringer (1977). *Looking Out for Number One*, 1st edition. Funk & Wagnalls.
5 Christopher Peterson and Martin Seligman (2004). *Character Strengths and Virtues: A Handbook and Classification*, 1st edition. American Psychological Association/Oxford University Press.
6 Fred Kiel (2015). *Return on Character: The Real Reason Leaders and Their Companies Win*. Harvard Business Review Press.
7 Ibid., p. 21.
8 Jean M. Twenge and W. Keith Campbell (2009). *The Narcissism Epidemic: Living in the Age of Entitlement*, 1st edition. Atria Books.
9 Emma Seppälä (2016). *The Happiness Track: How to Apply the Science of Happiness to Accelerate Your Success*, p. 144. HarperOne.
10 Ibid., p. 145.
11 Ibid. p. 155
12 Adam Grant (2013). *Give and Take: A Revolutionary Approach to Success*, first edition. Viking.

15

The Charismatic Dental Leader

"Empathy is full presence to what's alive in the other person at this moment."

John Cunningham

"My presence speaks volumes before I say a word."

Mos Def

"Be here now."

Ram Dass

I learned leadership through many sources, including books, mentors, and life experiences. Much of leadership comes through the wisdom of others, and being very sensitive to what works and what doesn't work. Being highly sensitive can be a blessing and a curse. Someone with high sensitivity can be described as having hypersensitivity to external stimuli and a greater depth of cognitive processing and high emotional reactivity, according to psychologist Elaine Aron, author of the book *The Highly Sensitive Person* [1]. Fred Kiel's description of the virtuoso leader in his book *Return on Character* explains how leaders develop. Most, through their own sensitivity, take the hero's journey in developing their self-awareness.

Virtuoso leaders spend a lot of time in self-reflection. They create versions of their story which include not only their outer journey, but their inner journey as well. They are described as mentally complex [2]. They are anchored in reality, and can relate to most things through their own life stories. I believe that it is that high sensitivity and emotional awareness and empathy that was responsible for much of L.D. Pankey's practical wisdom and philosophy. As they say, "all saints were sinners," and I believe that most wisdom is hard-earned.

That is why I get concerned when I speak with young dentists about the current state of dentistry. So many dismiss the leadership role, especially the emotional component, as being subordinate to the technical skills. Reducing dentistry to just the technical component can be a grave mistake. Maybe it's because there is so much confusion about how one learns leadership and communication skills. Unlike technical dentistry, leadership and communication cannot be taught in a step-by-step cookbook manner. And dentists love cookbooks.

I had a discussion recently with a young dentist about the topic of becoming a better dentist. He was so convinced that staying current with the latest technology and techniques were the key to his success. I argued that he would go farther through learning leadership and communication skills. He responded by saying, "that's a given." In other words, who doesn't know that? I guess that one might conclude that common sense is not equal to common doing. Descartes said, "Common sense is the most widely shared commodity in the world, for every man is

The Complete Dentist: Positive Leadership and Communication Skills for Success, First Edition. Barry Polansky.
© 2018 John Wiley & Sons, Inc. Published 2018 by John Wiley & Sons, Inc.

convinced that he is well supplied with it." As long as we know that leadership and communication are important, then the next step is to learn how to apply those skills. So many dentists certainly take the fixed mindset approach when it comes to learning the softer skills. Becoming a charismatic leader is a matter of applying the principles of pathos.

Recall the silent questions that every patient and staff member is silently asking us: "Can I trust you?" "Can you do the job?" and, "Do you have my best interests at heart?" The term I like to use for the leader who can always answer these questions in the affirmative is *charisma*. In the book *The Charisma Myth* [3], author Maria Fox Cabane explains that charisma consists of three components blended together: power, warmth, and presence. By power, she means that we have the ability and influence to help them; warmth refers to the trait of intention – that you are willing to help them; and presence means you listen to them without distraction. These three traits are a reflection of being other-focused.

Cabane cites research that shows that our reaction to power and warmth is deeply wired. We rely on instinct to assess people we encounter, as a survival mechanism. We get a gut reaction that tells us whether to like and trust another. The combination of power and warmth – or charisma, she claims – plays powerfully on our instincts. "From lab experiments to neuroimaging, research has consistently shown that they are the two dimensions we evaluate first and foremost in assessing other people."

In unrelated research, Dr. Leonard Berry of the Mays Business School at Texas A&M University, and author of numerous books on service, says that the five most important components of great service are: dependability, reliability, assuredness, empathy, and tangible items. It is interesting to note that being reliable, dependable and empathetic are all concerned with the intention of the service provider (warmth), and the assuredness factor is a reference to the skill and competence of the provider (power).

Cabane tells us that charisma can be learned, and that it is not something that is innate. It is interesting to note that understanding how to become charismatic requires many of the same principles that it takes not to only present well, but also to practice better dentistry at the same time. Dentists spend much of their career learning how to do better technical dentistry, and acquiring more knowledge via reading books and taking seminars. What they need to realize is that knowledge is not power; power is communicating knowledge. It is through a blend of empathic communication, and certainty of technical dentistry, that the power of leadership is expressed.

What sets charismatic leaders apart is that they are very good communicators. They are both verbally eloquent and also have the ability to communicate on a deep emotional level. Charismatic leadership depends on the leader's ability to inspire and motivate their followers. They also do not depend on power and autocratic behavior to motivate. Dentists who lead through autocracy and presenting doom-and-gloom scenarios are not using the traits of a charismatic leader.

Let's take a look at the three traits of charisma – warmth, power, and presence – all in the service of communicating a purposeful vision that goes beyond oneself. Warmth is the final expression of empathy. Empathy and compassion, rather than self-centeredness, is at the heart of who we are. Empathy is defined as the art of stepping imaginatively into the shoes of another person, understanding their feelings and perspectives, and using that understanding to guide our actions. One of the questions you may be asking is, "what if I am not a particularly warm person?" Not everyone has the gift of a warm personality, like Mother Theresa or Ronald Reagan. Personally, I am not the warmest of people. This begs the question of whether charisma can be learned, or is it something we are born with?

The first step in becoming a warm leader is to become other-focused. It is to look always at the other's point of view. For some people, this comes naturally. For others, like me, it takes some work. One of the things I did was to create a process where I was able to slow down and set aside time to truly listen to people. One of the reasons I developed my examination process was to get to understand people better, so that I could slow down and explore what dentistry means to them. This process is a never-ending course in compassion and empathy. It requires developing skills that go beyond listening. It requires us to know how to ask questions that reveal the deepest emotions and implications.

Truly understanding people is just the first part. The second part of developing warmth, compassion, and understanding is to be able to express what we have learned through empathic listening, in a manner that people understand – to express that we have truly listened, and that we can help them by providing solutions. I believe, as you will come to find out, that trust is the ultimate motivator. When trust is built, our lives become so much easier. Charismatic leaders place a great emphasis on how they communicate, and whether they can gain trust in order to influence change.

I hope I am not reducing this to a simple set of rules, like a recipe for success. One of the most difficult things to do in becoming more empathic is to become more vulnerable. There will be moments when our own emotions get in the way. We become impatient with people. Our inner voice wants to scream out and correct people. Our own personal curse of knowledge seems to get in our way. We need to let down our shields and live more in the world where others live, a world of their uncertainty, of their risk, and in a place where we realize their emotional exposure. Most of us do not understand that level of uncertainty, in a world where business and daily production mean everything.

I have learned to appreciate what Dr. Brené Brown, the author of *Daring Greatly* [40], says, *"My inability to lean into the discomfort of vulnerability limited the fullness of those important experiences that are wrought with uncertainty: Love, belonging, trust, joy, and creativity, to name a few. Learning how to be vulnerable has been a street fight for me, but it's been worth it."*

I suggest that leaders take the time to watch Brown's excellent Ted Talk, *The Power of Vulnerability.* Maybe this is why Aristotle included all three components of ethos, pathos, and logos in leadership development. Not one of the three, character, emotions, or work, exist in a vacuum. Developing the trait of being other-focused is deeply connected to self-awareness and self-control. Developing these traits requires a long-term commitment and practice. Deliberate practice, as mentioned earlier. I will describe the systems I use for practicing listening, questioning, and expression through presentation in the next few chapters.

The ultimate feedback that you are succeeding is not simply case acceptance. People accept your dentistry for any number of reasons that may, or may not, appear visible. They may be faced with no other choice than accepting your dentistry. They may accept your dentistry because you are the cheapest or most convenient option. They may accept your recommendations because they were referred by someone they trust. The key to great leadership is consistent acceptance over time. My practice is filled with patients and staff members who have stayed with me for many years, because I have learned how to build trust. You know when you have achieved it, because they tell you so.

Brian C. needed extensive restorative dentistry. He is a pipe fitter and an ex-drug addict. You have seen Brian in your practice, I am sure. From the moment he came in, we developed a relationship. He had not been to a dentist for many years. Slowly – and I mean slowly – I brought his mouth back to health, first through hygiene, and then with large, pin-retained, composite resin fillings. Yes, even a few root canals. Through it all, he never missed an appointment, always paid his bills, even after consuming every bit of his dental insurance, and never once accepted a prescription for anything more than Tylenol. Not only did we fix Brian's teeth, but we watched him develop into a healthy, responsible young man.

Recently, Brian came in for a check-up. I noted a small fracture on one of his older composites. I thought the tooth, at this point, would best be served with a crown. He responded by saying the words that say everything there is to say about pathos: "Whatever you say Doc,

I trust you." That moment of enlightenment, about the emotional aspect of what we do, should save you a lot of time and energy in developing your leadership skills.

In my first book, *The Art of the Examination*, I told a story of a patient, Audrey H. It was the story of an older diabetic patient who became a long-term patient. I completely restored her many years ago. I watched Audrey through the years, as her diabetes got the best of her. She loved to read. We shared that in common. Diabetes slowly took her sight away. She moved into a nursing home. She never missed an appointment. She had no family left, so she would take a taxi to the office, or we would send someone to pick her up. After 20 years, her upper restoration was beginning to fail and, at this point in her life, she could only afford a partial denture. We both had a lot invested in this relationship, so I replaced the fixed prosthesis with another fixed prosthesis. She paid us whatever she could afford. Audrey lived for another five years or so. I never regretted doing the *pro bono* dentistry.

I was on vacation when I received a call from my office manager, informing me that Audrey had remembered our kindness and left us 10,000 dollars in her will. I smiled when I heard the news. I truly do believe what Albert Einstein said: "The most important decision we make is whether we believe we live in a friendly or hostile universe." This is the kind of vulnerability we need as leaders. I am not suggesting that we give away our dentistry, or that dentistry is not a business. This is a book about leadership and communication. All of our dentistry does not have to end up on Facebook, nor do we have to prove ourselves by our production numbers. In the end, by investing in people, it will be the Brians and Audreys of your practice that make it all worthwhile.

If empathy, compassion, vulnerability, and humility help build trust, what hurts most leaders? If those qualities can be described as the warmth component of charisma, then what creates the coldness? The short answer is our own egos. Because of the nature of our profession, that we are generally the "go to" person in practice, it is easy for us to overdevelop our egos. Author Ryan Holiday defines ego as "an unhealthy belief in our own importance [5]." It creates an insatiable appetite for winning at any expense. It leads to arrogance, self-centeredness, and an excessive amount of micro-management. It is a sense of superiority that far exceeds any level of talent.

Ego can be our worst enemy, says Holiday, and it lives within all of us. When it comes to leadership, ego must be held in check, yet we see dental egoists all the time. The arrogant, self-centered dentist is very easy to spot. They gain a reputation in the dental community. What I am suggesting is not to squelch the ego, but to have a healthy sense of one's values and abilities. Being a highly skilled practitioner will not serve all of the requirements of being an effective leader. The majority of dentists are not spending most of their time doing highly difficult cases. Remember, people need both, the assurance that the leader cares about them, and the certainty that they can do the job.

I have seen dentists advertising their skills as if that is all that is important to their patients. One dentist I know used to advertise how he treated a few television stars. I referred a patient to him one time, and the patient came back to me, complaining how the dentist was so "full of himself," that he never once asked the patient about himself. Needless to say, I had to find a dentist who took a more human approach. Of course, this is the extreme, but it happens in dentistry all the time. It isn't restricted to patients either. Staff members get around; they tell stories of micro-management that travel quickly through the dental community. It is no secret that people want to work in warm, stress-free environments. Controlling the ego can go a long way.

Yet, the answer to the second question, "Can you do the job for me?" must be answered. That does take some level of ego – to develop and express the competence of doing good work. Becoming a competent dentist falls within the scope of "logos." Expressing competence so that patients and staff know that you have their best interests at heart falls under pathos. The charismatic leader has warmth, power and presence. Power and presence is a soft expression of the ego.

Harvard psychologist Amy Cuddy has become an expert on the subject of leadership presence. She has a widely viewed 2012 TED Talk on the topic, and a bestselling book, *Presence* [6]. She claims that "when we judge others – especially our leaders – we often look at two characteristics: how lovable they are (their warmth, communion or trustworthiness) and how fearsome they are (their strength, agency, or competence." Cuddy, then, when speaking of leadership presence, is describing charisma, and answering the same question that Machiavelli once asked: "Is it better to be feared or loved?" This may sound ambiguous, but it is a state that effective leaders must seek.

Cuddy tells us that presence is about moments. Being a child of the sixties, I have always tried to follow the advice of Ram Dass: "Be here now." This is easier said than done. When developing systems for my practice, I am always aware of those moments when my presence is fully required. I will discuss those systems in the next part of the book. I want to make it clear that practicing good leadership does not take a superhuman effort, or require being born with abilities that only a few people have. Presence, then, is a permanent state of being. It is these fleeting moments when leadership is necessary that we get to practice presence. Practicing dentistry can be full of daily distractions that remove our ability to lead effectively, unless we plan for them.

Nobody is present 100% of the time. Presence is about having the ability to access our best skills, knowledge, expertise, and core values, and bring them forth when they are most needed. Being present allows us to take the time to be there and to connect with our patients and staff – to understand where others are coming from, rather than to be wrapped up in our own worlds. It's all about building strong connections and relationships.

To most people, dentistry is a blind subject. They have their beliefs, thoughts, and opinions about teeth and dentists. We never truly know what is on the minds of most people. At times, we arrogantly think we understand what people feel, or what they are thinking. What we do know is that most people have objections to dentistry. The most common objections are fear, finances, time constraints, no sense of urgency, and a lack of trust. For most people, there is an element of risk when they become a patient. Who hasn't felt that risk when going to a new doctor or dentist? Our job is to reverse that risk, and the best way I know of doing that is by building trust. Trust is the basic unit of social glue that enables us to interact without fear.

"Can I trust you?"; "Do you care about me?"; "Can you do the job correctly?"; "Is it safe?" These are all questions people are asking of us. These questions are not fully formulated or actively thought about; they lie within the deepest recesses of the mind. They lie at the emotional center of the brain, far removed from conscious thought. When leaders promote and create a psychological safe zone, they communicate at a much more primal level. The charismatic dental leader projects the feeling that he has your back, because he communicates at an emotional level that touches the human universals that survive throughout time. These lie deep in our emotional centers: empathy; generosity; sadness; humor; music; aesthetics; fairness; reciprocity; pride; story; and leadership. This is the essence of pathos and the charismatic leader.

A dental practice can be a scary place. The leader's role is to create an environment of trust. Everything in his or her practice should radiate feelings of safety and trust. Organizations rise and fall on feelings of safety and trust, as mentioned earlier, in the chapter on building a culture of trust. This is true of all organizations, from the nuclear family, to schools, the military, hospitals, and businesses of all kinds. Leadership and communication are responsibilities we all must accept in order to function at an effective level. It has been said that being a parent is the most difficult job there is. Mothers and fathers accept the highest level of responsibility when they bring a child into the world. Parents are effective because they exhibit the very same traits of effective leadership, warmth, power and presence. They generally don't go to school to learn good parenting. It comes from a deep love for their children. Great leaders feel the same love.

It may sound a bit over-emotional and sentimental, but there is much truth and wisdom to developing the deep emotion of loving your patient. One of the principles of well-being is that of meaning and purpose. Doing our job with meaning and purpose always implies the "other." This is the all-important core of service. History is overflowing with wise teachers, from Einstein, Gandhi and Schweitzer, who have weighed in on the relationship of well-being, love and service to others as a prescription for a good life [7].

Leaders understand that it is never about them. It is always about the people they serve, just as a parent serves with unconditional love. I am fond of a Zen poem which exemplifies the evolution of a leader:

> In the beginning, there is only self, there is no other.
> And then, there is self, and there is other.
> Later on, self and other are one, there is no separation.
> Finally, there is no self, there is only other.

Leaders understand that in order to be effective, there must be trust. The practice must be a psychologically safe zone at every level, and this is especially true of a dental practice, where people feel they are taking risks. The dental practice should help patients to reverse the risk. If we nurture positive, trusting feelings, then patients and staff members will sense the deep trust and cooperation, and compliance will rise. The leader sets the tone in providing the psychological safety zones in the practice. Common sense practice management advises that we create a low fear-high trust atmosphere. This advice sounds like common sense, but it is generally not common behavior. Simon Sinek, in his wonderful book *Leaders Eat Last* [8], implies the responsibility of leadership compares with being a parent by providing circles of safety. When staff members and patients feel that they belong, and are part of a family, then cooperation, creativity, and compliance go way up. Feeling safe is a prerequisite of a high-trust environment.

Leaders must learn to take the hands of our patients and staff as exemplified by a story that I wrote about in my book, *The Art of Case Presentation* [9]:

> A little girl and her father were crossing a bridge. The father was kind of scared, so he asked his little daughter, "Sweetheart, please hold my hand so that you don't fall in the river."
> The little girl said, "No, Dad. You hold my hand."
> "What's the difference?" asked the puzzled father.
> "There's a big difference," replied the little girl. "If I hold your hand and something happens to me, chances are that I may let your hand go. But if you hold my hand, I know for sure that no matter what happens, you will never let my hand go."

The essence of trust is not in the bind, but in its bond. It's all about the relationship. In the following chapters, I will discuss the various steps that leaders use to build trust. I want to end this chapter by emphasizing just how important it is to develop the culture of trust through a mindset that has sound ethos as a foundation because, as Frances Hesselbein, the President and CEO of The Leadership Institute (formerly known as the Leader to Leader Institute and founded as the Peter F. Drucker Foundation for Nonprofit Management), says, "Leadership is a lot less about what you do, and much more about who you are."

Earlier I said that the five major objections to dentistry are fear, finances, time constraints, no sense of urgency and a lack of trust. All of these can act as resistance or roadblocks to compliance and cooperation. Trust building clears the way by removing the barriers. A simple way to think about trust building is to use the Trust Equation that I wrote about in *The Art of Case Presentation* [10]. There are four variables to trustworthiness: Credibility, Reliability, Intimacy and Self-orientation. The following equation expresses these variables:

$$Trust = \frac{Credibility + Reliability + Intimacy}{Self\text{-}focus}$$

When you increase the values in the numerator – credibility, reliability and intimacy – trust goes up. The flip-side is, when you increase the level of self-focus in the denominator, trustworthiness drops. The following chapters will further discuss how to improve the factors in the numerator.

Trust is central to human existence. It lies behind every one of the human universals that we I have continued to make a theme of this book. Trust is the constant. When we attempt to learn leadership and communication from others, we tend to copy their style and make it an issue of personality, rather than the human universals that are available to everyone. Ethos and pathos are traits that are available to every one of us, and that is why leadership and communication is accessible to all. Remember that, ultimately, trust is based on your care and competence. It is the fastest form of human motivation. Stephen Covey tells us that, "with people, fast is slow, and slow is fast." He is talking about trust-building. In the next chapter, we will see how time and timing is important to building trust.

References and Notes

1 Elaine Aron (1996). *The Highly Sensitive Person: How to Thrive When the World Overwhelms You*, 2nd edition. Citadel.
2 Fred Kiel (2015). *Return on Character: The Real Reason Leaders and Their Companies Win*, pp. 51–78. Harvard Business Review Press.
3 Olivia Fox Cabane (2012). *The Charisma Myth: How Anyone Can Master the Art and Science of Personal Magnetism*. Portfolio; uncorrected proof edition.
4 Brené Brown (1994). *Daring Greatly: How the Courage to Be Vulnerable Transforms the Way We Live, Love, Parent, and Lead*, 9th edition. Gotham.
5 Ryan Holiday (2016). *Ego is the Enemy*, p. 2. Portfolio.
6 Amy Cuddy (2015). *Presence: Bringing Your Boldest Self to Your Biggest Challenges*. Little, Brown and Company.
7 Gandhi: "*The best way to find yourself is to lose yourself in the service of others.*" Einstein: "*Only a life lived for others is a life worthwhile.*" Schweitzer: "*I don't know what your destiny will be, but one thing I know: the only ones among you who will be really happy are those who will have sought and found how to serve.*"
8 Simon Sinek (2014). *Leaders Eat Last: Why Some Teams Pull Together and Others Don't*. Portfolio.
9 Barry Polansky (2013). *The Art of Case Presentation*, p. 103. Word of Mouth Enterprises.
10 Ibid., p. 125.

16

Contact – The First Four Minutes

"You had me at hello."

Renee Zellweger (From the movie *Jerry Maguire*)

"It's not what you hear by listening that's important; it's what you say by listening that's important."

Thomas Friedman

"I learned that we can do anything, but we can't do everything ... at least not at the same time. So think of your priorities not in terms of what activities you do, but when you do them. Timing is everything."

Dan Millman

These days, a common complaint about doctors is that they don't spend enough time with patients. In a story I found circulating on the internet, a patient, Joan E., went for an appointment with a new ear nose and throat doctor [1]. She admitted that she didn't have a stopwatch on her, but the 66-year-old consultant claimed that she had never had a faster appointment in her life. By her estimate, she was examined and a given a prescription for an antibiotic in less than five minutes. I am sure many of us can relate to this situation, as many medical practices, as well as dental practices have kept their eyes on the clock and the data, rather than the patients, and the problems, beyond annoying the patients, can become significant.

Time and money are big factors in creating success, but so is the development of human relationships. Developing human relationships, specifically the doctor-patient relationship, takes time. As we head into the future, we will see more and more of the time crunch and the specific allocation of smaller amounts of time to get the production in the books. Inevitably, something will fall by the wayside, and it's generally the doctor-patient relationship that suffers. Shorter and more rushed appointment time can also lead to more mistakes in diagnosis and treatment. There is no doubt that rushed doctors listen less. That is a double-edged sword, because listening not only takes time, but also takes skill. And doctors are notoriously poor listeners.

A 1999 study of 29 family physician practices found that doctors let patients speak for only 23 seconds before redirecting them; only one in four patients got to finish their statement. A University of South Carolina study in 2001 found primary care patients were interrupted after 12 seconds, if not by the health care provider, then by a beeper or a knock on the door. It is interesting to note how most of us can identify with being on the receiving end of not being listened to, yet so many health care providers are the ones who do it. This sounds a little like the Lake Wobegon effect meeting the Curse of Knowledge. Making a patient feel heard is one of the most important aspects of being a doctor-leader.

The medical and dental communities have been looking at time allocation studies for years. Mostly, those studies have focused on how to get more production out of practice. In an April 2016 study [2], the online medical resource, Medscape, reported that the average amount of time a doctor spends with a patient is between 13 and 16 minutes. The problem, as I see it, seems to be getting worse as we go into the future. With a greater dependence on data and production, as well as a lack of training on the part of health care workers in communication skills, the human side of health care will diminish. I once posed this concern to a young dentist, and he replied, "My generation is different because we can't have the same relationships with patients as you did, we just don't have the time." "I'm sorry," I told him, "this isn't a problem of a generation gap, it's about being human and the human universals."

Most dentists do not take the necessary time to build trust and develop relationships, yet they constantly complain of not getting cases accepted, not getting compliance, not getting paid, cancellations, and other behavioral issues, when the answer is more about strong relationships than about poor patient behavior. "Medicine is an experiential learning experience," says Dr. Kathlyn Fletcher, an associate professor of medicine at the Clement J. Zablocki Veterans Administration Medical Center [3]. She goes on to say that, "there is no substitute for the doctor-patient relationship, efficiency is important but it isn't the end of the story." In other words, being effective, the main role of a leader, is more important than being efficient. The medical community is beginning to see this as a major problem. The dental community, too, needs to see this as a major flaw in dental education.

Not taking the time to get to know the patient is only part of the problem. Many dentists believe they spend the time. The other part of the equation is to structure the conversation around good listening skills that have the objective of building trust, or else much of the time could be spent on small talk about inconsequential topics. The next chapter will discuss how to structure the conversation. At this point, I want to make the dentist aware of the importance of the early stages – the rapport building and relationship building stage.

For those readers who have read *The Art of the Examination*, you know that I believe in the process. That everything has a structure. In that book, I wrote that it only takes four minutes to begin the process to know whether you have a patient's attention, and whether they are interested in what you have to say [4]. This is probably one of the most important moments in a doctor-patient relationship. It amazes me how many dentists delegate the earliest stage of the initial appointment. It amazes me even further that dental consultants suggest delegating this stage, for the sake of time and efficiency.

The *serial positioning effect*, also known as the rule of primacy and recency, tells us that a person has the tendency to recall the first and last items in a series best, and what happens in the middle, the worst. As far as the examination process, then, the most important moments are the "hello" and the "goodbye." Leaders who do any public speaking know how important the introduction and the conclusion are to the total effect. This is true of all presentations, including presenting oneself to a new patient.

One suggested reason for the primacy effect is that the initial items presented are most effectively stored in long-term memory, because of the greater amount of processing devoted to them. The example of Joan E. that began this chapter is a good example of what she remembered about her initial appointment. Think about the last time you saw a new doctor. How long did you wait in the waiting room? How much paperwork did you have to fill out, and was there any human contact? Who was the first person who spoke with you and, finally, when did you meet the doctor and how much time did they spend with you? I know what the expected norms are these days, but effective leaders break the norms.

The message the practice wants to convey is one of care and competence. Everything in the practice should be created to send the message of individual care and complete competence. The first chance to make that impression is even before the patient enters the practice, which is why word-of-mouth and referrals are the best way to bring patients into the practice. "Branding" is the marketing term for creating the consistent message that the dentist wants to send out to the public. In other words, dentists who want to be leaders understand the idea that they *are* the message. Their physical presence, as well as everything they say and do, is well thought out, in order to send the ultimate message of care and competence, because ultimately it leads to high trust.

Most dental practices focus on the competence side of the message. Yes, competence is very important, but the dentists who ultimately succeed more send out the message of caring as the first communication. When patients feel that they truly matter, that builds trust. Let's take a look at that word – *matter*. When something really matters, it means that it is important and it takes precedence. It is valued. Leaders understand the value of other people. Leaders send the message to everyone that the other matters more than even themselves. Other people are priority, and that is why other people become the first thing on their agenda. Today's corporate dental practices generally see production and efficiency as the number one priorities. This is another example of the insecure path being the secure path – in the end.

Acclaimed author Robert Cialdini, in his latest book, *Pre-Suasion* [5], writes about the traits of successful salespeople. Because influence and persuasion are indispensable communication tools for effective leadership, his research shows that it is the things that successful people do *before* they present their case that ultimately lead to success, by building trust. Most dentists do what I refer to as *present and persuade.* Many of them take courses to learn how to present cases better. They learn techniques that help to educate patients better, whether it is through better photography or storytelling. I agree that these are good ways to influence, educate and even motivate but, without the patient truly believing that the dentist really cares, acceptance is not guaranteed.

I am often astonished at the number of dentists who tell me how proficient they are at motivating patients to accept treatment, yet they still have patients send the radiographs to another practice, or the patient goes to a practice that accepts their insurance. I am not saying that trust-building will cure everything that is wrong with dentistry, but I have had patients stay in my practice when I don't accept their insurance. And since I have incorporated leadership and better communication into my practice, I rarely have to send radiographs to other dental practices.

Leadership and communication are not hard sciences. Becoming better leaders will not guarantee success at every turn. However, the dentist who studies these skills will enhance the likelihood of success in the long run. Cialdini says, "this is the inescapable reality of operating in the realm of human behavior [6]." No one is looking for one hundred percent success – just an edge.

Cialdini makes the point that successful people understand the concept of *privileged moments.* He defines these as "identifiable points in time when an individual is particularly receptive to a communicator's message [7]." In many cases, as noted earlier, this would be at the beginning and at the end of any presentation. Since the doctor/leader *is* the message, then the very first appointment can be considered a privileged moment. Smart dental leaders understand this subtle point – that trust must be implanted before we request that we actually place implants (pun intended). Psychologists, Cialdini tells us, call these moments, "frames or anchors or primes or mindsets or first impressions [8]". Dentists who are familiar with the work of Dr. Peter Dawson in occlusion understand the role of centric relation as a starting-point for restorative dentistry. Conceptually, this is a similar situation, and the results we get will be determined by how we begin.

My goal, and my hope with this book and, specifically, this chapter, is for dentists who choose to learn and understand leadership and communication to take it so seriously that they don't continue to deceive themselves into thinking they already know these apparently not-so-self-evident skills. As you will learn, there are many ways to build trust. The first lesson is to prepare to do it by planning for these sacred privileged moments, by building it into your process. Make the time to get to know your patients – not only by planning to put away enough time, but by structuring the process as well.

There are things that my practice does to help build a trusting image, even before the patient arrives. As stated earlier, our website tries to convey a very personal and caring message. When the patient arrives is when the rubber actually hits the road – in other words, at the point of contact. Within the first 15 minutes, after my office manager greets the patient and my assistant introduces herself, I enter the room. The patient is always sitting upright, without a bib. We prepare for our conversation. We *always* follow this procedure, and I believe that it has led me to complete some very sophisticated dentistry on the unlikeliest of patients, and also on their friends and families. More than anything I do, I believe that this one concept has led to most of my success as a dental leader. Through the years, my staff has learned to take on similar methods of building trust with all of our patients.

So many patients enter our practices in pain. Their major objective is to get out of pain. The dentist/leader understands that this is one of those moments when the patient is particularly receptive to the communicator's message – that privileged moment. What a time for powerfully influential conversation! Yet, so many dentists and patients get caught up in the heaviness and negativity of the moment. By staying positive, the dentist/leader can use this moment to create a patient for life and, better yet, to change one's views about dentistry and health. Staying positive, as I have already discussed, is a trait of leaders and a major factor in communication. Whether it's the pain of the moment, or the pain of the finances, it is the successful leaders that take that moment to build trust and to send the message that they care more about the patient than even the one tooth.

Julian is one such patient. He entered my practice with a furious toothache. He just wanted relief. I injected him immediately, and then we had a conversation. The specifics of the conversation will be discussed in the next chapter. What is important here is that I knew this was a critical point in the process to stop and build trust. Once Julian was out of pain, he was able to focus on the other problems he didn't even realize he had, because the pain had so clouded his mind. Those were his long-term problems. I always focus on long-term issues. What good is it to save a tooth and watch the entire forest burn down around it? There isn't a dentist who hasn't experienced that scenario. That is why this becomes the moment to begin that conversation.

Julian was comfortable. I learned a lot about him in a short period of time. He was a cook at a local eatery. His parents lived in Colorado. They had drug issues, and there were two things he was determined to do when he moved east: firstly, never take drugs; and secondly, never to end up like his dad, without teeth. Julian, though, found his own drug – Red Bull. Because he had created a situation where he practically lived in survival, the caffeine-laden drink became his crutch, and that crutch was killing his teeth. We talked about that. He also revealed that he was getting married, so I asked him about his future and whether he wanted to have kids. I think you are getting the idea. Our conversation was more about him and his future, and how I could help him in more ways than focusing on the offending tooth.

That was two years ago. Julian went on to get married, and we fixed his tooth, and his teeth. He needed two root canals and two crowns, in addition to extensive operative dentistry. There are many similar stories like Julian's in dentistry, but there are more stories about patients who never complete their dentistry. They show up in our practices every day with half-started work, only to end up with even more pitiful situations. These problems strike right to the heart of our profession and point to our biggest shortcomings – a lack of leadership and communication skills that lead to creating highly technical dentists, who understand what to do, how to do it, but not *why* we do things.

Ryan is another patient who came in many years ago. His history revealed that he had gone to a dentist that accepted his insurance from work. Like so many patients, Ryan sought advice from his friends and co-workers. Then Ryan got married and his wife, a long-time patient in my practice, sent him to us. As always, we began with a comprehensive examination, which begins the process with my "getting to know you" pre-clinical examination. Ryan's mouth was a mess. He needed operative dentistry on every tooth. The work was so extensive that we focused only on hygiene and large fillings. We never discussed anything more than that, even though I knew he would need numerous crowns and, possibly, implants. But not before ortho-gnathic surgery. I knew, in order for Ryan to keep his teeth for his whole life, that this complex surgery would be necessary. My exam gave me the opportunity to begin that process.

It was at that appointment that I let Ryan, with the help of his wife, know that I was there to help him, and that we would do things in sequential stages. After quite a few appointments, Ryan was looking and acting like a different person. It was time to revisit, with a new examination to take advantage of another privileged moment. At this appointment, we spoke about ortho-gnathic surgery. By now it was no surprise to Ryan. He understood the difficulty in keeping his mouth clean, with all of the crowding and overlapping. He always knew the cosmetic implications, but now he was seeing with new eyes that, in order to keep his teeth, he would need the surgery and orthodontics. I am pleased to say that Ryan has had his surgery and, at the time of writing this, he is in the middle of orthodontics. Stories like these exist in dentistry, but they will only happen when the dentist takes the time to lead the patient toward better, more optimal results, and that takes a process that centers around leadership and communication.

As I said earlier, I am proud that my career has been filled with success with the most unlikely patients, accomplishing some amazing dentistry. Doing a comprehensive examination on every patient is more than a moral obligation, as L.D. Pankey told us. It is a privileged moment that will lead to more fulfillment and success than anything else we do in dentistry. It is in those moments that we provide the meaning and purpose of what we do for our patients. It fulfills one of the key components of PERMA-V, meaning, in addition to achievement and positive relations.

The late Tom Leonard, who some consider to be the father of personal coaching, tells the story of how he first discovered the concept of personal and life coaching [9]. The one-time financial advisor was consulting with clients – a husband and wife who had been with him for years. Upon leaving a meeting, one day, the wife turned and asked him what color he thought they should choose for their new car. Leonard wondered what this question had to do with finances. He told them that he had a preference for red. Later on, he reflected on that moment. He realized that, whether he liked it or not, he had become their trusted advisor in more ways than one, and that position was enhanced by the trust he had built. Just think, if we are leading people toward decisions that take them to any more positive place, toward making healthy choices, it begins with trust. Trust tears down most of the obstacles people put up that get in their way.

References and Notes

1 Roni Caryn Rabin (2014). 15-Minute Visits Take A Toll On The Doctor-Patient Relationship. *Kaiser Heath News*, April, 21.

2 Erin Brodman and Dragan Radovanovic (2016). *Here's how many minutes the average doctor actually spends with each patient.* http://www.businessinsider.com/how-long-is-average-doctors-visit-2016-4.

3 Pauline Chen (2013). New Doctors, Eight Minutes per Patient. *NY Times* blog, May 20, 2013. http://well.blogs.nytimes.com/2013/05/30/for-new-doctors-8-minutes-per-patient/

4 Leonard M. Zunin (1972). *Contact: the first four minutes.* Nash Publishing.

5 Robert Cialdini (2016). *Pre-Suasion, A Revolutionary Way to Influence and Persuade*, p. 8. Simon & Schuster.

6 Ibid. p. 8

7 Ibid., p. 14.

8 Ibid., p. 8.

9 Thomas J. Leonard (1998). *The Portable Coach: Twenty-Eight Sure-Fire Strategies for Business and Personal Success*, 1st edition. Scribner.

17

Conversation With An Elephant

"Take advantage of every opportunity to practice your communication skills so that when important occasions arise, you will have the gift, the style, the sharpness, the clarity, and the emotions to affect other people."

Jim Rohn

"When dealing with people, remember you are not dealing with creatures of logic, but creatures of emotion."

Dale Carnegie

"Human rationality depends critically on sophisticated emotionality. It is only because our emotional brain works so well that our reasoning can work at all."

Jonathan Haidt

Ben Carson did not succeed in his quest to become the Republican presidential candidate in 2016. I supported the retired neurosurgeon in his quest because, he appeared to be one of the very few candidates on either side that had character, or ethos. Many of the other candidates, at least to my eyes, had issues of character. But Carson was doomed, because he didn't have what Aristotle believed was an essential ingredient of leadership. That was a strong ability to communicate who he was and what he stood for. His metaphors and analogies always seemed to miss their mark, and he didn't resonate with the public. On the other side of this argument stands Ronald Reagan, who was known as The Great Communicator. He appealed to the people through his ability to reach them at an emotional level. He had pathos.

The one thing that we all share in common is our humanity. We lean on our rational minds to help us make decisions but, as stated so many times in this book, it is the human universals that make us so similar, and the emotional brain, or our mind, is what makes the us human.

Jonathan Haidt, in his book *The Happiness Hypothesis* [1], gives an excellent description, through metaphor, of how the mind works. He defines the mind's operation as "intuition comes first, strategic reasoning second." This reminds me of the sales axiom about buying on emotion and justifying on logic. Haidt uses an apt metaphor of the mind being like a raging elephant (emotion), trying to be controlled by a rather small rider (reason). Quite a difficult task for the mind. People make their decisions when we appeal to their emotional brains. Too many facts tend to confuse them. Their minds are continually occupied with thoughts, beliefs, and memories of their own. Their minds determine how they each experience the world. Too much data can perplex and confuse them. The mind is continually looking for happiness. The elephant is always hunting.

The Complete Dentist: Positive Leadership and Communication Skills for Success, First Edition. Barry Polansky.
© 2018 John Wiley & Sons, Inc. Published 2018 by John Wiley & Sons, Inc.

In 1953, two scientists at McGill University, James Olds and Peter Milner, tried to elicit fear responses from rats by implanting electrodes into their brains. Expecting the rats to avoid anything associated with the shock, they were shocked themselves when the rats kept returning and hoping for another jolt. The rats gravitated in the exact direction of the shock, looking for more. What they found was that Olds had implanted the electrode in the wrong part of the brain, an as yet unexplored area. The new area, instead of producing shock, had produced pleasure. The rats were experiencing desire. This discovery lead to a series of experiments that opened the doors to our understanding of human cravings, temptation and addiction. Further studies showed that, when they placed food down, the rats would forego the food in favor of getting another hit of electricity. Then they starved the rats and, even at the risk of further starvation, the rats sought stimulation over food. Next, they placed self-stimulating levers in the cage, and the rats hit themselves every five seconds until the point of physical exhaustion.

Experiments progressed to humans at Tulane University, under the direction of Robert Heath. He found exactly the same thing; people would self-stimulate rather than eat. After hours of self-stimulation and not eating, a food tray was brought in. The subjects never looked up, and kept hitting the lever. One participant continued to hit the lever over 200 times after the current was turned off. How can we explain this behavior?

According to Kelly McGonigal, author of *The Willpower Instinct*, "*What if Olds and Milner's rats weren't self-stimulating to exhaustion because it felt so good that they didn't want to stop? What if the area of the brain they were stimulating wasn't rewarding them with the experience of profound pleasure, but simply promising them the experience of pleasure? Is it possible the rats were self-stimulating because their brains were telling them that if they just pressed that lever one more time, something wonderful was going to happen. Maybe what they discovered was the reward center rather than the pleasure center. Maybe they had discovered our most primitive motivational system.*" Maybe the stimuli were rendering a promise of happiness – a signal of hope and optimism, rather than the doom and gloom normally associated with dentistry.

Researchers have since discovered that the promise of happiness is associated with a release of the chemical dopamine. The emotional brain loves dopamine. That is why our communications, to be most effective, should speak to the elephant. That is why getting people out of pain is so satisfying for most dentists – because we do not have to do any convincing. The tooth is doing all of the communication directly to the elephant.

Think about how many things in dentistry have the opposite effect on our patients. How many of patients anticipate negative consequences when going to the dentist. Negative anticipation does not create dopamine release; it actually creates a different emotional response, a negative affect. It sets off the fight-or-flight response, and that is what positive leaders do not want. Our role is to help people to make healthy choices, to influence patients and staff in positive choices that lead to healthy outcomes. The positive psychologists call this *positive intervention*.

What makes this so difficult is that we have to do all of this within the context of teeth and technology. Dentists who are reading this may be saying to themselves that all of this is true, but "who has the time?" And it does take time. It also takes a willingness to learn and practice leadership skills. It takes a growth mindset and grit, as mentioned in Chapter 3. Add to the positivity that we must make our messages brief, simple and clear, and we have the recipe for effective communication. Many dentists do the opposite.

They communicate with jargon, highly technical language, and doom-and-gloom scenarios. Their language tends to frighten, promote anxiety, and confuse the patients. In today's accelerated world, people won't take the time for long complicated explanations. People want answers now, and leaders understand that we need to take the time to get people's attention and communicate effectively. Leaders don't communicate with CT scans, radiographs and laundry lists of technical things that need to done. They communicate through trust-building, storytelling and pictures.

There is a famous urban legend that comes out of the world of advertising. The story is very popular, due to a video reenactment that went viral on YouTube. The story is about Rosser Reeves, an iconic ad man who is the model for Don Draper, the main character on the popular TV show Mad Men. Reeves is famous for developing the idea of "unique selling proposition." As the video tells the story, a blind man is sitting on a step, begging for money. He has a cup next to him for donations. Beside the cup is a sign that states, "I am blind." People pass by without stopping. They glance at the sign and move on. There are very few coins in the cup. A man comes by, looks at the sign, and writes a few words on it. He places it back beside the cup and goes on his way. Some time passes, and the editor of the sign passes by again and now sees an overflowing cup. Legend tells us the man who passed by was Rosser Reeves. What changed? What did Reeves write that persuaded people to donate? The altered sign said, "It is springtime and I am blind."

What can we learn from this? First, it doesn't take a lot of explanation and thought to move people emotionally. Just a few well-placed words can be effective. Second, by adding the words, "It is springtime and, I am blind," Reeves developed the first component of a story – a setting. The rest of the story was completed in the mind's eye of passers-by. All of a sudden, the beggar was the main character of the story, because a human touch was added. The human face was added. The sign spoke to the elephant.

There have been many explanations about how Reeves reached the emotions of the people. Dan Pink explains it by referring to the "contrast principle", first explained by Robert Cialdini in his book *Influence: Science and Practice* [2]. The contrast principle says we understand something better when we see it in comparison to something else. Adding "springtime" makes blindness take on new meaning. Even in our own minds, we begin to have more appreciation for what is, compared with what might have been. It causes us to pause and be grateful for all that we have. Gratitude-building for all of our patients, our staff and mostly ourselves, adds to the leader's positive attitude. Positivity, as I mentioned earlier, is an essential principle for communication, influence and leadership. The contrast principle is a key in closing what I call the *emotional gap*.

Most dentists understand the contrast principle, through the currently popular use of digital photography to help people to understand why they should go forward with treatment. What is less known is that the contrasting that is going on in the patient's mind is more important than the actual photography. Understand that Jonathan Haidt's metaphor of the rider and the elephant is just a metaphor – a story, if you will, that helps us to understand better how the mind works. The human mind is difficult to define. Many scientists tell us that the mind is the brain's activities. "Mind," then, is both a noun and a verb. Everyone one of us has, moving within us, millions, even billions of thoughts, beliefs, memories, fears, experiences, values, and intangible messages that compete with one another at any given moment.

L.D. Pankey, in all of his wisdom, tried to codify this for dentists by telling them to get to know the patient by understanding their circumstances, objectives and temperament. When we take a closer look at the mind, this is a lot more difficult than it sounds. Business management people in all fields advise us to understand personalities better by studying personality and behavioral assessment tools, like the DISC system and the Meyers-Brigg Type Indicator. Although I do believe in the validity of these tools, I also believe that dentists who are trying to become effective communicators and leaders can get caught up in the daily application of these tools. I know I did. After all, at the most basic level, we are all human. I believe there is a better way to effectively close the emotional gap and improve our communication.

The answer is stories. Stories give your patients something to take home besides the bill. The human brain is hardwired to learn, and its best tool for learning is stories. Stories help us to de-clutter the mind. Storytelling helps to make things brief, simple and clear. Story organizes thought and helps the rider, the executive brain, to decipher everything for the elephant.

People come to us with their own stories. Their stories include their own personal circumstances, their own goals and objectives, all filtered through their own personality styles. In order to better understand their world, they confabulate, or fill in gaps in their memory with fabrications that one believes to be facts. Their stories include fearful stories of not being worthy enough, or not having enough. They include "why me?" stories, "why now?" stories, "who am I?" stories and "who do I want to be?" stories. The best communicators go through that maze of stories to get and maintain attention, in order to effectively communicate.

In my first years of dental practice, I hired a consultant who gave me a book to read. He told me this was L.D. Pankey's favorite book. It's title was *The Magic Power of Emotional Appeal*. I read it with great enthusiasm as if I had found the Lost Ark. But, once again, like the behavioral assessment tools, it was more descriptive than prescriptive – in other words, I had understood more about people's motivation, but didn't have a simple tool to actually apply my knowledge. What the book did teach was that pathos, or emotional appeal, is the key to communication. Storytelling is the much more simple answer – it's the prescription.

It is stories that our rider tells our elephant to explain why we feel the way we do. It is stories that calm the emotional brain to make rational decisions. The psychologist Jonathan Haidt explains it best, "The human mind is a story processor. Everyone loves a good story; every culture bathes its children in stories." I know this sounds counter-intuitive to most dentists. From dental school, and continuing into their formal careers, they are taught to sit down and rationally explain, at a technical and intellectual level, why patients should follow their advice. That is truly old school. It makes sense, but it just doesn't work.

Jonah Lehrer, author of *How We Decide*, explains that, ever since ancient Greece, as long as people have made decisions (case acceptance is a decision), the theory has been that the brain was responsible. Since the brain was an inaccessible "black box," they made the assumption that humans are rational. Thinkers like Plato, through Descartes ("I think therefore I am."), claimed that rationality defined us. However, as Lehrer tells us, and backs up with sound research, "They were wrong; it's not how the brain works." Hopefully, I have convinced you to communicate through stories, but that is only half of the answer. The most effective way to tell our stories is visually. Visual storytelling will really improve your effective communication.

The very best leaders speak with word pictures. I understand that some people are more gifted than others when it comes to using visual language. That is why, as dentists, we can take advantage of other tools to get our message across in a very positive manner. Even when I was in dental school, I would always take out my colored pencil and draw pictures, in order to explain what was happening. Occasionally, I would fall into using jargon, but I was quick to notice the bewildered and confused look on patient's faces. Today, I use my tools to tell a story. The tools include language, pencils and paper for drawing, professional illustrations, and the one tool, I believe, that no dental practice should be without – a digital camera. Of course, all of these tools will only be effective if they tell a story.

According to John Medina, author of the book *Brain Rules*, "We learn and remember best through pictures, not through written or spoken words." Yet our eyes aren't even accurate enough. We need our minds to make sense of what our eyes see. Our eyes do not act like cameras – they give us only the best representation of reality. What we see is what is delivered to our brains and processed in our visual cortex. How we interpret what we see is based on our past experiences and through the filter of subjectivity. Vision is intimately connected to memory and learning.

There is a phenomenon known as PSE, the Pictorial Superiority Effect. The more visual the input, the more likely it is to be recognized and recalled. In study after study, researchers have found that people can recall more than 2500 pictures with 90% accuracy, several days after exposure. A year later accuracy rates still hovers over 60%. When compared to the other common methods by which dentists present their cases, written and oral, pictures and photographs come out on top by a long shot. In fact, 90% of oral presentations are usually forgotten within 72 hours, unless there are images. If photographs are added to the oral presentation, retention rates increase to 65%. No matter what words we use, the brain will see them as pictures.

From what has been learned about storytelling, emotions, and PSE, I think there are many factors that go into case acceptance. I believe one main factor is building a high level of trust. I believe another one is transferring our information to the right place in our patient's mind, the emotional center. I believe the best way to do this by using pictures and very clear language, which helps patients form their own word pictures. The brain devotes a lot of real estate to vision, and it is the main way to get our patient's attention and keep it. Essentially, the dentist is an educator, a teacher, or a coach, a leader, and a communicator.

Comprehensive care has, as its goal, to help people keep their teeth for a lifetime; to create positive interventions. The mission is the "what" we do, the purpose is the "why" we do it, and the vision is the "where" we are taking our patients. This requires behavioral change. The purpose of education is behavioral change. To change people, we must reach them at an emotional level.

In the next section, on logos, I will go further into how to accomplish high level emotional communication. For now I want to make it clear that all of our messages should be brief, simple and clear. I see too many dentists attempting to get their messages across by being too long-winded, getting caught up in the minutiae of the case, forgetting why people are coming to us to begin with, and using jargon to explain themselves. In the last chapter, I discussed the importance of first impressions. The most important lesson that leaders need to understand about pathos is that everything matters. I want to close out this section of the book with a very famous quote by the poet Maya Angelou: "I've learned that people will forget what you said, people will forget what you did, but people will never forget how you made them feel." This is the essence of leadership pathos.

Reference

1 Jonathan Haidt (2005). *The Happiness Hypothesis: Finding Modern Truth in Ancient Wisdom*, 1st edition. Basic Books.
2 Robert B. Cialdini (2006). *Influence: The Psychology of Persuasion*, Revised edition. HarperBusiness.

Part V

Logos – Where the Rubber Meets the Road

"Science isn't about authority or white coats; it's about following a method."
Ben Goldacre

"The goal of climbing big, dangerous mountains should be to attain some sort of spiritual and personal growth, but this won't happen if you compromise away the entire process."
Yvon Chouinard

"A good system shortens the road to the goal."
Orison Sweet Marden

Logos is the starting and ending point of most dental education. It is where most dentists focus when creating their careers. Pankey's philosophy recognized the need for logos as one component of an overall system of thought for applying the principles of dentistry. Yet, like so many complex disciplines, we fail to hear the signal through the noise. Our entire careers center on the logos, rather than the ethos and pathos. The Greek word logos means "word," "reason" or "plan," and it refers to the idea of giving something form, order and meaning. The philosopher Heraclitus first used the term as a principle of order and knowledge. Aristotle applied the term to mean reasoned discourse. Pankey applied it to mean knowing our work at a rational level and, although he acknowledged character and human emotions in his philosophy, the main focus remains on the logos dentistry.

From a practical point of view, I believe that logos is how the dentist/leader puts all of the elements together, so that he or she can create methods to apply all of the components. It's what makes any philosophy work in the real world. For me, logos answers the question "how?" Not from the point of view of solely production or outcomes, where most dentists focus their efforts, but more from the perspective of learning a process, or an order of things that will lead to consistent, predictable outcomes in every phase of the profession – from excellent dentistry and approved case presentations, to positive, powerful and prosperous relationships. Author Robert Heinlein said, "One man's magic is another man's engineering." In other words, successful leaders get to create their careers through proper design, logos is the design.

One theme throughout this book has been on mindset and the work of Carol S. Dweck [1]. Earlier, I described her distinction between a fixed and growth mindset. If the dentist is going to put together all of the elements discussed in this book, then it must start with a growth mindset. Too many dentists operate with a fixed mindset, or they start with a growth mindset

The Complete Dentist: Positive Leadership and Communication Skills for Success, First Edition. Barry Polansky.
© 2018 John Wiley & Sons, Inc. Published 2018 by John Wiley & Sons, Inc.

and, after a few setbacks, fall into fixed mindset. One of the traits of a mindset is how we view goals: either *performance-oriented or learning-oriented* [2].

A dentist with a fixed mindset focuses on production and successful outcomes. There is danger lurking there, because behind that mindset is a quest for validation from others, and the sole purpose of achievement. Although achievement is one of the elements of the PERMA model of well-being, alone it does not lead to thriving. If goals are not met, or if outcomes fall short, the dentist tends to blame him/herself or others, which affects the entire culture of the practice. The tendency to judge or blame oneself leads the dentist to quit early, and possibly to fall into a state of apathy over time.

Instead of *performance goals*, the dentist with a growth mindset focuses on *learning goals*. With learning goals, the focus is on competence and mastery, rather than on simple production goals and winning. Mindsets can change everything. The growth mindset helps the dentist to sustain a long career, as new habits are created and continual long-term growth prolongs and preserves a fulfilling career. The growth mindset puts the idea of responsibility firmly in the daily obligations of the dentist. Responsibility means the ability to respond in a positive manner, rather than to react to every issue that presents itself every day. Reactivity is the source of the enslavement that dentists want to avoid, and responsibility is the source of freedom, happiness and success.

Sure, the fixed mindset can help with having a good month, or help to create a gorgeous cosmetic Facebook-worthy case, but it's not long-term success, fulfillment and personal well-being, which are the worthy goals. For those, the growth mindset is necessary. The growth mindset leads to a self-filling prophecy of mastery, and the development of passion for the profession. The fixed mindset may be one factor that can lead to burnout, because it does not equip the dentist with the tools to bounce back from the inevitable setbacks we all face.

Albert Einstein said, "If you can't explain it simply, you don't understand it well enough." It's in logos that the leader gets to apply everything that he or she has developed in building the mindset for leadership. The logos is where the leader gets to use the skills and tools for wellbeing and success. Too many professionals are what Texans call "all hat and no cattle." Leaders are the whole package, and they realize they can't fake their way to success over the long-term.

Before beginning the final section, I want to begin with a story:

> On a certain day, a bull and a pheasant were grazing on a field. The bull was grazing and the pheasant was picking ticks off of the bull – a perfect partnership. Looking at the huge tree at the edge of the field, the pheasant said, 'Alas, there was a time I could fly to the topmost branch of the tree. Now I do not have enough strength in my wing to even get to the first branch.'
>
> The bull said, nonchalantly, 'Just eat a littler bit of my dung every day, and watch what happens. Within two weeks, you'll get to the top.'
>
> The pheasant said, 'Oh come on, that's rubbish. What kind of nonsense is that?'
>
> The bull said, 'Try it and see. The whole of humanity is on to it.'
>
> Very hesitantly, the pheasant started pecking. And lo, on the very first day, he reached the first branch. Within a fortnight, he had reached the topmost branch. He sat there, just beginning to enjoy the scenery.
>
> The old farmer, rocking on his rocking chair, saw a fat old pheasant on top of the tree. He pulled out his shotgun and shot the bird off the tree.
>
> Moral of the story: bullshit may get you to the top, but it never lets you say there [3]."

We cannot account for what each day will bring. Dentists depend on working with other people. Our success depends on our ability to master technical, as well as behavioral, skills. Most important is our own well-being, which begins within ourselves. Logos is the structure that helps us create the systems and the processes to make practical use of the wisdom we learned in the earlier sections of this book.

References

1 Carol S. Dweck (2007). *Mindset: The New Psychology of Success*. Ballantine Books.
2 Kate Hefferon, and Ilona Boniwell (2011). *Positive Psychology Theory, Research and Application*, 1st edition, p. 152. Open University Press.
3 Sadhguru Jaggi Vasudev (2016). *Inner Engineering: A Yogi's Guide to Joy*, 1st edition, p. 30. Spiegel & Grau.

18

The Practical Wisdom of Systems and Processes

"A good system shortens the road to the goal."

Orison Sweet Marden

"If you can't describe what you are doing as a process, you don't know what you're doing."
W. Edwards Deming

"Practical wisdom is what's called for in situations that have a moral dimension to them."
Barry Schwartz

Let's try a little thought experiment, first proposed by James Paweleski, the director of education and senior scholar at the Penn Positive Psychology Center. He asked participants to imagine that a genie appears before them and says she will transform them into a superhero. There are two types of superheroes to choose from. One type would be a hero who would combat the negatives, or the things we don't like or want in the world, like poverty or inequality. If you were to become a dental superhero, your job would be to combat tooth decay and periodontal disease, like those TV ads that were popular many years ago, that made the "cavity creeps" the villains of the oral cavity. That superhero would be given a red cape. Then Pawelski describes another type of superhero: one who spends his time seeking out positives, like growth, harmony and justice, and the good things we want in our lives. These superheroes would wear a green cape. Which would you ask your tailor to make for you? Red cape? Or green cape?

If you choose the red cape, you look for problems and, in dentistry, as we know, there are plenty. The world certainly needs red-caped dentists. But if you're a green-caped dentist, you look for opportunities. I propose that dental leaders see these opportunities. Let me make it clear – and this is a dilemma. You can practice meaningful dentistry doing one or the other, but Pawelski suggests that we don't have to choose one or the other. We can tell our tailor to make our capes reversible. If we focus on one or the other, it changes the fundamental way we practice. Dental schools teach us to look for problems that need to be fixed. They teach red-cape dentistry. Certainly, a dentist will never go broke putting out fires.

Let me suggest that we take advantage of another of those cognitive biases that I wrote about in Chapter 9. This one is known as the attention bias, or the confirmation bias. This is a brain bias that occurs from the direct influence of desire on beliefs. When people would like a certain idea/concept to be true, they end up believing it to be true. In other words, our beliefs become the lens through which we see the world, and our brain has the potential to create our reality. Your perception is your reality. If you see yourself as a green-caped dentist, you will create the systems to help create the conditions for your patients to thrive by striving for complete

The Complete Dentist: Positive Leadership and Communication Skills for Success, First Edition. Barry Polansky.
© 2018 John Wiley & Sons, Inc. Published 2018 by John Wiley & Sons, Inc.

dentistry. If you see yourself as a red-caped dentist, you will be treating problems all day, and never taking the time to build successful, fruitful relationships that will be conducive to better long-term results for everyone.

Most dentists focus on what they don't want. Most dentists don the red cape daily.

It starts with a mindset on focusing on what you want, and creating the systems and policies to make it happen. Of course, the dentist can't retire his red cape, because problems are what generally bring patients into the practice. The leader's job is to fix the immediate problem and to have systems in place to start building long-term relationships. By focusing on the positive nature of green-cape dentistry, you will build the processes that lead to growth for all concerned. Doing the opposite does not involve the same processes.

Leaders understand that a lack of dental disease does not equate to dental health. Just because our patients do not have any cavities or periodontal disease does not mean that they have the optimal conditions to prevent future disease, or that they are functioning at the highest level. Leaders understand that most people are satisfied with their dental condition if there are no symptoms, but they also realize that there is a higher plane that reaches to a more favorable position. The same is true for the well-being of the dentist and staff. Red-caped dentists will gladly admit that they are happy taking care of problems, but they will never realize the potential to grow and flourish as a professional by taking the green-caped road. In other words, happiness is subjective, like dental health. Dentists who focus on their well-being by applying the elements of PERMA into their practice will thrive.

By creating processes that ensures the dentist builds a positive environment, spends most of his or her day doing engaging work, works with people who truly appreciate him and his efforts, and provides meaningful long-term dentistry and gets paid appropriately, the dentist will practice dentistry for many years, by creating a thriving and flourishing life and career.

Let me invoke another cognitive bias that may be working against us. It is the negativity bias. It says that negative thoughts are stronger than positive thoughts; thus, when left to its own devices, the mind defaults to the negative. From an evolution standpoint, this served the purpose of survival. We overlook the positive, because the results are long-term. In other words, problems scream and opportunities whisper.

Speaker and author Srikumar Rao said, "If you create your own reality, and the reality you're experiencing does not serve you, create a new one." One of the reasons that I used positive psychology as the foundation for leadership and communication is because creating your own world is more difficult than it sounds. It requires high levels of emotional intelligence, self-awareness and self-compassion. Building the systems to create a flourishing career requires that we understand the emotional requirements of leadership. It is through logos that we see our practice connected to the ideas of ethos and pathos. Character and communication skills get applied in our systems and processes.

The Scottish author Samuel Smiles said, "Practical wisdom is only to be learned in the school of experience. Precepts and instruction are useful so far as they go, but without the discipline of real life, they remain of the nature of theory only." I have found that to be true in my own life and career. Every day of practice began another adventure. No matter how hard I tried to be a good person and a good dentist, and no matter how many courses I took to learn the scripts of persuasion, it wasn't until I applied the use of processes and systems that I found any order to what I was doing. Things, through description, as Deming says in the quote at the start of this chapter says, began to make sense. As I created the systems and put them in place, we became better. We practiced the systems until systems became the highest quality of our practice. As Michael Gerber said in his book *The E-Myth Revisted* [1], "The system is the solution."

Gerber was a student of W. Edwards Deming, a mathematician and statistician who has been given the credit for reinventing Japanese management and business principles. Deming is the founder of TQM – total quality management – which helped to define the service industry in the 1980s. Here is a list of some of my favorite "Demingisms [2]" that imply the importance of process and systems:

1) "Management of outcome is a skill. It does not require knowledge."
2) "A rule should suit a purpose."
3) "By what method? Use the one that corresponds closest to your need."
4) "You should not tamper with the process."
5) "You cannot achieve an aim unless you have a method."
6) "It does not happen all at once. There is no instant pudding."
7) "A system must be managed, it will not manage itself."
8) "People care more for themselves when they contribute to the system."
9) "A goal without a method is nonsense."
10) "I am not reporting things about people. I am reporting things about practices."
11) "Without an aim, there is no system."
12) "A leader is a coach, not a judge."
13) "A system is articulated activities directed toward an aim."
14) "The beginning of the system begins with the patient (sic)."
15) "The problem is what most courses teach is wrong." (negative bias?)
16) "We are being ruined by the best efforts of people who are doing the wrong thing."
17) "We should work on our processes, not the outcome of our processes."
18) "There is a penalty for ignorance. We are paying through our nose."

Let's take a look at a few of these through the lens of ethos and pathos, and what we have learned so far.

In earlier chapters, I wrote about the importance of building a culture based on trust. I also mentioned the growth mindset and judgment. Deming claims that if we focus on the process, we can contribute toward a culture of trust. We learn that the process makes room for all contingencies, and becomes a living, changing guide to accomplish what we are setting out to do – high-quality, relationship-based dentistry. The method always keeps our mission in view, because everything is purpose-driven.

After writing *The Art of the Examination* [3], I had the opportunity to coach dentists. I found out how difficult it was to teach my process to them. In the interim, I understood the reasons why dentists have a difficult time applying a process. Some of these reasons are mentioned by Deming. "There is no instant pudding" is Deming's reference to the work necessary in putting the system together. The system isn't just thrown together without giving thought to the ethos and pathos of the practice. In other words, the dentist must create the specific goals and mission well before putting the system together. It took me over a year to create and implement my methods. Then I continued to improve it, by developing more and better technical and communication skills.

I focused on "process over product" where my colleagues and clients were placing more emphasis on the product. Whether the product was the production goals that were randomly set, or whether it was doing big, esthetic cases to present to their local study club, most had little tolerance for the process. I don't want you to think that this is a judgment. It is human nature to focus on the product, rather than the process. No one knows that better than writers. In writing this book, my mind continually drifts toward the result, or the published product. It takes effort to focus on the daily incremental advances that inevitably lead to success.

So, as Deming says, we are being ruined by putting our efforts toward the wrong thing (product over process), and we are being taught wrong. Dental schools don't focus on the process. The teachers are generally dentists who have been wearing the red cape throughout their entire careers. They never teach us about the negative bias that continually gets in the way of building positive strategies to get better outcomes all around.

One of those consequences is the well-being of the dentist, staff and the patients. That is the ignorance that Deming is referring to. We pay through our noses with poor dentistry, poor outcomes, staff turnover and burnout. It takes work to put high-quality systems in place; there is no instant pudding.

Let me give you an example. One of my coaching clients sent me a radiograph of two mandibular premolars that had severe caries below the gum-line. The teeth appeared hopeless. I asked him what his plan was going to be. He said his diagnosis was external resorption, and he made a referral to an oral surgeon, who was going to extract the two teeth and place two implants. My first thought was red-caped dentistry. On our coaching call, I asked about the patient. He reported that she was a patient of record for over 20 years. She had done everything asked of her, including some sophisticated cosmetic dentistry. I asked him how she felt about losing these two teeth, and he said she was upset, but she would have the implants placed.

I think this is fairly typical of the way dentistry is practiced. I asked him if he thought there may be any other differential diagnoses than external resorption. I just couldn't wrap my mind around external resorption localized to two teeth. I also didn't believe that, all of a sudden, we were dealing with severe caries on a patient who has good hygiene and has never missed an appointment. So I began to question him. Did he discuss any other reasons why this condition just popped up? Had she changed medications in the past six months? Is she aware of any new habits that she may have developed? Did she have any recent radiology treatments? In other words, I just wanted him to think in terms of process. Is that important? Yes, because I do believe that external resorption is one of the possibilities but, if it's not, does that change the final treatment plan? I think so.

This moment was a great opportunity to step back and re-examine the patient. To take her through the new patient examination again; a fresh start, because this is a new and significant development. Although the patient wasn't new, the finding was new, and it was significant enough to create a major treatment plan.

By re-interviewing the patient, we give the patient more of a sense of control in the process. We may find something different, or we may not. The second approach is a green-cape approach. We are not just "fixing teeth," we are involving patients in a process. The dental leader involves his patients and staff in all decisions and, whether people express it or not, having a sense of control in the decision-making process is important. As mentioned earlier, having autonomy is a human trait and, when autonomy is disregarded or omitted, people consider that a threat. Control is important. Sending the patient off to the oral surgeon or periodontist without a firm diagnosis and plan is red-caped dentistry, unless it's the diagnosis that is what is being requested. Green-cape dentistry is about the process of diagnosing the causes of the problem as well as the problem itself, then planning around the causes to prevent future occurrences.

Let's take a look at a classic experiment, conducted in a nursing home by psychologists Ellen Langer and Judith Rodin [4]. At the beginning of the experiment, the staff told all of the residents at a nursing home that they wanted them to have a pleasant experience while they were at the home. Hopefully, this is what we want for our patients. Part of the process, then, is to explain our intentions. For example, in a practice, we might explain that we want our patients to keep their teeth for their whole lives, and we want to do it appropriately, as we stated in our mission statement. It's sort of a promise. But those are words. How do we keep that promise? Through a high-quality process, which Langer and Rodin explained.

The experimenters divided the residents into two groups. One group was the *high responsibility group* and the other was the *low responsibility group*. The high responsibility group were told that they had a lot of responsibility in how they wanted to live their lives, whereas the low responsibility group was told that the staff would be taking care of them and making decisions for them. As an example, the high responsibility group was asked if they wanted a plant (they all did), and were told that it was up to them to take care of the plant as they saw fit. They were also told that they were going to see a movie and were asked what night they wanted to see the movie. The other group was just given a plant, and that the staff would take care of it for them. They were also told that they were going to see a movie on a specific night.

These were subtle differences in an approach, but they were different. Remember that both groups were told the intentions of the nursing home: to make sure that the residents had a comfortable stay and wanted them to be happy. The only difference was in the decision-making process; the staff in both cases were well-meaning. The short-term results were stunning. In three weeks, the researchers reported that the high responsibility group was significantly happier, more active and more alert than their counterparts in the low responsibility group. Eighteen months later, the results continued to go along the same path. The high responsibility group members became healthier and were less likely to die, relative to those in the low responsibility group.

These simple differences held very significant meaning for the recipients of the process. Part of the meaning has to do with the attributes of the process, meaning that the residents were subtly being told that they can and should take more responsibility for their lives. Isn't that what dentists complain about? That patients don't take enough responsibility for their health? The process should include the message that the dentist wants their patients to be involved, and that should be built into the process. The other thing about the high responsibility group is that the experience allowed them to be more involved and in control of the treatment. "Inclusive" is a word that comes up for me. If patients are given these feelings of control and autonomy throughout the process, cooperation and compliance will improve. One is a green-cape perspective and the other a red-cape perspective. This may be the difference between an overly clinical and a more human approach to healthcare.

In my examination process, which I will go over in more detail, so many people thank me for including them in the decision-making process. That is intentionally built into the system. Right from the start, they tell me how different it feels in my practice than anywhere they have been before. This is logos at work at every step of the way. The process I have put in place engages people to take part in their own health. If you have been paying attention, a leader builds systems that respects the human universals, not only for himself but for others as well. People appreciate the autonomy and engagement that the process allows. Here is another advantage; lawsuits and disputes will be lower. Studies show that physicians are more likely to be sued when a patient perceives that a procedure went badly and the doctor demonstrated poor bedside manner [5].

Dentistry is a complex profession. We just can't will desirable outcomes; we must create the processes to get there. When we get poor outcomes combined with a poor process, the results are highly combustible, like lawsuits, and the issues Deming referred to when we pay through our noses. Leaders can't bully their followers into submission. "My way or the highway" leadership doesn't work. Leaders understand the practical application of leadership. The practical wisdom of putting the ideas of ethos and pathos into systems that work is what the Greeks called "phronesis." or a type of wisdom relevant to practical things, requiring an ability to discern how or why to act virtuously and encourage practical virtue, or excellence of character, in others.

I understand that it is difficult to focus on process thinking, rather than results thinking. Sports psychologist Jason Selk advises his clients, "when the focus is only on results, you aren't necessarily learning the *whys* and *hows* that produce those results, which makes it hard for you to pull yourself out of a slump – and adds pressure you don't need [6]." Focusing on the results can actually make it harder to produce those results, and it makes any results you do produce take longer to achieve. Selk calls this a paradox, because the focus on results doesn't produce the results you truly want to produce: "Reformatting your thinking to emphasize the process is the only way to effectively set goals that will actually produce the results you want to see."

Most practice management people don't offer this advice. They push for production goals. When I began to create systems, I realized that I would have to also create behaviors that would eventually become habits, in order to effectively produce consistent results. In other words, the daily behaviors and habits are what led to the results I truly wanted. The good news is that both types of goals – production and process – can be monitored and tracked.

As a writer, I can tell you that spending at least two hours every day writing is a process goal. Athletes do it all the time as well. Football players who spend 30 minutes watching film after practice find that it makes them better. Those behaviors eventually become automatic. The nice thing about process goals is that they are always within your control, whereas production goals often become hopes and dreams. Daily actions are within your control and, preferably, they are being tracked daily. The most successful dentists and leaders I know devote much more focus on process goals. They never lose sight of their destination, their vision, or production, but they focus on the process. Maybe this is what Aristotle meant when he famously said, "We are what we repeatedly do. Excellence is not an act, but a habit."

Building habits is difficult. Dreaming about production is easy. Building habits is about doing the work and overcoming daily resistance. That is why the "quantified self" revolution has taken over. We understand how important it is to monitor our health, so we purchase devices to keep us on track. Here is what one dentist, a Faculty member of the Pankey Institute and principal of FunktionalTracker.com, has to say: "*Buying a better scale will not help you lose weight (outcome or product) … you have to track the behavioral changes in real time (process) with a Fit Bit or My Fitness Pal to help keep your cerebral cortex in charge. Our instinctual and emotional brains often trump the thinking brain and we give up. The same is true in our practices and in life. Knowing is not doing. We often confuse making a decision to do something with actually doing it.*"

Scott Adams, the creator of the popular comic strip *Dilbert*, says that "goals are for losers." He goes on to explain that, "If you study people who succeed, you will see that most of them follow systems, not goals [7]." He defines goals as "reach it and be done" objectives, and systems as what you do on a daily basis, with the general expectation of improvement. Examples include: losing weight is a goal, but eating right is a system; running a marathon in under four hours is a goal, but running daily is a system. Systems are flexible, and leave you open to newer and better ways of doing things. Goals aren't very useful for personal and career success because, by only focusing on goals, we miss other opportunities. Systems are skill-based and, essentially, just building and creating systems will improve your chances of long-term success.

Many dentists compare themselves to others, often blaming their success on luck. But success, Adams tells us, is nothing more than luck × skills = success. By developing and adhering to systems, we develop the skills that are necessary to help us see opportunities that are invisible to most. Author Richard Wiseman tells us that luck is the product of four basic principles: noticing and creating chance opportunities; making lucky decisions by listening to their intuition; creating self-fulfilling prophecies via positive expectations; and adopting a resilient attitude that transforms bad luck into good [8]. It all starts with systems that develop the skills that open us up to luck and success.

Recall the patient above with the external resorption? The green-cape approach would have brought her back into a new patient system, which may have led to different results. This is the power of positive psychology in creating our own luck. Hopefully, you have learned the importance of the difference in the processes of red-cape and green-cape dentistry. They are subtle, but they make all the difference. I also discussed the importance of habits and monitoring behaviors. In the next chapter, I will define the attributes of policies and systems, and the key skills that are needed to become a better dentist and leader.

References and Notes

1 Michael E. Gerber (1995). *The E-Myth Revisited: Why Most Small Businesses Don't Work and What to Do About It.* HarperCollins.

2 W. Edwards Deming (2012). *The Essential Deming: Leadership Principles from the Father of Quality*, 1st edition. McGraw-Hill Education.

3 Barry Polansky (2003). *The Art of the Examination*, pp. 154–155. Word of Mouth Enterprises.

4 Ellen Langer and Judith Rodin (1976). The Effects of Choice and Enhanced Personal Responsibility for the Aged: A Field Experiment in an Institutional Setting. *Journal of Personality and Social Psychology* **34**: 191–198.

5 W. Levinson, D. Rotor, J.P.Mullooly, V. Dull and R.Frankel (1997). Physician-Patient Communication: Relationship with Malpractice Claims among Primary Care Physicians and Surgeons. *Journal of the American Medical Association* **277**: 553–559.

6 J. Selk, T. Bartow, M. Rudy (2015). *Organize Tomorrow Today: 8 Ways to Retrain Your Mind to Optimize Performance at Work and in Life*, p. 93. Da Capo Lifelong Books.

7 Scott Adams (2013). *How to Fail at Almost Everything and Still Win Big: Kind of the Story of My Life*, 1st edition. Portfolio.

8 Richard Wiseman (2003). *The Luck Factor*. Miramax.

19

The Key Systems and Skills

"Communication is a skill that you can learn. It's like riding a bicycle or typing. If you're willing to work at it, you can rapidly improve the quality of every part of your life."

Brian Tracy

"There are good leaders who actively guide and bad leaders who actively misguide. Hence, leadership is about persuasion, presentation and people skills."

Shiv Khera

I recently had a coaching call with one of my clients. She was quite upset that she had to let someone go, and the firing was not pleasant. For the past two years, the employee had been asking for raises, and the dentist continued to give raises because she felt she was being held hostage by the employee. It was true that the employee had become an invaluable front desk person, but it was also true that the practice could not afford to pay excessive and exorbitant salaries. The employee, after working so many years, turned hostile and threatened to sue.

Needless to say, this episode caused the dentist major stress. I asked her if she had systems in place that were tied to the practice budget. I asked if there was a bonus system. The conversation turned to a discussion on the importance of policies and systems in the day-to-day running of a dental practice. The policies and systems are the ultimate expression of the information we use to run our practices. What is most important is that the systems inform every member of the team how everything is done, freeing the leader to pay attention to what is most important: the dentistry and the practice culture. Policies and systems answer the question: "How do things work around here?"

I hear stories like this all the time. It is no way to work. Things can quickly get out of control when there are no guides or governing rules. When there is no leadership based on guiding principles, there is chaos and stress. In the end, the way we work provides us with the energy to sustain our careers over a long period of time, rather than sucking the life and energy from us every day. Good leaders take the time to reflect on what it is that they want and how they want to practice, in order to satisfy all concerned: patients, staff, and the doctor.

Seth Lloyd, a professor of mechanical engineering and physics at the Massachusetts Institute of Technology, who refers to himself as a "quantum mechanic," says "One way of thinking about all of life and civilization is as being about how the world registers and processes information." His research area is the interplay of information with complex systems, especially quantum systems. Our practices are complex systems that integrate and communicate though the use of data and information. It is through building processes and systems that we can create a sustainable game plan for success.

The Complete Dentist: Positive Leadership and Communication Skills for Success, First Edition. Barry Polansky.
© 2018 John Wiley & Sons, Inc. Published 2018 by John Wiley & Sons, Inc.

Let me remind you of what I wrote in Chapter 1: "Psychologist Mihalyi Csikszentmihalyi [1] tells us that evolution has always favored complexity. By complexity, he means highly differentiated and integrated at the same time. If the components are not highly differentiated and integrated, then the result is too simple, and is not destined to hold up over time. If the components are not integrated, or do not properly communicate with one another, then the result breaks down, due to being overly complicated. It's the systems that are the solution. The systems give us the template to continually grow our careers over time, by providing us with the flexibility to grow in every way – financially, technically, and emotionally. Over time, the work provides us with a way to reach our highest potentials – what Maslow called self-actualization – rather than spending our whole lives and careers stuck in survival.

Policies and systems work together. A policy is a statement of intent, and is implemented as a procedure or protocol. Before building systems, the leader must think about "why" we will be doing what we do. The earlier parts of this book were concerned with my own particular philosophy, much of which was based on my life experiences and influencers in my life, like Peter Dawson, L.D. Pankey, and my parents and teachers. Creating policy takes self-reflection and self-awareness. We all must consider what Michael Gerber calls our "primary aim"; each system we create should be looked at through the lens of our primary aim or ultimate intentions. A policy is not set in stone. Policies must remain flexible, to guide actions toward those that are most likely to achieve a desired outcome. Deming said, "Without an aim, there is no system."

Things change. When I first began my journey, I started with self-reflection. *The E-Myth* [2] was one of the first business books I read that resonated with the plight of a small businessperson. Being somewhat philosophical, and considering that I was coming out of some of the worst years of my life, I focused on happiness as my primary aim. Yet, every time I sat down to reflect on how to make a "happy" life and career, I fell back to "production and collection" goals. In other words, I didn't have the mental or language tools to actually express how to get what I truly wanted. It took time. It took lots of reading, especially in the field of psychology and behavior. It took lots of conversations with trusted advisors. Some things worked; some did not. I met many people who gave me conflicting advice.

Discovering what you want in life is very personal. Most people buy into what the culture tells us we "should" want. Once we determine what it is we want, then the work really begins to figure out the systems, which become the roadmap to success. It was during these years that I began to feel and understand what Einstein meant when he said, "The significant problems we face cannot be solved at the same level of thinking we were at when we created them."

The vast majority of dentists give very little thought to the day-to-day operations of their practices. They usually solve all of their problems with two solutions that never get to the heart of most of their issues. They believe that all problems can be handled by building profit centers. They feel that building new profit centers by learning new skills, or that buying new technology will create growth. They also believe that measuring growth by increasing production will create success. They measure growth by setting daily and monthly production goals. That's where most dentists stop – by setting production goals, and giving no other thought on how to reach those goals, except by adding new profit centers. Goals are overrated. They only answer the question: "*What?*"

Every course I have ever taken has stressed the importance of goal-setting. They tell us the importance of setting goals through a story of the 1953 Harvard study, or the 1979 Yale study, on the effects of written goals of graduates on their long-term performance. Advice usually comes in the form of a story that sounds like this:

There was a study done at Harvard between 1979 and 1989. Graduates of the MBA program were asked, "Have you set clear written goals for your future and made plans to accomplish them?" The results that were reported said:

- Only 3% had written goals and plans;
- 13% had goals, but not in writing;
- 84% had no specific goals at all.

Ten years later, Harvard interviewed the members of that class again and found:

- The 13% who had goals, but not in writing, were earning on average twice as much as the 84% of those who had no goals at all.
- The 3% who had clear, written goals were earning, on average, ten times as much as the other 97% of graduates altogether. The only difference between the groups was the clarity of the goals they had for themselves.

If you haven't heard that story before, you may have heard a similar story of the 1953 Yale graduates, which concluded the 3% of graduates who set written goals out-produced the wealth of the remaining 97% of the class. The takeaway for generations of business people to come is that setting written goals causes or correlates with wealth and success. The problem is that no such studies were really ever done at Harvard or Yale [3].

This has become a point of fact, through a statement issues by Harvard a few years back:

> "It has been determined that no "goals study" of the Class of 1953 actually occurred. In recent years, we have received a number of requests for information on a reported study based on a survey administered to the Class of 1953 in their senior year and a follow-up study conducted ten years later. This study has been described as how one's goals at graduation related to success and annual incomes achieved during the period.
>
> The secretary of the Class of 1953, who had served in that capacity for many years, did not know of [the study], nor did any of the fellow class members he questioned. In addition, a number of Yale administrators were consulted and the records of various offices were examined in an effort to document the reported study. There was no relevant record, nor did anyone recall the purported study of the Class of 1953, or any other class."

In other words, this research, which has been reported and has spread virally since, never happened! It is another example of urban myth. There have since been further studies that substantiate the importance of goal-setting, but my point here is that just setting *what* you want to accomplish is not as important as *why* you want to accomplish it. Even the fictitious Harvard study said it was clarity of goals that made a difference.

The highest authority on goal-setting is Edwin Locke, who began to examine goal-setting in the mid-1960s, and continued researching goal-setting for more than 30 years. Locke derived the idea for goal-setting from Aristotle's form of final causality. Aristotle speculated that *purpose* can cause action; thus, Locke began researching the impact that goals have on human activity. He developed and refined his goal-setting theory in the 1960s, publishing his first article on the subject, "*Toward a Theory of Task Motivation and Incentives*", in 1968 [4]. This article established the positive relationship between clearly identified goals and performance. The article first described goal setting through quantification and measurement; hence, what gets measured, gets done. He wrote that setting goals affects outcomes in four ways:

1) Choice: goals narrow attention, directing efforts to goal-relevant activities, and away from perceived undesirable and goal-irrelevant actions.
2) Effort: goals can lead to more effort; for example, if one typically produces four widgets an hour, and has the goal of producing six, one may work more intensely towards the goal than one would otherwise.

3) Persistence: someone becomes more likely to work through setbacks if pursuing a goal.

4) Cognition: goals can lead individuals to develop and change their behavior.

Locke's research led to the science of goal-setting, which took a further step forward in 1981 with the work of George T. Doran, who first introduced the well-known goal-setting technique, S.M.A.R.T. goal-setting, in his article *"There's a S.M.A.R.T. Way to Write Management's Goals and Objectives* [5]" The acronym stands for **S**pecific, **M**easurable, **A**ttainable, **R**ealistic and Time-bound. The value of setting S.M.A.R.T. goals is that it helps the team to establish clarity in every area. It also provides a structure in which to set goals. One of the jobs of a leaders is to provide structure and organization to every area of practice, otherwise the objectives will be fuzzy. Clarity is the key to goals setting, not just setting a production or collection number and ending it there.

Creating policies is the first step in thinking about the way we want our lives to look. Policy study can refer to an actual process of making decisions at a personal, as well as an organizational, level. Policies can be understood as financial, health-related, managerial, administrative, or any other of the processes that guide how we do things and how we achieve our desired goals. Leaders are policy-driven. There are some policies and their accompanying systems that are more important than others. In my practice, I had policies that concerned how we operated on a daily basis, from doing an examination and writing lab prescriptions, to paying our monthly bills and bonuses. The total collection of policies and systems can be considered the office manual – or, even better, the constitution of our practice. Naturally, the very first policy and system to make is "The making of a policy and system."

How we determine what a policy should look like and how to implement it needs to be made into its own system. Let's take a run through how this works. The policy asks the question, "why?" Why do we do what we do? In the case of policy-making, for me, the answer was to provide me with a set of guiding principles and methods about how to organize the practice and carry out daily activities. Our policies and systems will answer every question that comes up during the course of our practice (see the Einstein quote above). This may take some time to get right but, more importantly, the policy will evolve into a working document that will guide the practice over time.

I have created forms which guide the process. Notice that the policy and systems ask every conceivable question we may have about the system. It guides us by telling us: who will carry out the system (responsibility and accountability); when and where the system will be carried out (right people in right places); why we do it one way or another (values based); what we are trying to accomplish (objectives and goals); and, most importantly, how the process will be carried out (directions). The example I gave in *The Art of Examination* is what I consider the most important policy and system in the practice: the New Patient System.

After some years of practice, I decided that the new patient process, for me, is the most important policy and system a dentist can apply in creating a great sustainable practice. By far the most important lesson I ever learned in dentistry – and one that changed my life even more outside the profession than within the profession – was committing to a comprehensive examination process. For that, I thank my mentors Peter Dawson and Irwin Becker. That one change in my philosophy led to the creation of more positive habits, more consistency in behavior, and the development of more necessary skills, which further led to more success through leadership than anything else I ever applied.

The key to putting an examination system together is to think in terms of intention. Who is it that we are putting the system in place for? The patient is first and foremost. If we want to consistently produce long-term predictable results, then it starts with the diagnosis, and the diagnosis starts with the examination. Skeptics may question this logic. However, I am just suggesting the examination as the starting-point for comprehensive care and predictable outcomes. The system is part of an overall thinking process that leads to quality, predictability and excellence.

Who else is the examination system created for? The doctor/leader. As the leader of the practice, the doctor needs to create a consistent structure for him/herself and the staff. The examination is the keystone system of the practice. All other systems in the practice, including the managerial, technical, and financial systems, are locked into the keystone. Everything is connected to the examination. Recall what Mike Csikszentmihalyi said about complexity – that evolution favors complexity, and that the more integrated the components, the more complex is the overall system. Like the brain or the heart in the human body, the examination process ties the entire practice of dentistry together. The examination process is the one that will sustain the practice of dentistry through the years.

The irony of the examination is that it is also a guide for developing all of the skills necessary to practice. Through excellence in diagnosis and treatment planning, we discover what skills we need to improve on, from the most technical, to the subtle communication skills that are necessary to motivate people toward the wonderful outcomes we envision. We learn to understand ourselves better by truly seeing where our strengths lie. We also see the strengths of our staff members, who can shine in certain areas of the examination process, for the comprehensive examination also brings out the very best in our auxiliaries.

The system that I created many years ago was presented in my previous books as an illustration of how I write a system. Of course, every dentist is different, and each of us has our own personal strengths, talents and personalities. This is the heart and soul of "knowing ourselves." Feel free to use this as a template to create your own process. You can find more detailed information in my two prior books, *The Art of the Examination* and the *Art of Case Presentation* [6]. Of course, there are so many working parts in a practice and a career, and all of those parts must work optimally and systematically to sustain over time. With the current emphasis on technical dentistry, and the innate inclination of people to want simple recipes for success, we are approaching a crossroads where our jobs will become more and more repetitive, and we will lose the human side of dentistry. Yes, the system is the solution.

What are some of the other systems the leader must consider in designing a career in dentistry? The heartbeat of life comes only after survival issues are met. We must create systems that provide us with the financial ability to sustain. Financial systems might include: how we budget our money; how we set our financial goals on a monthly or yearly basis; how we compensate our employees, in terms of salary and benefits; how we wish to get paid for our services; how we save for the future; and how we spend our money of education and equipment. Whatever dentists see as a way to help them move from the base of Maslow's Hierarchy of Needs (survival) is open for a system. I see many dentists who live their entire careers in survival.

Speaking of survival, time systems are important, as well. Time management, as I have learned, can be critical to the day-to-day operations. The next chapter will give you a different perspective on time management that I have found to be more useful for leaders.

Creating systems for every conceivable function in the practice becomes a progressive curriculum in designing a well-lived life and career. As most dentists know, form follows function. The systems allow us to operate optimally on a daily basis, and this is the heart and soul of our work – our logos.

Through our systems, we will learn to become more proficient in two major categories. We will improve our technical as well as our leadership and communication skills. Reading books and articles will not provide the dentist with the necessary skills. Taking courses will help, because hands-on is practical. Through the years, though, I have met many dentists who read the books, took the courses, but never get to apply the lessons. Why? Because practical application takes a playing field. We need the playground to get out and use what we learn. Consistently falling back on our processes gives us the playground to lower our learning curve, and get to proficiency, competency and mastery much quicker.

Let's look at a few key skill areas that a dentist needs in today's current state of the art. Digital photography is one that comes to mind. Many dentists buy the equipment and wait for the "big cases" to come in. The examination process improves over time, case acceptance continues to go up, and this provides the dentist with more opportunities to take a set of photographs. The more photos the dentist takes, the more discerning he becomes. The more photos the dentist takes, the more he creates interest from staff and patients, because photography, a visual communication tool, is highly communicative and is a great conversation builder.

Let's be real. In the end, it is the dentistry that pulls us along. It is our *raison d'être*, the justification for every dentist's existence. It is the reason why many dentists just want to skip all of the ethos and pathos, and get on with their work. Logos, as the Stoics told us, is the guiding reason of the world. In other words, logos is like the leash on a dog; at times, the leash will pull us in one direction and, at other times, the dog will take us where it wants to go. All three components help us to guide the dog.

Throughout our careers, we must master certain skills to guide our journey, or else we get stuck and fail to grow. It is human to grow. It is human to continue to get better and stay on the path to mastery. We all may not become masters, but what is important is that our careers continue to grow in an upward direction through improving skills. In order to improve skills, we must see our work as continually challenging. To many dentists, mastery is just when they get adequately proficient at a skill. For others, every skill becomes an exercise in continuous and never-ending improvement. In order to do that requires a commitment to practice, by taking on greater challenges that match the improving skill levels.

As discussed in Chapter 1 in this book, engagement is a component of the Well-Being Theory that requires us to do effortful learning through deliberate practice. The systems provide the guidelines that will guide our struggle to grow, through developing more and more interrelated skills that will lead to mastery. It will be a struggle to reach what the psychologists call unconscious competence. Once we take on the commitment to learn new skills, we will go through four levels of learning: being *unconsciously unskilled* as you left dental school; being *consciously unskilled*, as when you learn how much you don't know about the other skills necessary to be successful in practice; becoming *consciously skilled* where the growth begins to take shape; and, finally, reaching a level of mastery, which is becoming *unconsciously skilled*.

Many dentists spend their careers in the lower levels of skill development. The ones who succeed, and become the very best versions of themselves, understand the interconnectedness of skill development, deliberate practice, and creating that logos through developing a continuing guide of systems and policies.

As mentioned earlier, there are many systems that are key to developing a worthy practice. I began with the examination system. That led to developing skills in diagnosis, treatment planning, photography, listening, storytelling, case presentation, questioning (the art of), persuasion, scheduling and time management systems, and many others. As skills have developed, I have created new systems for case presentation, financial arrangements, marketing and branding, among the many coordinated systems that guide the logos of my practice. Putting all of these systems in place takes time, commitment and teamwork, and what I have found to be the greatest resource of all energy – positive energy.

Most dentists believe that managing time and money are the keys to a successful career. I have found that most dentists suffer from a lack of physical, mental, and emotional energy. I believe that the key to building leadership skills and developing mastery in technical dentistry requires energy management. The next chapter discusses how leaders can help themselves to get better by managing their energy.

References and Notes

1 Mihaly Csikszentmihaly (1997). *Creativity Flow and the Psychology of Discovery and Invention.* Harper Perennial.

2 Michael E. Gerber (1995). *The E-Myth Revisited: Why Most Small Businesses Don't Work and What to Do About It.* HarperCollins.

3 Mike Morrison (2010). *Harvard Yale Written Goals Study – fact or fiction?* www.rapidbi.com.

4 Edwin A. Locke (1968). Toward a theory of task motivation and incentives. *Organizational Behavior and Human Performance* **3**(2): 157–189.

5 Doran, GT (1981). There's a S.M.A.R.T. Way to Write Management's Goals and Objectives. *Management Review* **70**(11): 35–36.

6 Both of these books can be obtained from my website *AcademyofDentalLeadership.com,* or my blog *TAOofDentistry.com.*

20

Manage Your Energy, Not Your Time

"None of the other stuff is going to work if the animal that you live in is just a broken-down mess."

Elizabeth Gilbert

"While you're going through this process of trying to find the satisfaction in your work, pretend you feel satisfied. Tell yourself you had a good day. Walk through the corridors with a smile rather than a scowl. Your positive energy will radiate. If you act like you're having fun, you'll find you are having fun."

Jean Chatzky

"Things which matter most must never be at the mercy of things which matter least."

Johann Wolfgang von Goethe

David arrived for his 9 am root canal appointment on time. He was promptly seated. I could see the familiar patina forming on his face from his usual anxiety over dental appointments, and root canal held a special place in his range of emotions. I asked how he was doing since the last time I saw him, and in a half-joking manner he said, "Doc, you're on the clock today, I'm giving you 30 minutes." We both laughed and I told him I would do my best. So I numbed him up and began treatment.

There are some procedures that can be relaxing, even meditative for me. I enjoy packing cord, for example. I know there are more efficient ways to retract tissue, but I like to pack cord, and slow things down. My schedule, after all, is never rushed. We give people plenty of time. Often, not always, I feel the same about instrumenting a root canal. On this morning, I became pensive, and reflected on what David said about placing a limit on my time. I thought about time being a restraint, or a factor that can act either as a limitation or liberating factor, depending how it's used. After about 20 minutes, because I can be just as much of a kidder as David, I said, "Times up, Dave." He glanced at his watch. "Yes, it has only been 20 minutes, but I'm tired. I didn't sleep well last night, and I need a cup of coffee." We all got a good laugh at that, but it made me think more about our relationship with time and another important resource – energy.

The core problem with work, says author Tony Schwartz, is that "time is a finite source. Energy is a different story [1]." I couldn't agree more. This isn't a lesson that comes easy. When I was a younger dentist, I was concerned with success. My biggest problem was that I didn't know what success was. I, like most people, believed that success was measured in dollars. The more we make (and show the world), the more successful we are, so I placed an emphasis on making money – and you know what they say, "time is money." If you have read this far, you

The Complete Dentist: Positive Leadership and Communication Skills for Success, First Edition. Barry Polansky.
© 2018 John Wiley & Sons, Inc. Published 2018 by John Wiley & Sons, Inc.

know that my career was bumpy. At one point, after a few health setbacks, I decided that time was more important than money. Time with my kids, time with family and friends, and time for just about anything I valued more than working myself sick. So I spent many years making time a priority. I became an expert in time management. I read all the books and took all of the courses. I created a color-coded schedule, which I will discuss shortly. Years passed.

Things were pretty good in those years. Age, though, brings new perspectives and new wisdom. Just like in the example with David, what happens if you have become a master of time, is that you realize it was never time, because of its limited nature, but it was always all about energy management that leads to happiness – *that* is what will lead to success. Energy is a replenishable resource.

After years of dental practice, I can firmly say that it is energy depletion that gets to dentists every time. In the early years, they mostly complain about not having enough money, and not having enough time, or expertise, or the ability to nurture good relationships. When I speak with older dentists, the lament is that I am too old, and I just don't have the energy, or the will or resolve to do any more. It always amazes me how upset we get when someone, in a manner of speaking, steals our money, but we get less upset when people waste our time through unnecessary distractions, or waste our energy by doing things we do not necessarily have to do.

I believe there are three ways to run a dental practice. The first way is by volume – through using as much time as possible to see as many patients as the dentist can see. Such practices run by the numbers and are generally very busy. The most common questions asked about that mode of practice are, "How much did we produce today, this week or this month?" Or, how many new patients did we see this month, and how can we get more? In other words, this practice centers around money and time, with money being the priority.

The second type of practice centers around the frequency of appointments. This practice also views time as a major factor, but in a different manner. This is what I call the hygiene-driven practice. This practice tends to bring patients back more frequently. This, I feel, is a step in the right direction. Many dental practices use both methods as this, too, places time and money as priorities, but it adds in the value of long-term care and patient relationships.

There is a third way to practice other than volume and hygiene driven, and it is value-driven. Dentists who take the time to provide the highest value procedures to their patients will reap the rewards over time, and those rewards will be the intangible spiritual rewards, like less stress, happiness, and better health, to name a few. As a collateral benefit, they will also work shorter hours and make more money. It amazes me that most dentists choose the high-volume style of practice. Generally, the first questions I get asked by new coaching clients are concerned with getting new patients, marketing, and producing more per hour.

We need to remove ourselves from this factory mentality through better awareness and the creation of better policies and systems. Self-care, self-awareness, and self-compassion need to be brought into dental practice. If those three mindsets can become a reality, then I will guarantee that better patient care will follow. By becoming aware of how we drain our health and energy, and taking care of ourselves and our staff first, and noting over time how we are violating ourselves, our patients and the practice will benefit.

In Chapter 7, I discussed the concept of passion being the by-product of mastery. Mastery has three nutriments. A nutriment, the dictionary tells us, is a source of growth and development. To grow and to flourish is the promise that leadership makes. Leadership provides the beacon for a better future. In order to grow, we must continue to build passion, by providing ourselves with the nutriments of: *autonomy*, the control of our destiny; *competence*, the continual growth of our abilities; and *relationships*, because connection is the key to our lives, as Chris Peterson said when he said, "other people matter." In the end, we are social animals and we crave a need to belong.

As an example (for me, anyway), whenever I receive a letter from an insurance company that questions my treatment plan, or restricts what I feel is the best treatment for a patient, I get upset. I should know better than to get stressed about third party interference through restrictions, exclusions and, what I feel is the worst, the use of manipulative language to persuade people to make poor choices. I can't help it, because biology is working against me, as it is working against all professionals. Let me explain.

Anything that threatens the brain and produces negative emotions like anger or frustration is a threat to our overall well-being. When our well-being is affected, we tend to give up and become cynical. When our willpower becomes depleted, we slowly fall into a state of languishing, which effects our overall ability to grow. The leader creates an environment that promotes growth by creating conditions that support the continual production of positive energy. Positive energy in the dental practice can make or break a career.

This isn't breaking news, however; when I speak of energy, I am not only speaking of the physical energy that the dental staff needs to get through their days. I am speaking of the mental and emotional energy that is required to build a successful career – especially if the dentist has chosen to do relationship-based comprehensive dentistry. Going to the gym and eating right helps, but creating the right work environment will go further. The key is to create a schedule that does not deplete energy because, only then, can we benefit from the things that we can do to replete energy, like eating right, exercising, and getting enough sleep.

Where is the power source for the energy I am referring to? It is not the musculoskeletal system. The power source for our positive energy is the brain – specifically, the prefrontal cortex. That thin piece of tissue that is the brain's most recent evolutionary development is what separates us from the rest of the animal kingdom. Like muscle, the prefrontal cortex requires energy in the form of glucose. It also requires periods of rest and relaxation. We all know how a muscle feels when it becomes depleted and exhausted. The prefrontal cortex shows the effects of depletion by signs of brain fog, exhaustion, apathy, and the one thing that affects our day-to-day activities more than anything else: decision-making. In a relationship-based comprehensive practice, we need to make decisions based on numerous disparate pieces of information. We must also spend time developing positive relationships with people throughout our days. Essentially, we must become decision-making problem-solvers, and that requires brain power.

Our role as leaders is to create situations where we can minimize energy usage in order to maximize performance. During the course of our days, we are presented with many opportunities to make decisions and choices. Getting the letter from the insurance company that I mentioned above can be a drain on our energy, because the brain sees it as a threat. Social scientists have created a construct known as the SCARF model, which describes various threats that have applications for everyone, especially leaders [2]. The acronym stands for **S**tatus, **C**ertainty, **A**utonomy, **R**elatedness, and **F**airness.

My automatic response to letters like the one I referred to threatens me at every level of the SCARF model. My *status* is threatened, because patients tend to believe what comes from the insurance company. My *certainty* is threatened, because my treatment plan is based on predictable outcomes that I have been trained to perform. My *autonomy* is threatened, because my ability to make a rational decision based on my education is being contradicted. The *relatedness* is threatened because, after doing everything I can to invite the patient into my practice, the insurance company is applying pressure that is difficult to compete against and, finally, all of this can be considered un*fair*.

Of course, all this is counterbalanced by a rational disclosure statement from the insurance company, which claims that their assessment should not interfere with the doctor's or patient's freedom choice. But I am not talking about the rational mind. My automatic response is one of frustration, anger and, possibly, contempt. We have less control over those emotional responses. Over time they act to drain and deplete us. Once depleted, we have a difficult time making decisions and problem-solving. In the long term, this may lead to emotional exhaustion and burnout.

There are other things that deplete energy in the practice. I have discussed the importance of building positive relationships, but the other side is having toxic people in our practice. On a practical level, we all have had difficult patients in our practices. We know them. We joke that our fees should be higher for them, and we should charge for stomach lining and heart muscle. But really, it's no joke. Toxic people are dangerous. I call them energy-sucking vampires.

Throughout my career, I have made the mistake of taking on patients who turned out to become vampires, and the results were never good. My staff viewed me as someone who lacked judgment or showed weakness, because I took these people on as a challenge. I felt a certain amount of guilt that I may have been a sell-out. Treating toxic patients in my early years may have been one reason that I created a relationship-based practice, and followed Jim Collins axioms of "getting the right people on the bus," or "first who, then what." There may have been a little of that in my decision to treat them, but I also believe that healthcare professionals truly start out wanting to help patients – *all* patients. However, regardless of that, we need to survive and sustain our practice, or else we will become energy-deficient and possibly burn out.

Harry was a vampire. He neglected his teeth for years. He first entered my practice when he was 75. He told me he had waited for years to have a nice smile and now he could afford the best. He needed orthodontics, and he was willing to have braces. "Whatever it took," he said. He went through the complete diagnostic workup by my friend the orthodontist, only to revisit my original restorative treatment plan. That took numerous appointments, and time. The restorative case took more than time – it was exhausting. After a periodontist placed two implants, Harry settled on just restoring his upper six anterior teeth. That's when the problems started. It took over one year of Harry showing up in my practice, uninvited, to complain how the provisionals looked. He was never satisfied with the final case. He would sit in the lab for hours at a time, and tell the technician how things just were not right.

Finally, I sent Harry to Chicago, to a master ceramist who felt he could do the case. Harry spent two days sitting at the side of the master. When he returned home, I marveled at the result. I was still wary, and I wanted to make sure Harry and his wife were satisfied. I made them sign off before cementing the case. Things looked great. I called the ceramist and thanked him. But I didn't see Harry for over two years.

One day, while shopping in my local supermarket, I spotted Harry in the produce department, squeezing a honeydew melon. I laughed to myself that he was as fixated on that melon as he had been on his teeth. Because I wondered how things had been with him, I approached him and asked, in a friendly manner, "Hey Harry, how are you? how about those Phillies?" But Harry never looked up. Then he said, pointing to his teeth, "Charlie never got it right." I was shocked. That case was so nice that I presented it and put it on Facebook.

You might say that Harry was crazy, but that's not the point. Harry was a vampire, and my job as a leader was to protect myself, my staff and my technicians from vampires. It is easy to say that the rational mind can just nullify these incidents, but they add up. If we don't create the right working environment, we will find ourselves and our staff burning out right before our eyes. What's at stake is our well-being and survival. For that, we need systems and policies that help preserve our energy, rather than just being more time-efficient.

It should be clear that high volume and busyness do not equate to productivity and happiness. Busyness is not a formula for success. As a matter of fact, it may be a formula for disaster. Working long hours on many patients can actually subtract from productivity, becoming less effective by draining attention and energy. Stephen Covey, in his wonderful book on time management, *First Things First* [3], uses the allegory of the *Goose and the Golden Egg* to make some of these points.

In my book *The Art of the Examination* [4], I explain how I use the allegory to explain how dentists can justify a two-hour examination by comparing production to production capability. My explanation at the time was based on time and money management. I explained that by focusing only on production, and not on the production capability, we sacrifice our production. This is very much like the farmer in the story killing the golden goose and losing the production of the golden eggs. Today, 14 years later, I look at that metaphor through the lens of energy and well-being.

If we take care of ourselves first, then we will have the production capability through energy reserves, rather than working through time constraints. Our ability to prioritize what really matters, to build habits that will not drain us, enables us to become clear on how to reconcile the biggest question of the paradox of duty and desire. With that in mind, let's take a look at a color-coded time management system that is set up to preserve and use energy more effectively.

The tasks that require the most energy are the tasks that require the most focus. They are the tasks that can't be interrupted, because task-switching is draining. As a matter of fact, all multitasking is less effective and is energy-depleting [5]. The color-coded system should focus on the health and well-being of the doctor and the staff. The system should never leave the staff depleted at the end of the day. Nothing will go further in building a culture of trust than creating a system that prioritizes the health and well-being of staff members first. With that in mind, let's take a look at some of our daily tasks.

The morning huddle is the first scheduled task. It sets our day. The huddle is like eating a good breakfast. The next tasks are the ones that require the most energy. These are generally the most productive and have the most potential to create future production. In my previous books, I used the color green to signify the most productive time of the day, and the color yellow for the times that had the highest production capability – large cases and examinations. I would always place these blocks of time at the beginning of the day, or directly after lunch. Why? Because that is when our energy levels are at their highest. It also requires us to take care of ourselves so that we get enough rest and eat properly. This is not a book on personal health care, but I want to make the correlation that all success truly depends on personal development. Diet and exercise matter at a practical level.

These two color-coded blocks of time are the ones that will create your effectiveness. Still, there are many tasks that need to be done during the course of the day. Emergencies always come up, but they usually can be handled quickly and without too much problem, if they are scheduled in the system. We put this red time at the end of our mornings. In my practice, that ends up being extra time for personal replenishment, which is mostly appreciated by all. When an emergency does occur, we are ready and willing. Routine operative visits, which I call blue time, are scheduled at the end of the day or in the afternoons, after an examination. These are the times that the less taxing procedures can be more easily handled.

Before leaving this section on color-coded time management, I want to remind readers that maintaining this system requires discipline. Yet, maintaining discipline is, in itself, an energy driven task. My advice is to continue to follow the system until it becomes a habit. It is what philosopher Aristotle meant when he said, "We are what we repeatedly do. Excellence, then, is not an act, but a habit". By relegating certain daily tasks to our subconscious mind, through habit formation, we are preserving energy for our more demanding tasks, as well as for the other portion of our work-life balance.

Have you ever left work feeling totally exhausted? On days when we are busy and highly productive, we can certainly expect nothing less. When exhausting days pile up, we can physically burn out. But have you ever had a day when you weren't particularly busy, but felt even more exhausted than on the more active and engaging days? By now, we realize that energy is the fundamental currency of high performance. Our conscious capacity for self-regulation is limited and easily depleted. The problem is that our energy must be evaluated on four levels: the physical, the emotional, the mental and the spiritual. If any one of these areas is depleted, then the brain itself lacks energy, and that leads to all of the problems noted above that are associated with poor performance.

At the beginning of the book, I made reference to the Cross of Life that L.D. Pankey used to create his philosophy. The Cross of Life, originally created by Dr. Richard Cabot in his book *What Men Live By* [6], mentioned keeping the four components of the cross – work, love, play and worship – in balance. They still teach the Cross of Life at the Pankey Institute. As mentioned in an earlier chapter, students are continually reminded to keep their "cross in balance" when life is just not working out, or when the student is having a problem with reconciling that paradox between duty and desire.

The problem is that keeping anything in balance is a myth. Your cross will always be out of balance, because nothing in life ever achieves complete balance – especially life itself. Balancing our "cross" is just an idea. Balancing is something we constantly do, it isn't something we can go home and just fix to make it right. To balance is a verb, and the balanced life is a construct. The idea was first taught by Aristotle, with his concept of the "golden mean," which was his way of telling students to avoid extremes and keep things in moderation. So what about the nouns in the cross: work, love, play and worship? How do we keep these things from getting out of balance?

If we view these four elements in terms of energy, then it can make sense. We can take specific action, rather than just staking a claim to a balanced life. When we speak in terms of energy, we know when we are depleted, and how we must replenish the energy. We measure physical energy capacity in terms of quantity (low to high) and emotional capacity in quality (negative to positive). According to Tony Schwartz, "these are our most fundamental sources of energy because without sufficient high-octane fuel no mission can be accomplished [1]." Let's take a look at the Cross of Life through these four forms of energy.

Physical Energy = Play

This is the obvious one, and the one most talked about in all industries. We certainly have learned the benefit of diet, exercise and good sleep habits. Physically, dentistry is a demanding profession. It is easier today than in years past, with the advent of four-handed, and even six-handed dentistry. There was a time when dentists stood all day long. Committing to good health and fitness habits go a long way in preserving the physical energy to be a productive dentist and leader. Scheduling patients properly, as discussed earlier, helps. So does getting restful and complete sleep. Dentists today are very concerned with sleep for their patients. Sleep hygiene is just as important for them. The recommended time for sleep is between 7–9 hours per night.

One thing that helps me is to eat a big breakfast every morning, consisting of low-glycemic carbohydrates. I eat oatmeal and berries every morning. I can go till at least 11 am without feeling hungry. No breakfast is the worst breakfast. Commit to this, and you will notice immediate energy returns. Another way to preserve energy is to build short breaks into your schedule. Get rid of your roller-skates. Low-volume practices are not only less stressful, but they also preserve energy. Lastly, everyone knows the benefits of regular exercise. For years, I have been going to the gym three days per week, and doing Bikram Yoga three days per week. My gym routine is one hour of cardio-training on the treadmill, and one hour of weight training. I have been doing this routine for six years. I have been working out for 25 years, consistently. When I speak to dentists my age, they are astonished that I can still work and do the things I was physically capable of 20 years ago. Commit to physical fitness – it goes a long way.

Emotional Energy = Love

It may be a stretch, but I equate the love element to our emotional energy levels. Relationships, inside and outside of work, can be either energizing or depleting. The brain only knows positivity and negativity. In our careers, we must manage our relationships with staff and patients, or we won't have enough energy to come home and take care of our most important relationships. Too many personal lives have suffered at the hands of poor relationships at home. Leaving work with enough energy, by controlling emotions, can go a long way in building reserves for what really matters. Emotional energy is measured by positive and negative feelings. Creating systems and schedules with this in mind is what good leaders do. Too many dental practices suffer from stress and overwhelm. How many stories have we heard about the moody, irritable, and anxious dentist? These states of mind cause the dentist to become emotionally dysfunctional and apathetic. They suffer from brain fog.

Relationship-based dentistry accounts for the feelings of the dentist, the patients and the staff. The systems are built to spend time with people to discuss very sensitive issues, like fear and money. We have already discussed some of the leadership and communication skills that dentists need to learn in order to serve their patients better, but it is just as important for self-preservation.

Committing to learn better listening skills, questioning skills, and storytelling skills can help slow down the daily practice, so we can create the best responses for any situation. Understanding that we all tend to place ourselves into the drama of life means we need to realize what role we play in the lives of the people we come into contact with. We must be able to use proper language, so that we stay away from blame and criticism toward those we serve. We must also stay away from blame and criticism toward ourselves. In other words, the phrase, "the buck stops here," is necessary for all leaders. The key, as the PERMA model explains, is to stay positive, and to keep positive energy high.

There are many ways to build our reserves. Two habits that I have created include a gratitude journal and meditation. Every morning, I write in my digital journal (I use an app called *Day One*) three things that I am thankful for. This is a bit more difficult than it sounds, because of the brain's natural tendency toward negative bias, but a trick I have learned is to look around at contrasts: being thankful for my health; being thankful for still having the energy and passion at my late age; being thankful for my wonderful family. You get the idea.

By far one of the most energy replenishing things I do is mindfulness meditation. For the past several years, I have been meditating twice per day. I block out 20 minutes in the morning and 20 minutes in the evening. There are times I miss the evening session, but I have meditated at least once per day for over a year. Nothing I have done has given me more benefits in terms of rejuvenation. It gives me energy by creating more emotional stability and calmness throughout my day. Mostly, it has extended the gap between stimulus and response. I take the time to make sure my response in every situation is a deliberate and thoughtful response. Creating this habit was a bit more difficult than my gym habit, but it is certainly doable, because there is no right or wrong way to meditate. My suggestion is to start with five minutes per day and grow from there.

If you find yourself feeling irritable or anxious, it may be time to consider emotional energy. Remember the first sign of burnout is emotional exhaustion. If you find that the things you enjoy the most, especially your family, are suffering, then it's time for emotional replenishment. And lastly, if you have taken for granted everything you have done in dentistry, it may be time to stop and give thanks to your patients and your staff.

Mental Energy = Work

Creating a successful and flourishing career, where you create positivity through engaging and energizing work, requires a good environment. A practice that does not allow time to think can become exhausting to work in everyday. High-volume practices, where everyone is looking for the dentist to solve their problems, can be draining for all. The dentist should be allowed to practice what he has been trained to do. I hear from so many of my doctor friends who are leaving medicine because, after a full day, they go home and enter data into a computer. I know dentists who also take administrative work home to complete instead of playing with their kids.

Understand that it takes the mind approximately 23 minutes to get up to speed on any subject we work on. Most work environments, research shows, have interruptions every 7–9 minutes. Our systems need to build in sacred time, for example during long difficult appointments and the pre-clinical examinations. That means no distractions. That is why those appointments are made when our energy is at its highest level and we are in the best moods – when our ability to focus and concentrate is high.

Multitasking actually lowers performance. Numerous studies have shown that multitaskers perform much worse at everything than focused workers. Multitasking can be likened to what the Buddhists called "Monkey Mind". When the mind switches from one task to another, both tasks are at risk of being done wrong. Yet, many sell out effectiveness for what they believe is efficiency. A Russian proverb says this best: "If you chase two rabbits … you will not catch either one." Most important is that distractions and interruptions from any source, like cell phones, email, messages, texts, and social media, play havoc with our capacity to self-regulate. Our willpower diminishes, and everything suffers.

Let me give you a simple example. Someone in my office loves those little mini-pretzels. Every week, she brings in a large see-through plastic container of those delightful little treats. When I walk by the lunchroom, I see them staring at me. For a while, I gave in and grabbed a handful. Do you know how many times I walk by the lunchroom each day? Those little pretzels in those little handfuls add up. The worst thing, though, even more than the calories, is that I can feel the resistance of saying "no" and losing the battle. That inability to self-regulate eventually affects my performance. Once again, willpower is a limited resource. My solution was to move the container out of sight, until I found out who was bringing in the pretzels. It was my wife! Now that's another issue.

If you are finding yourself being rushed all day, never having time to see patients on time or seeing way too many emergencies, it may be time to look more closely at a deficiency in mental energy. If there isn't enough time to sit back and smell the coffee without worrying about when the next patient will be in, or what you are going to be doing on that patient, it may be time to slow down. And if you're taking work home, then maybe new systems are in order.

Spiritual Energy = Worship

When I first went to the Pankey Institute, I was a bit confused about this word "spiritual." I was not the only one who was confused about it. Through my speaking career, I have been asked to explain what this means many times. There was a time when an administrator asked me to remove the word "worship" before my presentation. I replaced it with the word "service." When I looked at the Cross of Life through the lens of energy, these issues took on a different meaning. I now believe that my burnout, more than anything, was an existential crisis that depleted my spiritual energy. Many people today are walking around with a sense of malaise caused by a lack of meaning and purpose in their lives. In dentistry, it's easy to ask ourselves why we are doing this work. For me, although I wasn't able to adequately express this idea to myself, even when I was exposed to the Cross of Life, creating a meaningful and purposeful way to practice probably save my life.

When we do work that really matters, we typically feel more positive energy, we focus better, and we demonstrate much more perseverance, resilience and overall grit. Self-reflection and introspection came to me when I continually asked myself, "Is that all there is?" When

I asked myself what it was that I wanted my patients to remember me for, I decided that I would build my practice around doing meaningful dentistry.

Accessing this deep reservoir of positive energy is the message of this book. It takes time to reflect on our character issues (ethos), and to learn the methods of communication that produce trust and growth (pathos), and then to put it all together into systems that make things work (logos). When our work is aligned with our values, our purpose, and our mission, our energy continues to grow and we flourish.

You may be having a spiritual crisis, as I did, if you are not enjoying dentistry, or you are spending time on work and with people you truly don't enjoy. You may be in crisis if you have a double standard, and are doing work that you truly do not believe is worthwhile, or there is a gap between your beliefs and values and what you are doing every day. You may be in a spiritual crisis if you are only focused on the material rewards, without giving any consideration to the importance of what really matters – making a difference in the lives of others.

In the final chapter, I want to revisit the idea of the culture of trust through the lens of organization and teamwork. Our success always depends on others. We must look at our leadership, not only to create a thriving career for ourselves, but to also realize that our success depends on a happy team. I am often asked how I have employed many of the same people from a minimum of 15 years to 40 years. I don't think it was me, as much as it was the culture.

References and Notes

1 Tony Schwartz and Catherine McCarthy (2007). Manage Your Energy, Not Your Time. *Harvard Business Review,* October, 2007.

2 David Rock (2008). SCARF:a brain-based model for collaborating with and influencing others. *NeuroLeadership Journal* **1**: www.neuroleadership.org.

3 Stephen Covey, A. Roger Merrill and Rebecca Merrill (1994). *First Things First,* 1st edition. Simon & Schuster.

4 Barry Polansky (2003). *The Art of the Examination,* p. 32. Word of Mouth Enterprises.

5 Gary Keller (2013). *The One Thing: The Surprisingly Simple Truth Behind Extraordinary Results,* 1st edition, pp. 61–72. Bard Press.

6 Richard C. Cabot (2012). *What Men Live By – Work Play Love Worship.* Forgotten Books.

21

Master of the Intangibles – It Takes a Team

"Your first and foremost job as a leader is to take charge of your own energy and then help to orchestrate the energy of those around you."

Peter Drucker

"When "i" is replaced by "we," even illness becomes wellness."

Be_inspired

"Teamwork makes the dream work, but a vision becomes a nightmare when the leader has a big dream and a bad team."

John C. Maxwell

I am an incurable New York Giants football fan. The 2007 New York Giants won the Super Bowl in an incredible four-game winning streak that featured many improbable moments. They came in as a wildcard team, they won every game on the road, and the Super Bowl game itself was marked by beating an undefeated New England Patriots team with a catch on the helmet of wide receiver David Tyree. Most people will forget the details of that run to the Super Bowl, but no one forgets the catch. Football is the ultimate team sport. It takes 53 men coming together as one for 20 weeks. Most Super Bowl teams are about the greatness of teamwork, and I am sure that most people have stories about their own individual team, but that particular team stands out to me.

I attended the game in Phoenix that year. I witnessed "the helmet catch" first hand. After the game, I ran into the renowned football analyst, Chris Collingsworth, as he waited for his flight back home to Cincinnati. I approached him, and reminded him that he, as well as most of the pundits, had picked the Patriots to win in a romp. I will never forget his response to me. With a look of astonishment he replied, "Who woulda thunk it?" I remember saying, "I would – because Tom Coughlin was a master of the intangibles." Teamwork is about the intangibles.

If you recall the story I told in Chapter 6, later that year, I wrote an article for the industry magazine, *Dental Economics* [1]. The article concluded that it was leadership and communication that resulted in the winning moment. From July to January, teams take on daily obstacles, opponents and roadblocks that they must overcome on their road to success. Only one team gets there. In the post-game interviews, the players speak about the chemistry and the love they have for one another as the reason why they prevailed. I sent a copy of my published article to the Giants' coach, Tom Coughlin.

A few months later, I received a package at my office. The return address read, "New York Football Giants, East Rutherford, New Jersey." It was a signed photograph of the coach accepting

The Complete Dentist: Positive Leadership and Communication Skills for Success, First Edition. Barry Polansky.
© 2018 John Wiley & Sons, Inc. Published 2018 by John Wiley & Sons, Inc.

the coveted Lombardi Trophy. There was also a personal letter enclosed, which essentially told me all I had to know about the importance of leadership and communication for creating successful teams, it is worth revisiting that letter:

Dear Barry,

Thank you for your letter and a copy of your article. I really enjoyed your admission, "I am a die-hard, hard core, Blue Bleeding Giant fan."

<u>Realize</u> one other thing, perhaps the biggest accomplishment was the "Art of Communication – and through the Leadership Council – we improved communication – but with that ownership – responsibility – and the veteran players drew the younger players into the Web of Accountability, and the entire team, "would not let the other guys down!"

Sincerely,
Tom Coughlin

It was a short letter, but I can draw some conclusions about the coach, the organization and the team. Winning a Super Bowl is not easy. Winning four Super Bowls is even more difficult. The Giants organization is one of a handful of NFL teams that have done that. It showed me a lot that the coach would take the time to even write that letter. It was not the first time I had received a communication from the Giants. Many years ago, I sent a letter to the late owner, Wellington Mara. He, too, responded with a return handwritten letter. They care. Care is an intangible that can be made tangible.

We take language for granted. If we read Coughlin's letter and note the language – communication, Leadership Council, responsibility, ownership, accomplishment, and team, we can begin to see how all of the philosophy we learned in the earlier part of this book, applies to teams as well. The Lombardi Trophy became the tangible evidence of all of the intangibles that leadership puts together. As the owner of our professional lives, our careers and our practices, it is our responsibility to build great teams, because no one can do it alone.

Leaders build the environment to enable the team to succeed. It first starts with self-management, because everyone on the team needs someone whom they believe in. In other words, it starts with character and ethos. The leader always remembers his or her responsibility to teach, motivate, and provide the resources to create excellent dentistry. The team needs the right education, equipment and supplies. They also need positivity, to carry them through when things don't go according to plan. Dentistry, as all fields, in fraught with setbacks and disappointments. Team members need some hand-holding; leaders also need to cultivate other leaders. So many of these intangibles are based around the theme of the culture of trust, appreciation, and ownership, that was discussed in Chapter 13.

It is also the responsibility of the leader to build a great team. The leader is the one constant that will continue to be there throughout the life of the practice. A famous meditation teacher once said, "wherever you go, there you are." That is why it is so important to work on the self first. The first thing to do in building a great team is to choose the right people. It's always nice to have competent team members. I hear so much about choosing team members who can do various skills. Throughout my career, I have always trained my assistants to handle the technical skills. The areas I had problems with were the very same character and communication issues that we all have. I found these skills much tougher to teach than how to pass the right instrument, or how to pour impeccable models. By the way, pouring impeccable models may just be a character issue.

Another aspect of building a team of superstars is that many are not team players. They overvalue their worth. Some can even cause dissension on the team. "Me first" teammates are trouble. Remember, trust is based on care and competence. One of the best things a football player can say about another player is that he is a great teammate. How many dental practices are sabotaged by the selfishness of overly competent staff members? No *one* is smarter than all of us; that is why there is no "I" in team. Thriving dental practices flourish because team members feel that they are part of something bigger than themselves. That is why creating a mission is so important. Mission is other-focused, and it provides a sense of meaning and purpose beyond the self. Meaning and purpose are essential for the well-being of individuals, as well as for organizations.

A healthy relationship between staff and a dental practice begins with a shared mission, meaning, and purpose. We draw our well-being from the idea that we are making a difference in the world. As reported by Tom Rath from the Gallup Organization, the author of *Strengthsfinder 2.0*, "a 2013 study of more than 12 000 workers worldwide found that employees who derive meaning and understand the importance of their work are more than three times as likely to stay with their organization [2]." He went on to claim that shared mission and purpose and providing meaningful work has the highest single impact of any other single variable. In my practice, getting to know the patient through our new patient examination plays a big role in teaching and applying meaningful work, by clarifying our long-term goals and providing a method to get our patients on the road to complete dentistry.

In my coaching, I find that dentists who do not commit to the new patient examination process fail to reach their long-term goals beyond the production goals. When production becomes the only focus, they fail to provide the meaning of the dentistry to their patients. By starting a proactive conversation, the dentist and the staff can guide their patients toward complete dentistry which is what I have called a positive intervention that truly makes a difference. Most dentists react to the situation at hand rather than taking the time to proactively change directions with their patients. This early proactive conversation can lead to much of the effectiveness that Covey calls his 7 Habits [3]: being proactive by having the conversation; beginning with the end in mind by thinking about long-term health; putting first things first by introducing the process that will create complete dentistry; thinking win-win by laying out the treatment plan that considers the total patient and their circumstances; and seeking first to understand before being understood by showing empathy.

Once applied, the staff rallies around these long-term goals, rather than just production and collection. Most dentists concern themselves with just being busy, rather than making real progress toward goals that really matter. A dental practice, as Tom Rath and the Gallup Organization tells us, is a purpose, not a place.

Team members know each other, just as leaders know their patients. They also know their staff, and their staff knows everyone on the team. There is nothing more disruptive to a practice than teammates bickering with one another, and there is nothing more pleasant than when teammates come together to help one another. One of the hallmarks of good relationships is that people know one another's personal stories. They know the little things about one another that provides the depth needed for the *esprit de corps* that creates team effectiveness. They know about one another's families and pets. They relate, and build deep personal relationships that last over time. They cover for one another, so the practice goes on without interruption. Deep positive relationships are a big component of successful teams, just as they are a big contributing factor in the well-being of individuals.

There is a trending thought, these days, that Millennials are more self-centered and more entitled than previous generations. In an interview, I heard Simon Sinek, author of the books *Leaders Eat Last* and *Start With Why*, say that there are four reasons why this may be true. He believed that parenting, technology, impatience, and the corporate world are responsible for this apparent trend. He claims that parents make our children somehow feel "special" by giving everyone a trophy. He also believes that technology has created a certain amount of mindlessness, especially around relationships, because face-to-face communication is diminished. He feels that impatience has created more instant gratification, instead of delayed gratification, and feels that corporations focus more on short-term results instead of setting more noble long-term goals.

The first lines of the song *In the Living Years* state: *"Every generation – Blames the one before – And all of their frustrations – Come beating on your door."* I believe that is what is behind Sinek's opinion. We can't sit back and blame a whole generation for the results of cultural evolution. Positive psychology teaches the answer to the basic question of *"how to live the good life,"* which is why I have chosen it as the foundation of leadership in this book.

In each of Sinek's reasons, there is an answer that comes from the world of positive psychology which makes philosophy practical:

- On parenting: we must all develop the growth mindset that Carolyn Dweck described. Students are not special, and everyone does not get a trophy. We must celebrate effort. Students who choose to learn, rather than get things handed to them, will reap the rewards.
- On technology: we must understand that digital devices can't replace the depth of human relationships.
- On impatience: delayed gratification is one of the standards of success, as noted by the famous Stanford marshmallow studies that were discussed in Chapter 6.
- On corporate greed: long-term thinkers have always done better than short-term thinking.

In other words, today's generation still needs to learn and apply the principles that have taught people *"how to live"* throughout time, whether it be L.D. Pankey's philosophy, the stoicism of Marcus Aurelius, or Seligman's Well-Being Theory. The principles are ageless, timeless and perennial.

It may appear that we live in a new "me generation," but that term is used for every generation. "There is no 'I' in team" means we must be other-focused to live with more meaning and purpose. What Sinek goes on to say in his interview is that today's generation must learn the ultimate lesson: that there is no shortcut to creating meaningful work and job satisfaction, and there is no shortcut to developing meaningful and profoundly significant relationships. Learning leadership and communication provides the practical application to create the life worth living and a fulfilling career in dentistry. Building a team is one of the practical applications of that philosophy.

Building a culture of trust also means that the leader must develop other leaders. There will be times when feelings, and misinterpretation of events, will create tense moments that will test any organization. Leaders see the big picture. They understand that their success depends on a commitment to their beliefs, values, and mission. They inspire others to be better. They handle conflict because they understand the sacredness of high-quality connections. They use the language of care, rather than the language of conflict, which results in very peaceful, low-stress days, adding up to long careers with very little turnover. The practice becomes that psychological safe zone that is the hallmark of the culture of trust.

Great teams are also focused on goals. It's easy to set high production goals. Great teams also set goals that stretch each person as individuals, as well as setting team goals. Goals can be created at any level. Assistants and hygienists can set quality goals. The team can set goals for education. Lab assistants can set capability goals. By achieving goals, we cause our self-esteem to go up, and we become part of something greater than ourselves.

Another question that comes up is "Who is on our team?" The UPS ad slogan, *"What can Brown do for you?"* says it all. Amusingly, our FedEx driver, Glen, who has been with us for years, used to greet us every day with that expression. Glen recently retired, but our new driver hasn't missed a beat. Both of them would send me texts when they had a package they thought was important and no one was in the office. They might actually deliver it to my house. Our FedEx drivers are part of our team. So is our dental laboratory, our suppliers, our clean-up crew, our accountant and lawyer, and anyone else we can think of that helps us get our job done. Most of us get this concept and yet, as the owner of a dental laboratory, I can tell you that there is a problem in this industry with the dentist and laboratory relationship. I see it all of the time.

Sometimes, that relationship is strained by a disconnect on basic business principles, but mostly it occurs because of a difference in technical philosophies. Sure, it can break down on either side, but leaders understand their role in building the relationship. The leader must provide the lab with the very best in communication, from the prescription to the models, treatment plans that make sense, and the impressions and bite registration. The lab tech must also become a leader, so that all of the information that is sent is properly applied and, if there is a problem, the lines of communication are wide open.

Of all of the relationships that a dentist engages in, this may be the most sensitive. When a dentist is only looking at price, because the other areas of his or her practice isn't working optimally, then the dentist-lab relationship will suffer. Work will come back late, the work won't fit correctly, and it will feel and look as if the person who did it did so without care. My advice is to nurture this very special relationship, in order to create a better life and career.

So is this all about a mindset of teamwork, or are there practical things we can do to create this psychologically safe culture of trust? The answer may lie in science. Recall how the neurotransmitter oxytocin is what author Paul Zak calls the "moral molecule" because, when it is secreted, it helps us to build trust. I have been guilty of avoiding this idea for years. I am not what people might call a "warm and fuzzy guy." When I used to go to courses, many years ago, and the lecturer would tell us to stand up and hug the person next to you, I would get uncomfortable. I'm just not a hugger. Well, it seems that hugging causes a secretion of oxytocin. Since I learned that, I have become a bit more touchy-feely. Does it work? I don't know, but I sure am envious of those happy practices where a lot of hugging is going on. So if we begin to understand that whatever causes us to even want to hug another, that will increase oxytocin secretion, and trust will rise. One thing Zak says is that "trust begets trust."

In Zak's most recent book, *Trust Factor: The Science of Creating High-Performance Companies* [4], he describes a few applications that may be useful in developing our own trusting organizations, which become cultures of high engagement, optimal function, and high performance. Let's look at a few that dentists can apply to build better teams. Building a great culture and a great team takes hard work, constant learning, and renewal, but it's worth it.

The first area of positive intervention is in the area of *appreciation*. Zak claims that 67% of a culture's trust level comes from appreciation and celebrating the efforts of team members. It is not surprising that in a survey of over 100,000 workers worldwide, 79% said that "a lack of appreciation" was the primary reason they quit their jobs [5]. Imagine those who disengaged, rather than actually quitting. Imagine also what a little appreciation can do.

Zak recommends that appreciation should come in specific ways. It should be unexpected, tangible, and personal. It should also comes as a surprise, not the obligatory "staff member of the week awards," that lose their meaning after a little while. A real, heartfelt, public "thank you" for a job well done goes a long way in building trust. Praising people in public also goes a long way in building trust. However, the praise should also be very specific; rather than praising the person, praise the specific effort. Tell the employee, or even the patient, exactly what they did in order to deserve the praise. In public, this sends the message that others, too, can be worthy of the same recognition, through hard work and intentional effort. In other words, we build teams by letting each member know that appreciation is earned, rather than just through showing up.

"Leadership is about developing the human potential around you," says Zak. Whether it is a staff member or a patient, our main goal is to build better people. It is never our job to break people down. We praise in public, but we criticize in private. When staff members see us lose control, and start yelling at other staff members for doing something wrong, it sends a clear negative message that will undermine the team in the long run. Positive psychology's Martin Seligman's earliest research centered around learned helplessness [6]. He proved that dogs can be demotivated from actually going after treats when they know they will be punished. We can teach people to become helpless through creating a negative environment. Learned helplessness is the opposite of optimism and motivation. Fear will undermine trust. That is something that every dentist should understand and practice.

Building a culture of trust is an ongoing process; leaders need to continually praise people for their efforts, rather than withholding praise until a performance review. Daily hits of positive feedback create eustress and the desire to do better, while silence and criticism create chronic stress among staff members. It is no wonder that staff members will sometimes just leave for no apparent reason.

Positive leadership, with constructive feedback in public, goes far in keeping a team together. As I said earlier, the challenges that we give to the staff members are important, too. When I discussed the concept of *flow*, earlier, I made a point of including that the challenges we face should equal the skill level, or else we will become bored with the job or become too stressed by the job. The leader's job is to continually challenge the team with more difficult projects, and to provide the proper training for continued improvement. This is a reward that many team members enjoy even more than bonuses. Bonuses are extrinsic rewards, and they usually take a backseat to the intrinsic rewards of learning and growth. According to Paul Zak, a recent study showed that 89% of employees leave because of pay issues. The study showed that the actual number who leave is 12%. "Work is not about pay", he says. "People need a paycheck, but they do not put their passion into work because of money [7]." Further research concludes that when there is a belief that the work is mission-based and in a high-trust culture, the feeling of "we're all in this together" takes precedence.

Setting high goals is important. Research at Harvard University by Teresa Amabile has shown that making progress toward one's goals was the most important motivator at work [8]. The research also showed that people had their best days at work when they applied what they learned, and they did it together with other team members. Team members reported being in better moods when approaching their goals. Pride in accomplishment, in addition to a positive environment, enhances trust. Leaders fully appreciate the capabilities of staff members. Very early in my practice, I challenged staff members to learn new skills, like laboratory skills and dental photography. There is nothing more pleasing to a leader than when a staff member comes to them beaming with the pride of a job well done.

Morning huddles are a good place to review any projects that need to be addressed. The leader should offer any assistance that is necessary, if asked. It's also a good time to ask questions about whether projects and challenges are moving along. Leaders constantly ask questions in order to get the proper feedback and to take the temperature of the team. The temperature the leader is always looking for is positivity. Start every day with a positive and uplifting morning huddle. Be transparent and inclusive. Staff members enjoy being part of the decision-making process, from the creation of the mission statement to the creation of specific policies and systems. This is a team effort.

One of the biggest problems I see with dental practices is that the dentist becomes the "go to guy" whenever any problem arises, from scheduling to equipment to changing light bulbs. Most dentists would prefer to be doing their jobs and delegating other tasks to people who can do them. This is the essence of teamwork. The dentist should be left to do what he or she does best: dentistry. But the dentist who is also a leader understands that the job requires building a team, by designing and organizing the strategies that will make sure the organizations flourish over time. Most dentists tend to micro-manage. When dentists can fully focus on what is truly important rather than being distracted, their well-being goes way up, their dentistry improves, and levels of satisfaction throughout the practice rises.

Teamwork allows for all members to have the freedom to choose their own destinies – it's a human right that should never be violated. Leaders take that risk, and allow people to make mistakes, fall down, and recover better next time. Southwest Airlines founder Herb Kellerher says, "You build self-confidence when you give people room to take risks and you give them room to fail, you don't condemn them when they fail, you just say 'that's an educational experience.'"

No one is perfect. I get to see how dentists respond or react when my lab sends out work that doesn't meet the dentist's expectations. I get to observe all kinds of responses. I believe that how a person does anything is how they do everything. When I sense anger and frustration on the part of the dentist or a staff member, I conclude that is part of their leadership style. Some offices can make the lab feel good about what happened, if that is possible, and everyone learns and grows from the experience. The ones who react negatively seem to continue to have issues, until they take their business elsewhere, where they continue to wreak havoc. This is micromanagement, not leadership.

We all learn through mistakes, or we don't learn. This is how teams grow and, in a field like dentistry, we need to continually keep up with new technology and new cultural shifts. Circumstances will always change but, if we protect our freedom to choose our own responses, we will thrive. As mentioned earlier, I have had virtually no staff turnover in over 20 years. How this shows up is incredible. There are times that I don't know if a problem arises, because someone is on it before it gets out of hand. What a wonderful place to be. This is one of the long-term rewards of successful leadership, other than greater efficiency and productivity. When we create a team that is more like a group of associates, rather than a top-down organization of bosses and subordinates, that's when the magic happens.

One of the more meaningful problems that I have faced in my long career is what Paul Zak describes as the *lead-singer syndrome* [9]. It was originally described by Keith Richards's assessment of Mick Jagger's self-indulgent behavior as the lead singer of the Rolling Stones. For many of us, including myself, getting thrust into a leadership position – especially without training – can cause a rise in testosterone levels. Elevated testosterone can make anyone into a jerk because, as Zak tells us, "testosterone tells your brain that the world revolves around you [10]."

In the past, I have heard this called the "doctor syndrome", or the "white coat syndrome." In other words, it's an overblown sense of importance. The funny thing that I have learned is that, although it can be very counterproductive, people expect it and almost welcome it. More and more, people will come to depend on the "lead singer" or, at least, this is what I have experienced. Zak tells us that the more testosterone that is secreted, the less oxytocin we have available. Without oxytocin, our levels of care and trust go down. Thus, there is science that tells us to recognize the downside of being the lead singer. Caring and trust are the essential ingredients of the culture of trust. Understanding that our biology can sometimes put us in compromising situations is very important. Everyone has the ability to change and to become a better, more caring and considerate leader. A student once asked Peter Drucker to reduce business management down to its most fundamental idea, and his response was, "Good manners."

I want to close this chapter with a story about how these forces are ubiquitous, and how we must be vigilant in order to maintain our leadership role. A little while ago, I came in for an early morning crown and bridge appointment. The patient was scheduled from 7:30 am until noon. We were prepared, and ready to spend a very productive morning. She was our first patient, and she had a habit of coming in a few minutes late. When 30 minutes had passed by, my receptionist called her, then called her at every telephone number we had in her chart. No response. One hour after her appointed time, she was still a no-show and a no-call. To say we were frustrated would be an understatement; our morning was shot. I know about the "practice management tip sheet advice", to always have a call list on hand in case situations like this arise. In my younger years, we had such a list, but I am slowing down considerably, and I don't do all of the "management" things I used to do. Believe me, they are just band-aids for times like this.

The situation got the best of me. My staff couldn't reach her, and I was brooding (not recommended). I went on my computer and found her on social media. I sent her a message (really not recommended) and told her I didn't want her back in the office. This isn't the behavior of a leader. I was being emotionally hijacked.

I am writing about this now because I feel it is instructional to illustrate the resistance we need to garner in order to become leaders. I also want to make the point that we are all human, and we must exhibit self-compassion. We grow from our mistakes, and we must learn every lesson in order to grow.

The patient was highly insulted that I used social media to contact her. In the end, she apologized and I apologized as well. It was a mistake. Even more, the mistake extended to my team. I became the lead singer. I took over their responsibilities, and may have caused more damage in the future. Making decisions that involve patient relations, from appointments to fees and discounts, can undermine teamwork. Situations like these occur all the time. Circumstances change, but having control over our own minds should always be the constant, regardless of the situation.

Later on, when I calmed down (another reason for mindfulness practice), I asked myself why I got so upset. It wasn't the production loss, or the loss of time, that bothered me – after so many years, I could afford those losses. What bothered me most was the message I received, whether intended or not (because feelings are facts to the people who have them), that I didn't matter. For me, and I suspect for most people, when they feel that their time and effort doesn't matter, it hits a hot button. We are all human. So the lesson I learned, and continue to learn, has a lot to do with the theme of this book and positive psychology. It is that, in life, for our own well-being, remember one thing. Other people matter – because we are *all* other people.

References and Notes

1 Barry Polansky (2006). *Bring a Super Bowl to Your Practice*. www.dentaleconomics.com/.../bring-a-super-bowl-victory-to-your-practice.

2 Tom Rath (2015). *Are You Fully Charged? The 3 Keys to Energizing Your Work and Life*, p. 30. Silicon Guild.

3 Stephen R. Covey (1989). *The Seven Habits of Highly Effective People*, p. 18. Fireside Book, Simon and Schuster.

4 Paul J. Zak (2017). *Trust Factor: The Science of Creating High-Performance Companies*. AMACOM.

5 http://www.octanner.com/blog/category/leadership.

6 Martin Seligman (1991). *Learned Optimism*, 1st edition. Alfred A. Knopf.

7 Paul J. Zak (2017). *Trust Factor: The Science of Creating High-Performance Companies*, p. 60. AMACOM.

8 Teresa Amiable and Steven Kramer (2011). *The Progress Principle: Using Small Wins to Ignite Joy, Engagement, and Creativity at Work*, 1st edition. Harvard Business Review Press.

9 Paul J. Zak (2017). *Trust Factor: The Science of Creating High-Performance Companies*, p. 128. AMACOM.

10 Ibid.

Part VI

Epilogue

"A master in the art of living makes little distinction between his work and his play, his labor and his leisure, his mind and his body, his education and his recreation, his love and his religion. He hardly knows which is which. He simply pursues his vision of excellence through whatever he does, leaving others to decide whether he is working or playing. To him, he is always doing both."

Lawrence Pearsall Jacks

A Master in the Art of Living

In the recent bestselling book, *The Undoing Project*, author Michael Lewis tells the story of Daniel Kahneman and Amos Tversky, two Israeli psychologists who are credited with developing the field of behavioral economics. Although they were the best of friends, only one, Kahneman, was awarded the Nobel Prize in 2003. Kahneman was a behavioral psychologist and an introvert, while Tversky was a mathematical psychologist and quite extroverted. They were an enigmatic pair who founded an enigmatic science about how people decide. Their work has left many of us questioning the concept of certainty.

Tversky stood for the side of certainty – the economic side of behavioral economics. He had a strong personality, while Kahneman was always doubting. He was the one who symbolized the behavioral, or softer, side of behavioral economics. Their work has become the basis of many bestsellers in recent years that discuss the irrationality of decision-making. Their work opened the eyes of many in academia as to the importance of psychology in all fields. Schools began to put together courses and curricula that included both economics and psychology. However, there was a problem: they didn't want to get to know each other better. The economists craved predictability, while the behaviorists understood uncertainty. According to Lewis, "the economists were brash and self-assured, while the behaviorists were nuanced and doubtful."

Harvard psychologist Amy Cuddy explained the difficulty of bringing these two factions together as, "the psychologists think economists are immoral and economists think that psychologists are stupid." Tversky, the economist, did not like emotion as a subject he wanted to deal with and, at times, he could be rude. I find a similar situation in dentistry.

The Complete Dentist: Positive Leadership and Communication Skills for Success, First Edition. Barry Polansky.
© 2018 John Wiley & Sons, Inc. Published 2018 by John Wiley & Sons, Inc.

There is a technical side to dentistry, as well as a behavioral side. In order to be successful, the dentist-leaders must have an appreciation for both. Throughout my career, I have seen dentists argue about everything, from philosophies of occlusion to materials and impression techniques. And sometimes, these arguments bordered on being more than rude. I have seen highly technical dentists walk out on behavioral and practice management lectures. It is the rare dentist that who has an appreciation for both the technical and the behavioral.

Dental leaders need to change this. Hopefully, this book can act as an impetus to bring the whole of dentistry into dental education, and we can then learn complete dentistry.

Index

The Complete Dentist: Positive Leadership and Communication Skills for Success, First Edition. Barry Polansky.
© 2018 John Wiley & Sons, Inc. Published 2018 by John Wiley & Sons, Inc.